"Fatigue drains women of their total spirit, but Holly Atkinson's *WOMEN AND FATIGUE* tells how to put spark back into our lives."

—Sonya Friedman

"Don't walk around exhausted! . . . Dr. Holly Atkinson reveals strategies for banishing fatigue."

—*The Star*

"*WOMEN AND FATIGUE* outlines major contributors to fatigue . . . then lists concrete suggestions for dealing with these fatigue causers . . . A commonsensical illumination of a very real problem."

—*Roanoke Times and World News*

"Dr. Atkinson strikes out such responses as 'There's nothing wrong' and 'It's all in your head,' and offers all women everywhere hope and reassurance, facts and solutions."

—*The Macon Beacon*

"Practically every woman I know is *tired*, be she wife, mother, employee or all those things combined. Thank heaven for *WOMEN AND FATIGUE,* because it helps!"

—Jane Bryant Quinn

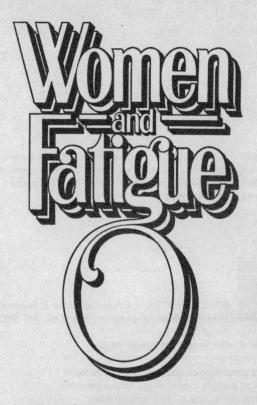

Women and Fatigue

HOLLY ATKINSON, M.D.

POCKET BOOKS

New York　London　Toronto　Sydney　Tokyo　Singapore

POCKET BOOKS, a division of Simon & Schuster Inc.
1230 Avenue of the Americas, New York, NY 10020

ISBN: 0-671-69216-X

First Pocket Books printing January 1987

10 9 8 7 6

ACKNOWLEDGMENTS

A countless number of people deserve to be thanked for their support and guidance in the writing of this book. The most important people influencing it were the women who shared their life stories with me. I withhold their names to protect their privacy but extend my heartfelt appreciation to each and every one of them for giving so freely of themselves. I also wish to extend my thanks to all the physicians, psychologists, and other professionals who contributed to my understanding of fatigue through either personal conversation or published research.

A special word of appreciation goes to my agent, Bill Adler, and to Diane Reverand, formerly of G. P. Putnam's Sons, for their inception of *Women and Fatigue*. I am deeply grateful to Christine Schillig, my editor, for her support, enthusiasm, and guidance throughout the writing of the book and her masterful editing on the final revisions. She has contributed enormously to *Women and Fatigue*.

Two very special people deserve more credit and praise than I can possibly express in this short space: my sister, Karen Ann Atkinson, Ph.D., and my husband, R. Grant Tate. Both were a never-ending source of constructive criticism and emotional support.

Karen's illustrations grace these pages. Her attention to detail and concern for accuracy have earned my deepest respect. I can't thank her enough for all the time and effort she devoted to this project.

v

ACKNOWLEDGMENTS

Last, I must try to acknowledge my husband's invaluable contribution to *Women and Fatigue*. I simply do not have words sufficient for thanks. Grant has supported me with endless words of encouragement, lengthy conversations, generous nurturing, and hours of editorial assistance. My deepest gratitude goes to him for sharing this book and his life with me.

To Grant,
with love

CONTENTS

CONTENTS

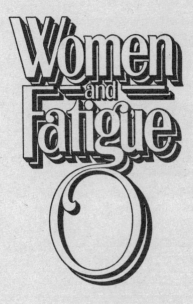

Introduction

Chronic fatigue has been a part of most of my life. I had become so accustomed to being tired, I simply assumed that I had been born that way. I imagine that the first few steps I took as a child absolutely exhausted me. Nevertheless, I pushed on into life.

Some people may be surprised to hear me, now a physician, journalist, and wife, admit that I have known chronic fatigue so intimately. In fact, I know it quite well. My mother, too, struggled with fatigue at times in her life. At one time she was going back to school to get her college degree, caring for a new baby at home, and carrying the other responsibilities of the cooking, cleaning, laundry, and shopping. I understand her feelings better today than I did then. To me and the rest of the family, Ma was just doing what she was supposed to do, and then a little bit more on the side. Her fatigue? I thought tiredness was in my family's genes. She had it, I had it, and that was that.

I often cursed those genes as I struggled with fatigue as a student in high school, in college, in medical school, as a medical intern, and as a reporter covering stories for CBS News. I thought I had received a bigger "dose" of tiredness than most people; it seemed that others had a lot more energy. It is true that some people do have greater reserves of energy than others. Individual metabolisms and, to a certain extent, energy levels are inherited from parents. Yet tiredness is not in our genes. It is a symptom of having too many demands made upon our minds and bodies.

WOMEN AND FATIGUE

I finally confronted my fatigue when I got married. Until then, I had been able to devote most of my precious energy to my work. Marriage created a tug-of-war. There just did not seem to be enough energy to do my job, take care of a home, and develop a good marriage. And we didn't even have children! I can remember thinking to myself, ". . . and if I had kids to care for on top of all this, I just couldn't do it!"

One of two things had to happen: Either my energy had to increase or the demands on me had to decrease. Demands never seemed to go away, so I decided to look for ways to increase my energy. But my study of the problem of fatigue has taught me that one truly can increase energy and decrease demands. My old assumption, that chronic fatigue was a necessary part of my life, was wrong.

One afternoon, a few months after my intensive struggle to overcome my own fatigue began, I had lunch in New York with my book agent, Bill Adler. After we had been chatting a while, Bill said, referring to my busy schedule, "How do you do it, Holly?"

"Oh, I have some secrets," I teased. "I have learned some things about myself. For instance, I don't drink alcohol when I can't afford to be tired. And I take naps whenever I can." Somewhere in that conversation was the beginning of this book.

I wrote it not only as a physician concerned about the health of women but as one who has personally struggled with chronic fatigue—and won! I have discovered that the causes of fatigue can be found and, furthermore, that something can be done about them. I can now look back at various points in my life and attribute my fatigue to real causes. In high school, I had hypothyroidism; in college, mononucleosis (famous for causing fatigue). In medical school, role conflict, overwork, sexual harassment, and sex discrimination took their tolls—all factors that are common experiences today for women in the work force. The fatigue of my medical internship was purely and simply overwork and no sleep. The list goes on. But, you see, my fatigue was not just one big long stretch of endless tiredness; there were identifiable causes for each situation.

Perhaps the most important question regarding those

situations is: If I had known the cause of the fatigue, could something have been done about it? YES. I could have handled all of those situations better if I had been more knowledgeable about fatigue. Even during medical internship, when one has so little control over her or his life, I could have acted to alleviate the agony of the long hours and the constant fatigue. For one thing, I could have exercised more consistently. When daily exercise was part of my routine, I felt great in spite of the demands placed on me. Something can always be done about fatigue.

Why should something be done about fatigue? Does it really deserve the attention I have devoted to it? YES. Chronic fatigue causes a lack of well-being, a loss of good health. It is a signal that something is wrong with your life. Fatigue can make you feel "sick" just like any other symptom; although fatigue itself cannot kill you, some of its underlying causes can.

When I finally came to grips with my personal fatigue, I found many things "wrong" in my life. As a result, I quit smoking, I stopped drinking alcohol, I started exercising regularly, I totally changed my diet (from Cokes and chocolate-chip cookies) to a low-fat, high complex-carbohydrate diet, and I started carefully watching my sleeping habits. I changed jobs, my husband and I worked out a schedule to share the responsibilities of home, and I began working to overcome my negative internal voices (those voices that say you're too fat, too short, not pretty).

Many of these changes came about as the book was evolving. Researching, reading, interviewing, and writing led me to examine my own life in detail. I began to realize how much fatigue pervaded my life and the lives of most women. It affects our moods, our thinking, our ability to concentrate, our productivity, our relationships, our loves. It takes away our sense of wellness and our joy in life. When I started to discover just how much chronic fatigue robs us of pleasure and productivity, I decided that the changes were worth it— and that others should have the benefit of these findings.

Women around me have changed too. One of my close friends, whose voice you will meet somewhere in these pages, called me late one night as I was writing. She said, "I just want to say thanks—thanks for doing the book." I was taken quite by surprise and deeply touched by her comment. I replied, "How can you say that, you haven't even read it yet." "I don't have to," she retorted. "It has already changed my life. Just by asking the questions, you got me thinking, and I have realized so much about myself that I never knew before. It's made a big difference in my life."

The questions to which she referred came from a questionnaire that I prepared to help collect information from women about their fatigue. It was short: only three questions. But those three questions started women thinking. I got feedback from other women long after they had mailed their written answers to me. Most of them had the same message: They were thinking about their fatigue and its causes in a way they had never done before. No longer were they accepting chronic fatigue as a way of life.

The first question was: *Have you ever suffered from chronic fatigue at any period in your life? If yes, when and for how long? Please describe how you felt and your life circumstances at that time.* Often, women began by saying no, but then went on to explain all of the responsibilities and burdens they were carrying. After painting a picture of their life circumstances, they would close by saying, "I was exhausted all the time," or "I didn't realize how tired I was, I'd never really thought about it until I wrote this." Quite a few of them were shocked by what they had written.

The second question on the questionnaire was: *Have you ever consulted a doctor about feeling tired? If yes, what was the diagnosis and treatment? Do you think the doctor was responsive to your condition?* Of those women who visited a physician, all of them reported that when a physical cause was found to explain their fatigue, the doctor was sympathetic. If no physical cause was found, the women were left to fend on their own. One woman wrote, "In discussing fatigue as a general topic with doctors I have gotten the impression that, with women anyway, if they find no obvious physical cause for the problem, they either (a) humor you and tell you to get more sleep, (b) prescribe iron (all women need iron), or (c) ignore you." Unfortunately, she is right.

Answers to the third question—*Whether or not you consulted a doctor, did you discover any ways to alleviate your fatigue?*—were very revealing. I felt the anger and frustration seeping from the answers. Many women saw no way of changing their lives and yet they were exasperated by the sheer load of work they were carrying. Unfortunately, many women are so overworked that they essentially have no personal time. Others have succeeded in lightening their burdens and talked about fatigue in retrospect. These women were able to offer some good tips.

Whatever the circumstances, one major theme permeated most of the women's answers—the issue of control over one's life. I was amazed at how many women talked about control or, more pointedly, the lack thereof.

Those who felt they did not have control of their lives were being pulled and pushed by endless demands upon their emotions and time, demands from their husbands, the kids, the in-laws, the boss, the local committee, the church. There was always somebody who needed nurturing and always something to be done. Consequently there was fatigue in their lives too. These women had not learned to set limits, to say no without feeling guilty.

Interestingly enough, the women who testified that they had control over their lives said that a crisis forced them to realize what was going on. They were so overloaded that life became unmanageable and they were forced to do something. Those "somethings" included, for example, going to a counselor to resolve conflicts, getting divorced, going back to school to train for a better job, and saying good-bye to their high housekeeping standards. Something had to give. But when something did give in these women's lives, they were able to learn to set limits and say no to those persons making demands. They stopped trying to do it all and trying to satisfy everyone else's needs. These women reported that they are much happier and healthier than they had been.

You will hear the voices of these women in the following pages. Many of their stories are very touching; the answers to the questionnaires deeply moved me. I had sent out a simple questionnaire about fatigue, and I was jolted by the testimonies that came back. Some made me cry, such as the story about a young mother with eight children whose husband just walked out on her, and she had nothing but sheer willpower and love for her children on which to survive.

Women were so honest about their burdens and struggles. My respect grew for the women I know as I learned about their difficulties in life. I have always thought that women are great, but after writing this book, I know women are magnificent creatures. I cannot believe what women are doing today. They are doing more than half of the work in this world and more than half of the loving. Because of that, I think women also have more than half the fatigue and suffering in this world.

In this era of transition, women must now strive to strike a balance between those values that are highly cherished yet seem to be pulling us in opposite directions. We must struggle for changes in our social institutions that will facilitate the integration of various aspects of our lives, particularly the family and the workplace. Perhaps we can use our own personal fatigue as an indicator of how well we are faring in achieving these goals. Fatigue is an excellent gauge of well-being because it is a very hard symptom to mask. The only way to get rid of it is to treat the underlying causes. Fatigue has many faces, but they all say the same thing—the mental or physical load is too great. I hope this book helps you to become aware of your fatigue, to learn to listen to what it is trying to tell you, and most of all, to provide you with guidance on what to do about it.

Part One
KNOW YOUR FATIGUE

1
FATIGUE IS REAL

American women are exhausted. Fatigue is one of the most common complaints voiced by women workers.[1] In one study, 70 percent of women managers listed tiredness as their main symptom, outranking both anxiety and tension.[2] Mothers with an infant or young children at home are especially weary. Doctors report that fatigue is one of the most frequent complaints they hear from their patients.

It seems that women are talking about fatigue more and more each day. I overhear conversations at lunch, in offices, on street corners, and in elevators. The first two women to step on an elevator I was riding last week were discussing their day's work. One said, "You know, I just can't do a better job when I'm so overworked and tired." A few floors later, two other women got on as one was saying, "I know I'm right, but I am just too exhausted to confront him."

It is ironic that in this age of labor-saving devices women are more exhausted than ever. We have our washing machines, dishwashers, vacuum cleaners, and microwave ovens (I cannot wait for the robot who knows how to use them all) to help at home, yet we cannot seem to find the energy to get all of our work done, to develop a good relationship with our spouse, and to give quality time to the children. Our grandmothers may have known exhaustion after a long, hard day of work, but rare is the grandmother who experienced the chronic fatigue that plagues women today. Why?

As a doctor, I have been in the privileged position of hearing the most intimate details of women's lives. As a result of listening to the stories of countless tired women, there are three recurring themes that I believe are the primary causes (in addition to, of course, medical illnesses) of chronic fatigue. First, women today have acquired many bad habits: smoking, drinking too much alcohol, fad dieting, sedentary living, and drug abuse. Second, many women are (justifiably) in conflict about their roles. Such conflict can be good if it leads to personal improvement. But for many women, the conflict is never resolved, resulting in a constant energy drain. Third, women have taken on new work burdens without being able to give up or to get help with their traditional responsibilities in the home. Most women are substantially overworked.

Consider the story of fifty-nine-year-old Abby. For the last ten years or so, Abby has been tired upon rising in the morning and feels she has to push herself through the rest of the day with the help of coffee and tea. She works five days a week in a very busy local government office, answering telephones and waiting on the public. Abby also does most of the housework: shopping, cooking, cleaning, laundry, and bookkeeping. In short, she is both the breadwinner and the breadmaker. Her husband is not able to help as much as he would like because, at age fifty-two, he is retired after having had two serious heart attacks and coronary bypass surgery.

Abby is resigned to a life full of fatigue. "I do not feel I have much to look forward to," she said. "I know of no way to alleviate my fatigue other than to inherit a million."

Like Abby, many other women feel that there is no way to alleviate their fatigue. They see their lives as presenting no options. However, options and choices always exist, although sometimes they are hard to see. That is what this book is all about, helping Abby and you to see your options and choices. Your first choice is to decide whether or not you are willing to fight chronic fatigue.

Ah, I can hear you sighing now, "She wants me to *fight* fatigue—why, I don't have the energy to fight anything anymore, let alone fatigue. I'm too tired." I know that when one is tired, especially chronically tired, it is almost impossible to mobilize whatever energy you have left and direct it into making changes. But if you can take the first step, then all the others will follow. You will find that when you direct energy into something you truly find rewarding, you will not mind the tired feeling that follows. On the other hand, we become frustrated and discouraged if we are tired without receiving personal gain or without understanding the source of our languor.

You do not have to accept chronic tiredness. You can beat your fatigue! This book will be your guide. By the time you finish reading it, you will be more aware of your fatigue, you will have pinpointed its causes, and you will know the changes that are necessary to increase your vital energy. You will discover, too, that these energy-boosting changes have many added benefits; you will love the overall results. As you are fighting fatigue, you will notice yourself becoming thinner, more attractive, healthier, and happier.

WHAT IS FATIGUE?

What is fatigue? Fatigue is the feeling of having "insufficient energy to carry on and a strong desire to stop, rest, or sleep."[3] It is the weariness that comes from either physical or mental exertion. It can be a short-term or a chronic feeling. And, obviously, there are different degrees of fatigue. Because fatigue is a feeling, it can represent different sensations to different people. We have over one hundred words in the English language that describe a feeling like the one I just labeled "fatigue"—tired, exhausted, weary, flagging, weak, haggard, lethargic, bushed, languid, listless, drowsy, sleepy, sluggish, pooped, worn out.

Actually, fatigue is well described and is composed of a subjective *feeling* and several predictable behavioral effects:

> Aside from feeling weary tired persons are unable to deal effectively with complex problems and tend to be unreasonable, often about trivialities. The number and quality of their associations in psychologic tests are reduced. The ability to deliberate and

to reach judgment is impaired; decisions made late at night may appear unsound the next day. The worker after a long, hard day is unable to perform adequately his or her duties as head of a household; the example of the tired business person who becomes the proverbial tyrant of the family circle is well known. A disinclination to try and the appearance of ideas of inferiority are other characteristics of the fatigued mind.[4]

Physical sensations are part of fatigue too, including headache, dizziness, nausea, and tremulousness. Some people may feel more physical sensations associated with their fatigue, while others may feel more mental ones. Each person has her or his own particular composite fatigue.

Because fatigue is such a normal part of daily life, it is something we do not think about often. We may only realize we feel too much of it at certain times. At other times, we may not even be fully aware that we are fatigued. Getting to know your own fatigue (and the fatigue of those close to you) can really help your life run more smoothly. Start paying close attention to all the sensations (mental and physical) that make up your feeling of fatigue. This is the first step to alleviating it: You must learn to recognize your personal fatigue sensations and become consciously aware of them when you are feeling tired.

You should begin to think of fatigue as a signal of an energy imbalance; too much energy is being expended and not enough energy is being conserved. The energy-balance concept is much like money in the bank. If you keep taking money out of your account without depositing any back in, you will eventually overdraw your account. The bank may cover a small overdraft, but if you continue to overdraw, the bank will cut off your cash flow. So it goes with energy. Your body will forgive you for a while, but if you constantly utilize energy without restoring it sufficiently, you will soon begin to recognize that you are not functioning properly, and you will feel chronically fatigued.

Another way to think of the concept is to imagine an

energy pool as shown in figures 1 and 2. Each pool represents the amount of energy on which we might have to draw during the day. We start out with a certain level of energy, which comes from our natural reserve. By natural reserve, I mean the baseline amount of energy inherent within the living body. To a certain extent, our natural reserve is dictated by heredity. Some people seem to need only a few hours of sleep, while others need more; some are always bursting with energy, while others tend to drag through life.

You can increase your energy pool and be less tired if you have more energy boosters than energy drainers in your life. The boosters are good nutrition, physical fitness, restful sleep, a sense of pleasure, and a sense of mastery (see Figure 1).

On the other hand, more energy drainers than energy boosters leaves you with a smaller energy pool, so you will be more tired. The energy drainers are bad habits (smoking,

THE BOOSTED ENERGY POOL

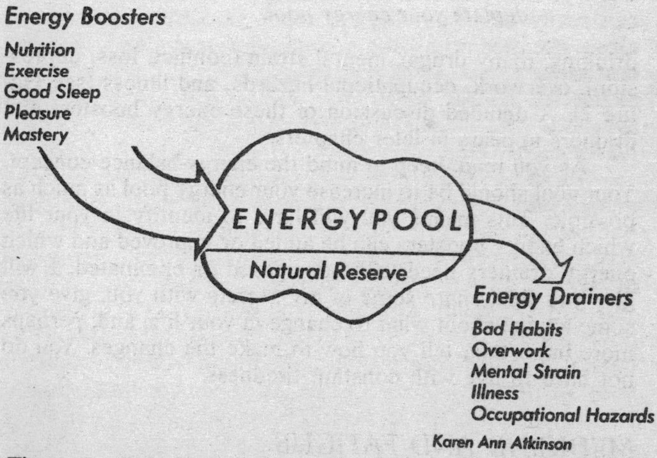

Energy Boosters

Nutrition
Exercise
Good Sleep
Pleasure
Mastery

ENERGY POOL

Natural Reserve

Energy Drainers

Bad Habits
Overwork
Mental Strain
Illness
Occupational Hazards

Karen Ann Atkinson

Figure 1: *More energy boosters than energy drainers will replenish your energy pool.*

13

THE DRAINED ENERGY POOL

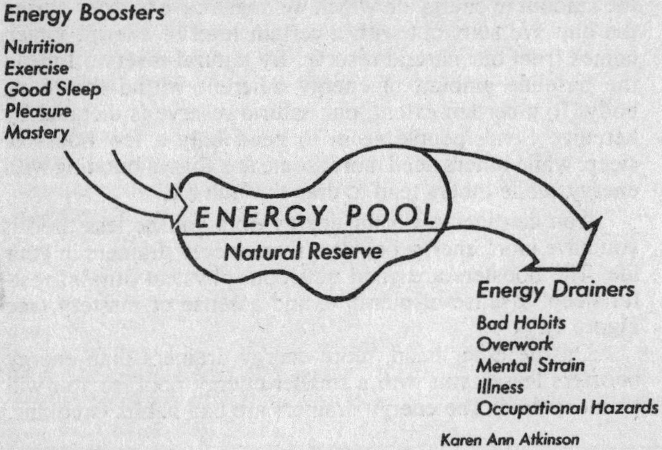

Energy Boosters

Nutrition
Exercise
Good Sleep
Pleasure
Mastery

ENERGY POOL
Natural Reserve

Energy Drainers

Bad Habits
Overwork
Mental Strain
Illness
Occupational Hazards

Karen Ann Atkinson

Figure 2: *More energy drainers than energy boosters will deplete your energy pool.*

drinking, many drugs), mental strain (conflict, loss, depression), overwork, occupational hazards, and illness (see Figure 2). A detailed discussion of these energy boosters and drainers appears in later chapters.

As you read, keep in mind the energy-balance concept. Your goal should be to increase your energy pool as much as possible. This means you will have to identify in your life which energy boosters can be added or improved and which energy drainers need to be decreased or eliminated. I will give you tips, share some of my secrets with you, give you some advice about what to change in your life, and, perhaps more important, tell you how to make the changes. You do not have to live with constant tiredness.

MEDICINE AND FATIGUE

First and foremost, fatigue is the loss of well-being. Many people do not think of it that way, but fatigue can make us feel "sick" just like any other malady. It is not a dramatic symptom, but it can be one of the most disruptive in life. Fatigue can disturb our moods, our concentration, our perceptions, our capacity to do work, and our capacity to love, often without us even being aware that something is wrong. It takes the sparkle out of life.

When does fatigue become such a severe symptom? Obviously, fatigue, or tiredness, is a daily part of living. Fatigue that is alleviated after a night's sleep can be considered normal. Dr. George L. Engel explains when fatigue is a signal that something is wrong:

> Fatigue may be considered a symptom when it becomes the occasion for complaint, as when one becomes fatigued with less effort or at unusual times of the day; or when rest is no longer recuperative or diversion as distracting. *Fatigue is probably the most prevalent symptom of illness, physical as well as mental, and is often its first indication.* [italics mine][5]

Fatigue is part of the body's alarm system. When the symptom is present, it is telling us that the body needs to conserve its strength. Fatigue is a protective mechanism that immobilizes the body so it cannot be driven to sheer exhaustion and death. People who try to override their alarm systems and work in spite of their fatigue may suffer dire consequences. They become more susceptible to the development of serious illness. Fatigue is a symptom that should be heeded; its cause should be sought.

Unfortunately, women's complaints of fatigue are rarely taken seriously. Many doctors write off the symptom after only a few simple tests. Yet even if the doctor takes the time to conduct a battery of physical tests to rule out any major infection, disease, or chronic condition, the cause of the fatigue may be very difficult to pinpoint.

Too often when no physiological conditions are detected, the patient may be told that she is perfectly healthy and that there is no reason to be concerned. Although the woman may feel better to find out that there is no apparent physical condition causing her fatigue, she is left to deal with the situation on her own. She suffers in silence.

All doctors are not this insensitive. According to one psychiatrist writing on the symptom of chronic pain,

> . . . everyone benefits from the knowledge that a thorough physical examination is negative as long as the patient is then skillfully taken to the psychological side of the matter and not left dangling with the impression that there is nothing wrong or that the patient should pull himself together and get rid of the pain by his own efforts.[6]

The same is true for fatigue. I have been told by so many women that this is the precise treatment they have received from doctors for the complaint of fatigue. After the laboratory tests came back normal, they heard "nothing is wrong" from the doctor. This phrase simply means that no serious physical illness can be found. As far as I am concerned, though, that does not mean "nothing is wrong."

I think such a statement does a severe injustice to a patient because it instills in her the notion that the fatigue is "only in your head." Some doctors may not only imply that, they actually may come out and say it! What does this phrase mean? It is usually taken one of two ways: The cause of the fatigue is psychological (and therefore not important) or the fatigue is a figment of your imagination (in other words, not real, totally made up).

It is appropriate to suggest the cause of fatigue may be psychological, but not with phrases such as "nothing is wrong" and "it is only in your head." The doctor who does not take psychological fatigue seriously and fails to initiate follow-up treatment adds insult to injury. Too often, the woman ends up feeling worse. She may feel that her fatigue does not deserve treatment. She may feel that the doctor is saying she was either untruthful or incorrect in reporting her symptom. She may feel embarrassed about wasting the doctor's time, guilty about her condition, or downright crazy. This is a deplorable situation, but, unfortunately, all too often the case.

In Chapter 14, "Discuss Your Fatigue," I will give you some advice on what to do when you hear those phrases in a doctor's office, but for right now I want you to understand that psychological causes of fatigue are just as important as physical causes and need to be treated. Whatever the source, fatigue disrupts life.

I have great respect for anybody with a psychological problem who seeks help for it. Getting help demonstrates a strength of character and concern for yourself and those around you. Too many people who could be helped do not seek psychological assistance because of social attitudes and myths. If you have unresolved psychological problems, I do not want you to be one of them. I will discuss some of the typical issues with which women are struggling in later chapters.

Some women assume from the beginning that their fatigue is caused by a psychological problem; they do not wait for a doctor to tell them. Unfortunately, many never visit a doctor, thinking either that the symptom is not important enough or that nothing can be done. If you are one of these women, I hope to change your assumptions.

Chronic fatigue is probably the most prevalent and often the first symptom in disease. Some studies show that if you are chronically fatigued, there is a one-in-three to one-in-four chance that a physical illness is responsible. Some people who suspect psychological problems are to blame for their symptoms find that they actually have a physical disorder. Their assumptions lead to unnecessary delay in diagnosis and to prolonged suffering. *A woman with chronic fatigue should see a doctor.*

The point to remember here is that the symptom of fatigue itself does not tell us what is causing it. Even if you think you know what is causing your fatigue, keep an open mind. You might be mistaken.

Fatigue is a very common complaint, and yet there are no clear estimates on exactly how prevalent it is. We have statistics for almost everything, and yet, I could not find any estimates on the frequency of fatigue in the general population, let alone in women. A few studies, however, show that fatigue is more common in women than in men, perhaps by as great as a two-to-one ratio.[7]

Are women more susceptible to fatigue than men? Yes. Our natural constitutions as females make us more vulnerable. First, women have smaller bodies with less muscle mass than men, leading them to suffer from physical exhaustion sooner than the average male. Second, hormonal changes during different stages in a woman's life, such as menstruation, pregnancy, and menopause, are often accompanied by periods of fatigue. It is normal for a woman to feel some fatigue at these times, and we will examine these times in detail in the next chapter.

But I also believe that women simply have more about which to be sick and tired. I think that women's fatigue problem is primarily caused by the pressures of today's world. It is, for the most part, a result of the life-styles women are living and the psychological burdens they are carrying.

The causes of chronic fatigue can be divided into three categories: life-style causes, psychological causes, and physical causes. There is a section of the book devoted to each of the three categories. It is helpful to break down the causes of fatigue in this way, so that you can determine the area (or areas) that need change.

LIFE-STYLE CAUSES

We live in an era of rapid personal and social change. The last decade probably saw a greater change in the form and life-style of the American family than any other decade in history. The percentage of American women who hold full-time jobs increased from 35 percent in 1960 to 51 percent in 1980. In the decade from 1970 to 1980, the number of women running households alone increased by 24 percent. The divorce rate skyrocketed 141 percent between 1960 and 1980. These numbers reflect what too many women already know—that they are juggling both family and job. The responsibility for raising children has fallen exclusively to women, many of whom receive no alimony or child-support payments. Working has become an economic necessity for most women.

Most people will agree that the more hours one works and the more stress one feels, the more likely it is that fatigue will appear. Women fit the bill in both cases. One study reported that a mother with preschool children who has a forty-hour-a-week job outside the home, "works an average of seventy-seven hours a week."[8] Those additional thirty-seven hours a week are spent doing household chores: the laundry, cooking, cleaning, shopping, caring for children, and other tasks. (Thirty-seven hours a week for household chores is at the low end of the scale. Other studies have shown that even the housewife who does not work outside the home spends about one hundred hours a week working at twelve different chores.[9])

While women have expanded their responsibilities, they have not been able to give up or receive help with their traditional chores. The same study reported that the amount of time husbands spend doing housework has increased by less than thirty minutes a week in the last ten years! Other studies show that men are helping more than that, but male attitudes and behavior, for the most part, seem to have changed little.

We will deal with work-related problems throughout the book; there are so many issues we face on the job that can drain us of energy. Poor pay; sexual harassment; child-care problems; discrimination; job-related conflicts, such as career-versus-family or fear of success; and occupational hazards are only a sampling of the types of work issues that can add to your fatigue. I will discuss all of them in the appropriate chapters and make some suggestions about how you can solve some of your problems.

Unfortunately, many women cope with their problems in ways that only compound the fatigue of overwork. Women often use eating, smoking, drinking, and medications to deal with tension, anxiety, and dissatisfaction. All of these coping mechanisms cause fatigue. In the life-style section of the book, I will examine diets in detail and explain why exercise is essential in your life. We will look at why smoking, drinking alcohol, and even taking prescription drugs make you tired, and we will investigate your sleeping habits.

PSYCHOLOGICAL CAUSES

Women have good reason to be struggling with psychological issues today. Traditionally, we were socialized in a very narrow role, one that said that the key to happiness and fulfillment for a woman was through marriage and childbearing. A woman's satisfaction in life was to be gained by living vicariously through her husband and children. She was a wife and mother—rarely an individual with her own aspirations and goals.

This nurturing role, as wife and mother, is fatiguing for numerous reasons. It is a role defined by self-abnegation and self-denial. The nurturer is always attending to the endless needs and demands of the family; however, no one is charged with taking care of her. The job of chief nurturer in the family can be exhausting.

The domestic work involved in the job never ends either. Millions of women have cared for families, children, and homes for years, providing a social and psychological framework for the country and society. Yet housework is often degraded by our culture; it is not assigned a dollar value (although that is changing), and it does not provide its practitioners a sense of mastery of the outside world. Because of this denigration, housewives often suffer from poor self-esteem, boredom, lack of satisfaction, and low motivation. All of these feelings are usually accompanied by a good dose of chronic fatigue.

These rigid sex-role stereotypes are changing. Women are in a period of rapid transition, leaving the old roles behind and discovering the new. It is a time of experimentation. Women are gaining new freedoms, but at the same time encountering discrimination that is even more entrenched and insidious. Every new barrier that is challenged brings new tests to the women at the forefront of change. But change generates insecurity and endless types of conflict, many of which are variations on the same theme: Our old concept of what is good and feminine is clashing with our newly formed ideas of what is healthy and feminine: Family versus career. We are fighting internal and external battles of the old role pitted against the new role. And battles, whether mental or physical, leave women exhausted.

In the psychological section, I will discuss the changing role of women and the conflict it is generating. The response to this change has been an increase in the physical and psychological stress levels for women. Women feel overworked, women feel anxious, women feel tired. Women also feel tired because of the psychological losses they endure and because of the depressions they suffer. We will cover loss and depression in detail because fatigue is a dominant symptom in both of them.

PHYSICAL CAUSES

When we are sick, we naturally have less energy. The body uses resources to fight illness. Almost every major disease will cause tiredness in one form or another. Certainly, a person suffering from a heart condition or cancer can be expected to have less energy than someone who is not. There are a variety of conditions that are more subtle, often not diagnosed, that can cause a tremendous drain of energy. Low-grade urinary-tract infections or reproductive-tract infections can quietly sap your strength. Endocrine disorders, such as hypothyroidism, often begin with an insidious fatigue, as can diabetes or iron-deficiency anemia. This is just a sampling. Many of these maladies, if left untreated, can go on to do serious harm. Yet most can be easily diagnosed. The good news is that there are treatments, very successful ones. Let your fatigue be a signal in your life, and get it checked.

In the physical section of the book, I will explain how a doctor views fatigue, why it is important for you to see one, which doctor to go to, and what to expect in the typical workup for fatigue. I will also teach you how to talk to your doctor about fatigue in such a way that your complaint will not be ignored. We will spend time reviewing the more common diseases that cause fatigue, identifying their symptoms, and determining if you have any of them. Finally, we will examine the work in your life and pinpoint the five factors that are important contributors to fatigue on the job. Many people, especially doctors, tend to underestimate the important impact of occupational hazards on physical and mental fatigue.

How to deal with factors in your life that contribute to your fatigue is what this book is all about. Remember Abby, who thinks that only a million dollars can alleviate her fatigue? Abby and you will learn that most chronic fatigue is beatable. Most of the causes of fatigue—whether they fall in the life-style category, the psychological category, or even the physical category—are under your control. You should not accept fatigue as a way of life.

Take a lesson from successful people. Rarely do they set out on a path without having a sense of where they are going and more important, what they want to achieve or where they want to go. Successful people visualize, daydream, and fantasize about how they want to be. While you work on your fatigue problem as you read through the book, I want you to start dreaming of how you want to be, the things you want to get done, the energy you want to have. Just close your eyes and begin to paint a picture in your mind of yourself without fatigue, doing things, going places. If you are too tired to do it in real life, that is okay for now; use your imagination to start to form the new you. You will have a much better chance of becoming that image, if you know what person you want to be. Remember: Your fatigue is not a figment of your imagination, but the "new you" should be—for starters.

YOUR GOALS

1. Learn to recognize your fatigue symptoms.

Everybody manifests their fatigue in a very personal way. Some will experience more physical symptoms, while others will feel more mental symptoms. It is important for you to learn how you feel when you are fatigued, so you can recognize when fatigue is creeping in on you and then figure out which symptoms give you the most difficulty (for example, irritability with the children in the evening).

2. Develop new ways to cope with fatigue.

Once you know your fatigue symptoms, you should try to develop skills to combat those symptoms. You will find suggestions on how to cope scattered throughout the book. Initially, you might respond by feeling some of these activities are too selfish or that there is no time available to squeeze them in; for example, taking a nap, devoting an hour and a half to yourself every day, taking a walk, et cetera. Try to think of these activities as well-invested time. You can make room in your day, and time-outs will eventually give you a big payoff in that you will have more energy and feel better.

3. Identify the factors in your life that are causing your fatigue.

You cannot eradicate chronic fatigue from your life unless you get a firm grasp on what is causing it. You may already have a good idea of some of the factors, although I hope this book triggers you to think about other areas of your life. Decide which areas in your life need improving and concentrate on those. Make a list.

4. Decide what to do to promote a life free of chronic fatigue.

You can do something about most causes of fatigue once you have identified them. Remember the energy-pool concept; your goal should be to maximize your energy pool. Identify the energy boosters missing from your life and the energy drainers that are in your life and make a change.

At the end of each chapter is a section called "What to Do." In it you will find a list of suggestions on how to increase your energy store and decrease your energy drain. This book is filled with ideas on how to beat fatigue. Some will apply to your life, while others will not. Once you have identified the fatigue factors in your life, you can begin to implement the suggestions that will help you most.

CYCLES OF FATIGUE

All of us have experienced fatigue. It is usually a normal state of the human condition, especially after a long hard day of work or after physical exertion. The fatigue that sets in after such a day is telling us something; it is a signal from our mind and body that says, "rest." We understand that signal; it tells us that we have worked, we expect to be tired, and we welcome the night's sleep.

Recently my husband and I faced that awful chore of moving a household by ourselves with one of those do-it-yourself trucks (every time we move that way, I always swear never to do it again). We packed box after box after box (the medical books and journals alone consumed about one hundred boxes), and then lifted box after box after box. It took us almost a full day to unload the truck. When I sank into my reading chair on the Saturday night we finished, I was moaning—exhausted from all the hard physical labor, muscles aching with pain, and stomach hungry. But as I moaned, there was a smile on my face; it was that feeling of "Ohhhh. I am so sore, but it hurts so good." The physical exhaustion and the tightness in my muscles felt great; it was a wonderful fatigue. I slept soundly that night and awoke the next morning feeling refreshed and invigorated.

We do not worry about this type of exhaustion. Often there is a sense of well-being and a feeling of reward that go along with it. We may have achieved a lot in the course of our exertion and we all know that physical exercise is good for us. Our sore muscles remind us of a job well done. The fatigue represents an accomplishment of some sort. I think people feel frustrated with their fatigue when the source of it is not apparent, when they cannot see any accomplishments gained from their energy spent, or when they see no end in sight.

Fatigue, then, can make us feel good about ourselves or it can make us worry about ourselves; it can represent a normal body process or it can be a symptom of an imbalance in life. This chapter will help you understand and identify your times of normal fatigue.

We can expect to feel fatigued not only after physical exertion, but also at certain points during the day, during the month, and at other special times during our lives. Once you learn when these times occur, and particularly when they happen in you, you will be able to distinguish normal fatigue (and cope with it) from abnormal fatigue.

THE DAILY CYCLE AND FATIGUE

Let us look at the cycle of a normal day, assuming for a moment we do not suffer from chronic fatigue. When we awake in the morning, we start the day with a given pool of energy. We can increase the pool by eating the proper food and exercising. As the day wears on, we expend some of the energy through physical and mental exertion, but not all of it. (We are never totally depleted of energy. And to prove it to you, just imagine yourself being told at eleven o'clock some night that you just won a million dollars in the lottery. No matter how exhausted you felt, I bet you would have the energy to jump up and down.)

Nevertheless, as we go through the day we generally feel more tired. We finally go to bed and sleep, letting the restorative processes go to work. When we get up the next morning, our energy pool is full again.

I have been describing a cycle, a circadian (daily) rhythm. Most organisms on the earth, including humans, live their life in cycles of activity and rest. The sleep/wake cycle is the most obvious rhythm we live by, but we have hundreds of others. Each of these rhythms has a peak and a valley; the high point of activity occurs at about the same time in each daily cycle. The same is true for the low point. The time it takes to complete the entire cycle remains the same.

A set of sophisticated internal "clocks" determines how long each cycle will take; some are completed in minutes, others repeat themselves daily, while others take weeks or months to run their courses. Where these clocks are located in our bodies and how they work is not yet known. However, we do know that our internal clocks synchronize with the external world by reading cues such as the light/dark cycle of the planet, the intensity of the sunlight, and the seasonal changes.

When we are in harmony with our environment and with ourselves, all of our biological rhythms are synchronized, interacting smoothly like the meshing of gear teeth. Our biological functions—such as body temperature, blood pressure, pulse, respiration, sleepiness, and hormone levels—are all operating in cycles in a manner that makes us perform in the best possible way and gives us the best chance of survival.

Complex body functions—such as alertness, visual acuity, mood, and energy level—rise and fall in coordinated cycles too. People perform differently on physical and mental tests administered at different hours of the day. It is important for you to realize that your strength or weakness, your happiness or sadness depend, in part, on the biological time of day. Understanding your internal clocks and biological rhythms will help you begin to understand your fatigue.

You may feel especially fatigued if your internal clocks get out of synchronization. This can happen by traveling to different time zones, switching work shifts, or changing your sleeping patterns just a few hours. It may take three weeks for all your clocks to get synchronized again and for you to feel energetic.

Unfortunately, we tend to live in a world that ignores personal biological rhythms. It is the clock on the wall, not our internal clocks, that gets us out of bed, hastens us to work, tells us when to eat, and allows us to go home. We may all look relatively constant to one another from the outside, but if we stop to think about how we really feel from minute to minute, hour to hour, day to day, we know that we constantly change in energy, mood, alertness, and many other functions.

Maria, a twenty-year-old woman, was able to describe her daily energy changes to me. She said:

> "Usually every day between 1 P.M. and 3 P.M., I become 'lazy' and feel sluggish. Some days I will take a short nap and other days I will wait the tiredness out. The short naps do help, although I wouldn't say they are necessary to revive me. Like I said, the tired feeling will last only a short while and, whether I take a nap or not, it will eventually fade off to the point where I feel completely awake again."

Maria has provided us with a lovely description of the "afternoon slump." Researchers have learned that most people usually have such a slump for a few hours sometime after lunch. Although a big noon meal can make it worse, the afternoon slump cannot be blamed on food alone. It is a valley in our daily cycle when energy wanes, sleepiness creeps in, and mental abilities flag.

Do you notice an afternoon slump? When is your best time of day? Are you a "morning" person or a "night" person? Have you paid enough attention to what your body is telling you? Many people do know whether they are the proverbial owl or lark. Larks find that their best time of day is morning; they are brighter, more alert, more energetic, and more creative. It may take them an hour or two in the morning to do what it would take them four hours to do in the afternoon. On the other hand, owls are just getting a running start in the afternoon, and can go until late at night. Learning your natural daily rhythms will help you predict your peak performance, best mood, and high-energy time so that you can plan your day accordingly.

If you do not know when you are at your best, you can find out by keeping daily notes. Decide every night before you go to bed:

1. At what hour of the day did you have the most energy?
2. At what hour of the day did you feel most fatigued?
3. At what hour of the day were you in the best mood?
4. At what hour of the day were you in the worst mood?

I have found that the simplest way to keep a record is on a three-by-five-inch index card. Note the four questions on the left hand side of the card and make a column for each day of the week. One week fits quite nicely on one card. The example in Figure 3 shows how to use such a card.

Keep notes for at least four weeks. Once you have completed a month, analyze your answers to see if you can recognize a pattern. When is your best time of day? Are you answering the first question with morning hours or evening hours? Do you have an afternoon slump? When are you in the best mood?

Questions	Days of Week						
	S	M	T	W	T	F	S
1. Most energy?	9 am						
2. Most fatigue?	1 pm						
3. Best mood?	7 pm						
4. Worst mood?	2 pm						
Week of: October 20-26							

Karen Ann Atkinson

Figure 3: *Learn when your daily mood and energy rhythms occur by keeping notes on a three-by-five-inch card.*

If you can identify a good time of day, take advantage of it. Plan work that requires patience, alertness, or creativity for your best time; use good periods for tackling the more difficult tasks. Chores that do not require concentration or energy can be more easily done during low periods. If you are fortunate enough to be able to select the time you begin work or the shift you work, then you can live more of your life according to your inner clocks. A certain amount of minimal fatigue is normal in your life because of your rhythms. One of your goals should be to learn your highs and lows and plan your days with them in mind.

THE MONTHLY CYCLE AND FATIGUE

> "I suffer fatigue a few days before my period nearly every month. The best way to alleviate this fatigue is to do something nice for myself, go to a movie, play, out to dinner, et cetera."

Like this forty-year-old married homemaker, millions of women experience fatigue as part of their monthly cycles. The menstrual cycle, which has a great effect upon our energy, is a body rhythm to which almost all women can relate quite easily. Getting to know your monthly rhythm a little better will help you predict your periods of fatigue so that you can plan accordingly.

Many women who schedule around their periods find they can alleviate some of their tiredness. A thirty-six-year-old single government employee said this:

> "When I'm in my period I find myself a little bit more emotionally susceptible. The first day or two of my period I'm drained, is the best way to put it; I feel slowed down, I feel pressure in my belly, sometimes I have a backache. I usually plan for it, though. Maybe a long time ago I could have talked about being really tired, but now that I have learned my body better, I make sure things happen so I do not get tired. I sleep a little bit more, I get plenty of

exercise, I stay away from drinking, and I do not expect as much out of myself."

For most women, the menstrual cycle brings a variety of symptoms: backaches, cramps, headache, bloating, depression, irritability, anxiety, and fatigue. Somewhere around 40 percent of women have symptoms (called premenstrual syndrome, or PMS) before their periods begin and anywhere from 25 percent to 100 percent (depending on which study you read) of women suffer some discomfort during the menstrual period.

Medical researchers are discovering that some of the physical symptoms women feel before or during their periods, such as cramps and bloating, are attributable to chemical changes occurring in the body. Hormonelike substances called prostaglandins are now thought to be the culprits behind menstrual cramps, and drugs that block prostaglandin activity are quite effective in reducing pain.

Whether or not prostaglandins are involved in causing the fatigue associated with the menstrual cycle is another matter. Fatigue is often lumped together with other symptoms, such as depression, nervousness, and irritability, in a category called "behavioral symptoms." Relatively little research has been aimed at finding the cause of such symptoms.

Some doctors think fatigue and other behavioral symptoms associated with the menstrual cycle are the result of psychological conflicts. Others disagree and believe hormonal fluctuations are responsible for the mood changes most women feel before or during their periods. Still others claim that life-style (poor diet, lack of exercise) and life stresses are to blame for the mood changes.

We know that fatigue is a symptom that is the result of numerous complex bodily processes, including both physical and psychological ones, that are triggered by a variety of causes. In the next chapter, I will examine those underlying processes in detail. However, the point to be made here is that probably all of the aforementioned theories, to a certain extent, are true. Although no one specific theory explains all premenstrual or menstrual fatigue, it is likely that life-style factors and psychological issues can interact to intensify a hormonally caused fatigue.

Fatigue during the premenstrual or menstrual phases is not only the direct result of the physical and psychological changes occurring during this time of month; fatigue can also grow out of secondary problems that are exacerbated by the period. A medical condition, a poor diet, lack of physical exercise, side effects of drugs, or minor depression can surface as fatigue during your premenstrual time or during your period.

Janice, now fifty-six, remembers the fatigue she suffered for a couple of years in her late-thirties because of an underlying medical condition associated with her periods. Besides having to deal with her physical illness, Janice was under considerable stress at this time in her life. She was adjusting from a move across the country, taking care of her sick father, and very busy with three school-age children. She recalls:

"I had anemia due to frequent hemorrhaging during my periods, which finally ended up in a hysterectomy. It started out very slowly, at first it was sort of insidious, and my periods were getting longer. I was sort of tired all the time. But then, after a year or two, I really got to hemorrhaging and I was weak and dizzy. . . . I got very tired and thin, and my mood was fluctuating. I was up or down, and we'd [she and her husband] have fights. We had more fights then than we ever did."

Janice was hemorrhaging so severely each month that she finally made the decision to have a hysterectomy. She said that she felt like a new person after she had fully recuperated from the operation. With no more hemorrhaging, her anemia was slowly corrected and her fatigue subsequently vanished. As awful as the memory of this time is to her, Janice told me that she learned a very valuable lesson from the whole experience. She said:

"In those days, in the sixties, they'd give you pills for the walking patients. The GYN guys [the gynecology doctors] gave me D———, that had aspirin, amphetamine, and phenobarbital in it, which is enough to make a junkie out of anybody. I mean, you felt a lot better—you could run around and do everything—and then you'd come home and practically faint, you'd be so exhausted. So that is why, after the hysterectomy, I listened to the advice the doctors gave me, 'When you are tired—REST.' They insisted that I set aside a structured time to rest every day and not push myself the way I had been doing. I really took them very seriously, and I did—I did rest. I didn't run around as much or try to do as much as I had before—almost wildly, every minute of the day, I had been doing something. They said take it easy for medical reasons, and I *had* to, and I *did,* and then I realized what a difference it made in my life; that I didn't have to do all the things and that if I didn't do them, it was okay."

Now, I do not recommend Janice's solution, a hysterectomy, for everyone with menstrual difficulties. However, I do recommend her style of coping. It is important for women to rest and not push themselves in the face of fatigue. Remember that fatigue is a signal from your body that says your energy balance is tipping.

Menstruation is an added physical burden to the body (and sometimes an added psychological burden), if only because lost blood must be replaced. The menstrual cycle consumes a certain amount of energy, which means there is less energy at that time of month to expend on other activities. Your routine activities, which may not fatigue you most of the month, may exhaust you during the menstrual period. The period is enough to tip the energy balance.

Any life stress at this time of month can make the situation even worse. For instance, dealing with a crisis consumes even more energy, leaving a person less fit to cope with premenstrual and menstrual discomfort. If there exists less energy to cope with the discomforts, the symptoms of that particular cycle may be perceived as particularly troublesome.

Some fatigue can be expected during the premenstrual and/or menstrual time. But this fatigue does not have to be, nor should be, overwhelming or incapacitating. First, your goal should be to learn what to expect from your menstrual cycles. All you have to do is add two more questions to the left-hand column on your daily note card:

5. Are you menstruating?
6. What other symptoms do you have today?

List symptoms such as anxiety, irritability, hostility, depression, nausea, diarrhea, cramps, backache, headache, and bloating. Use abbreviations on the card to represent your individual symptoms; for example, use *D* for depression, *I* for irritability, *C* for cramps, *B* for backache, and so on.

You should keep track of your menstrual cycle and symptoms for at least three consecutive months. No one is the same from month to month, so it will take a few cycles before you begin to see a pattern emerge. Once you have a few months completed, ask yourself whether your daily rhythms (you should already be in touch with these) are

Questions	Days of Week						
	S	M	T	W	T	F	S
1. Most energy?	9 am						
2. Most fatigue?	1 pm						
3. Best mood?	7 pm						
4. Worst mood?	2 pm						
5. Period?	Yes						
6. Symptoms?	DI						
	CB						
Week of: October 20–26							

Karen Ann Atkinson

Figure 4: *Learn how your monthly rhythms affect your daily rhythms.*

affected by your coming period. Do you have symptoms before your period? Do your mood and your energy sink? Do they flag during your period? Do you ever end up on the couch or in bed? Why? Do you have serious symptoms that are preventing you from functioning?

If you experience fatigue, cramps, pain, or any other symptoms that prevent you from going to work, or put you to bed, or really interfere with your functioning, you should see a doctor who specializes in obstetrics and gynecology. You could have an underlying medical condition like Janice did, which could explain the severity of your symptoms. Fighting pain or discomfort can cause fatigue. You may have to get these symptoms under control before you can abolish your fatigue.

You can minimize the fatigue of menstruation by taking steps to increase your energy pool and decrease your energy drain. This means eating well, getting exercise, curtailing your use of alcohol and other drugs, and decreasing your expectations for the short time period. If you do suffer fatigue during menstruation, learn what to expect from your body and then plan around it as best you can. You have control over more than you think you do. If you learn to predict your daily and monthly rhythms, you can schedule around them in advance. If I have a choice, I avoid luncheon engagements, business meetings, important decisions, serious conversations, et cetera, during a few down days. Obviously, some things cannot be scheduled, but if you take advantage of those that can, they really make a difference in your energy drain.

Fatigue During Other Special Times

There are other special times in a woman's life when she is especially prone to fatigue—during pregnancy and menopause. Both of these conditions have several characteristics in common. They are events that mark milestones and profoundly change the way a woman views herself and her relationships with other people. Because these events are major happenings in life, they are also capable of raising emotions and conflicts that previously had laid buried, resulting in added psychological turmoil, which causes fatigue. And, of course, pregnancy and menopause are also physiological processes marked by extreme fluctuations in hormones and other body changes. As we have seen earlier, whenever hormones are fluctuating, fatigue seems to show up on the scene.

Pregnancy and Fatigue

Pregnancy and fatigue go hand in hand. So much so, that easy fatigability in a woman of childbearing age should make one consider that she may be pregnant. Pregnant women often report a profound sense of fatigue in the first trimester, only to have it disappear in the second and return full-blown in the third. Liz, a mother of eight children, knows about pregnancy and fatigue:

> "With the first pregnancy, the body is feeling the demands of the pregnancy and, because there are no other obligations (if you are not a working mother, like I was not), why, you can just indulge it; if you get the chance, you just lay down and sleep. But with the following children—now the body does get just as tired, but you can't indulge it quite as much—when you do feel the need to sleep, boy, you take it whenever you can get it. I used to just lay down on the floor wherever I was and go to sleep. I remember my neighbors walking in and thinking I was dead. They would walk into the house and here there were three or four little kids running around and me flat out on the floor. You just learn to go to sleep at the drop of a hat and wake up at the first sign of trouble—usually silence."

Liz told me that the tiredness of pregnancy never went away—she had it with all eight pregnancies. However, she said that the first was the most difficult one because everything about the experience was "new." With the subsequent pregnancies, she learned how to cope better with the constant fatigue:

"I learned to sleep when I could. You know, you don't have to wait until night to go to bed. If you are tired and you've got fifteen minutes, or if you're a working mother and you've got an hour lunch break, eat your lunch for fifteen minutes and sleep for forty-five. Do it when you can do it—and don't feel guilty about it. You need your rest and you've got to have it."

Women do need extra rest during pregnancy. This is because the body is expending a tremendous amount of energy to support the fetus. Just carrying the additional weight is tiring. Furthermore, the mother's heart and lungs must work extra hard to deliver blood, oxygen, and all the necessary nutrients to the fetus and carry away the wastes. All of this is very hard work, which understandably leaves one exhausted.

The work of pregnancy increases as the months pass. After the seventh month, the fetus consumes so much of a mother's energy that there is really very little reserve left to cope with pressures from the outside. One study has investigated the life changes and stresses suffered by various pregnant women and the number of symptoms they experienced in each month of pregnancy.[1] The results showed that pregnant women tolerate stress less and develop fatigue and other symptoms faster with every passing month. The study found that the eighth month of pregnancy was the most difficult for women psychologically and warned that a woman should be extra-careful about her stresses during the last trimester.

The authors of the study suggest that the reason the eighth and final months are so taxing is because the physical energy needed to carry and support the fetus is so great that there is no energy left over to cope with other physical and mental problems. With no energy available to fight outside pressures, the pregnant woman can be significantly stressed by almost anything. The energy imbalance leaves one exhausted; it is a result of the state of pregnancy itself.

What is the significance of the fatigue? Does it hurt mother or infant to ignore fatigue as a signal that energy is being depleted? Unfortunately, we have little data to answer such an important question. I have seen some studies however, that suggest premature delivery can be attributed to fatigue. I do believe that fatigue does mean something. It is a protective mechanism that the body has developed to slow us down when we are depleting our energy stores. The fatigue is meant to stand in the way of our overexerting ourselves.

It is especially important to recognize that pregnancy places very special and taxing demands on the body. You can expect to feel more fatigue, especially in the first and third trimesters. In the third trimester, you should try to listen to your fatigue and use it as a gauge as to when you have had enough. You must be ready to accept the fact that you will need more rest and you should try to get it. Do not overcommit yourself to work, family, or social events. Set an even pace and allow yourself enough time to get your needed rest. Take naps whenever you can and try to get one more hour of sleep than usual every night. If you are excessively tired, pay attention to the signal—discuss your fatigue with your doctor. Fatigue can be a signal that something is wrong.

Nutrition and exercise are especially important during pregnancy. Good nutrition will assure the proper nutrients to the growing fetus, and exercise will help keep muscles strong. Exercise may seem counterproductive at first glance because it takes energy to do. However, in the long run exercise creates energy and improves muscle strength. You can reduce your risk of fatigue by planning and sticking to a well-organized exercise routine, eating the right foods, getting the proper rest, and, yes—pampering yourself a bit!

Menopause and Fatigue

Menopause, like pregnancy, is a milestone in a woman's life. It is an event that brings about many changes—changes in body function and appearance, changes in relationships, and changes in self-image. All of these make menopause a special time of adjustment.

Menopause actually refers to the last menstrual period, although the word is frequently used to signify the range of time when the change of life is occurring. *Climacteric* is the word that properly denotes this range of years during which ovarian function declines. For some women the climacteric is noneventful, but for others it can be extremely debilitating.

Several factors determine how difficult this time will be for any particular woman, including (1) the rate of decline of the female sex hormones, estrogen and progesterone, (2) the final degree of hormone depletion, (3) genetic factors, (4) life-style factors, such as diet and exercise, and (5) psychological preconceptions about the menopause, many of which are culturally determined.[2] All of these factors directly affect our energy pool and, hence, how tired we will feel during menopause.

The cessation of the menstrual period, and thus the loss of reproductive ability, occurs because of a decline in the ovaries' ability to produce estrogen and progesterone. The falloff of estrogen and progesterone leads to the changes and symptoms usually associated with the menopause. What are the changes and symptoms clearly linked with hormonal decline? Is fatigue one of them? The answer is still debated in the medical literature, but I am convinced that much of menopausal fatigue is from the fluctuating hormones.

In the past, it seemed as if any symptom in a menopausal woman was attributed to fluctuating hormones. Today, although there is still some debate over a few symptoms, the list has been pruned significantly. Symptoms known to be caused by hormonal decline include hot flashes, sweats, vaginal dryness, urinary incontinence, insomnia, and, perhaps for some women, fatigue and psychological difficulties, including depression, anxiety, and irritability.

I say "perhaps" because the symptoms that fall within the behavioral category have not been clearly shown to be directly caused by the hormonal fluctuations. There is still debate over this. However, studies have linked hormonal changes at other times in a woman's life, such as before the menstrual cycle and after childbirth, with "psychological" symptoms. It seems reasonable that fluctuations in hormones during menopause would do the same. Furthermore, some doctors have reported that the use of hormone-replacement therapy does alleviate the depression, irritability, insomnia, and fatigue of menopause.

Yet other studies suggest that these symptoms may be caused by the psychological difficulties menopause brings for some women. There is, I am sure, truth in this theory as well. Cross-cultural studies have suggested that the menopause need not be a difficult time. One researcher found that Indian women in Rajasthan had no symptoms at all and were eagerly awaiting the event. In Indian society, women are rewarded for reaching the menopause and are allowed new social freedoms.[3] In contrast, our society is preoccupied with youth and there is no reward for aging. Menopause, in America, is a time of tremendous loss, which must be grieved.

In our culture we may view menopause as a period of mourning. Mourning brings with it all kinds of predictable symptoms—fatigue is one of the most common. If women begin to understand that menopause is an important transition time that involves losses, it might be easier to cope with its feelings and symptoms.

We understand that when we lose a loved one, we go through a period of grieving our loss. But the same is true for any type of loss. We grieve all losses, some more than others, whether we are aware of it or not. Menopause is a time of major loss, either real or feared, and these losses too must be grieved.

What exactly do women lose during menopause? First, the physical capacity to bear children is lost, and although one may not desire more children, the ability to do so is intrinsically linked to most women's senses of identity. Many women feel a loss of confidence during menopause, and much of this has to do with a shaken identity.

Furthermore, menopause forces a woman to confront her age—the loss of youth. Very closely linked to the loss of youth and childbearing capacity, is the loss of beauty and sexuality. In a culture that is obsessed with youth and sex, it is understandable that a woman would equate growing older with losing one's attractiveness and sexual desirability. All of these losses have something to do with one's sense of femininity, one's basic womanhood. That is why the losses can be so disturbing.

Of course, different women react different ways. For some the loss may be greater than for others. The grieving process varies accordingly. (In Chapter 12, we will examine loss and the grieving process in more detail, learn why grief causes fatigue, and see what to do about it.) Whether the fatigue of menopause is more a result of the hormonal decline or of the psychological grief reaction is far from clear. Most likely, it is a combination of both, with the balance differing from woman to woman.

Fatigue can also result indirectly from other symptoms during menopause. For instance, sometimes hot flashes will be severe enough to disturb sleep, leading to daytime sleepiness and chronic fatigue; heavy bleeding is common and frequently leads to severe iron-deficiency anemia; chronic pain from backaches or headaches often causes poor sleep and chronic fatigue. Or fatigue can be the result of family problems during this time, including a sick parent or spouse, a newly retired spouse, rebellious teenage children, or children leaving the nest. All of the symptoms and issues, in addition to the underlying hormonal fluctuations of menopause, must be considered as potential causes of chronic fatigue and treated appropriately.

Treatment for symptoms during menopause and beyond is very successful today. Hormone-replacement therapy has been made much safer by administering estrogen and progesterone in a cyclical fashion to replicate the body's rhythm. Hormone-replacement therapy has been shown to ameliorate such symptoms as hot flashes, sweats, vaginal dryness, and some urinary difficulties, and to help prevent heart disease and osteoporosis, or bone thinning.

Some doctors think hormonal therapy helps with psychological symptoms, while others do not. Dr. Penny Wise Budoff reported the following in her book *No More Hot Flashes:*

> De Lignieres found that depressive symptoms in postmenopausal women, including sleep disturbance, loss of energy, pessimism, and fatigue are often correlated with a drop in blood levels of estrogen or its precursors (androstenedione). He also found that these symptoms were reversed with HRT [hormone-replacement therapy].[4]

In conclusion, I believe that some of the fatigue that women experience during menopause is caused directly by the decline in estrogen and progesterone. Some fatigue is also a result of the grieving process, while the remainder is probably a result of coping with other symptoms. You should consider hormone-replacement therapy. It will alleviate any fatigue that is resulting directly from the lack of hormones, and it will also alleviate other symptoms that may be affecting one's rest.

Some degree of fatigue should be accepted as normal for this period in one's life, and besides getting symptoms properly treated, you should learn about your fatigue, identify those times when you feel it the most, and develop new coping skills.

My discussion of fatigue during pregnancy and menopause has been brief. But in later chapters we will be discussing many of the problems that can arise during these times that could be causing your fatigue, such as sleep disorders, psychological conflicts and depression, and iron-deficiency anemia. The good habits you will learn in the other sections of the book will be just as applicable to fatigue brought on by pregnancy and menopause as they will to general chronic fatigue.

A certain amount of fatigue is wedded to our daily cycles, our monthly cycles, and our life cycles. This fatigue should not be incapacitating, although at times in our fast-paced world, it is annoying. By becoming aware of your fatigue, accepting it, and planning for it, you can alleviate much of the discomfort it causes. You should also attempt to make your life as fatigue-free as possible from other causes, which is what the rest of this book is all about.

I have learned that through determined effort we can reduce our fatigue. Compared to past years, I have very little fatigue in my life. I used to be tired all the time, but I have changed in many ways, ways that you will learn throughout the following chapters. I have all but abolished my fatigue. One of the most important things I learned was when to expect my daily fatigue, and what to expect from my monthly cycle. I give in to those valleys now; I do not even try to do demanding tasks between one and three o'clock in the afternoon, and my husband and I do not engage in serious conversations during those few down days a month. My husband is fully aware of the ticking of my internal clocks. Sometimes he can see the low points coming before I do. If the day permits, he is the one who sends me to bed for a nap. And you know what? I finally do not feel guilty for doing it anymore.

WHAT TO DO

1. Recognize some fatigue as normal.

After reading this chapter, you should know that it is normal to feel some fatigue as part of your daily, monthly, and life cycles. This fatigue is most likely caused by hormonal fluctuations and secondary events associated with the fluctuations: blood loss, pregnancy, grieving, et cetera. Your fatigue is real. Allow yourself to feel tired and down during these times; do not waste energy fighting your body's natural inclinations. It is okay to feel tired, and it is okay to do something about it, such as take a nap or sleep more.

2. Discover your own rhythms and learn about your body.

Learning about the particulars of your own body really does make a difference. The key is to get in touch with your daily and monthly rhythms, determine your highs and lows, and move with them instead of against them. This way, you will maximize your energy and lessen your fatigue.

You can also gain a much greater sense of control during pregnancy and menopause if you learn what to expect from your body. Just knowing what is happening to you will reassure you that nothing is seriously wrong and you will feel less overwhelmed by your symptoms. Ask questions of your doctor or nurse, or read women's health books. You will not feel so buffeted about by unknown forces. You will be in control.

3. Organize your life according to your rhythms.

Once you can predict your periods of fatigue, you can adjust your schedule accordingly. Plan to do your heavy work or your most difficult tasks at your best time of day and during your best time of month. When you are in one of your low periods, do not try to do as much as you normally would.

Decide what must be done and then forget about the rest. Many women set their expectations of themselves far too high and consequently end up dissatisfied and exhausted.

Also, try not to take on major decisions during your low points. Save important and serious conversations for when you are feeling more energetic. Call time-outs when you need them, and do not feel guilty for doing it! Do not be hesitant to seek physical and emotional support from your spouse, your family, your friends, and your doctor. People cannot read your mind; let them in on how you are feeling. It will make for easier interactions and help you feel better.

And finally, pamper yourself during your daily and monthly valleys, and during pregnancy and menopause. Doing little things for yourself is a good coping mechanism during these times. Pleasure raises the threshold for fatigue! This is difficult for many women because they often feel guilty when they indulge themselves. Women have been raised to be self-sacrificing and to take care of everybody else's needs. But sometimes women do a poor job of taking care of themselves. If this rings a bell, you have to start working on pampering yourself. Make a list of "My Favorite Things to Do" when you are in a good mood, then when you hit a slump, you can pull out the list and try some of the things you have listed.

4. Get other symptoms treated.

Other symptoms during the menstrual period, pregnancy, and menopause can compound the usual fatigue felt at these times. Fighting pain—whether it's from cramps, backaches, headaches, or other causes—can be draining and can disturb sleep. Heavy bleeding causes anemia. Hot flashes interrupt sleep. It is mandatory to get other symptoms you experience during these times under control so you can prevent big energy drains.

5. Examine your attitudes about menstruation, pregnancy, or menopause.

These are very important times in a woman's life. They mark milestones and bring changes in our bodies, our minds, and our hearts. Because these changes concern our core identities, our femininity and womanhood, they also have the potential for stirring up conflicts over many issues. Menstruation can precipitate feelings of shame and uncleanliness. Pregnancy can raise conflicts about one's own mother and one's potential to be a good mother. Menopause, as we saw, can be marked by the sense of loss of youth, beauty, attractiveness, and sexuality. It is not surprising then that women often suffer distress and depression during these times. Ask yourself what your attitude is about these events. If you do discover that you are harboring some negative thoughts, work on eradicating them.

3

WAVES OF FATIGUE

For most of us, fatigue is a feeling—composed of *both* physical and mental sensations—that is experienced throughout the whole of our being. Because fatigue is a nonspecific symptom that affects both mind and body, it has not been sufficiently studied. Fatigue cannot be broken down into neat little packages to study under the microscope in the laboratory.

The cause of fatigue can be elusive and its search frustrating to a doctor who is accustomed to dealing with concrete physical evidence. The phrases "It's all in your head," or "There's nothing wrong" arise from some doctors' overemphasis on the purely physical. If a physical cause can be found, then the complaint of fatigue becomes "legitimate." But if the doctor cannot discover any physical illness, the patient is often made to feel as if she were a hypochondriac and not to be taken seriously. Perhaps this is why so many people go to the doctor with a secret hope that the physician will find something physically wrong that is "fixable" with some drug. The patient's complaint then finds legitimacy with herself and others.

On the other hand, many psychologists and psychiatrists overemphasize the mental, neglecting the fact that biological processes underlie all of our thoughts, feelings, and perceptions. Certain symptoms—such as anxiety, depression, irritability, memory loss, and fatigue—have earned a reputation for being of psychological origin. Many doctors are all too quick to attribute these kinds of symptoms to pschological problems, and so they fail to test for physical ailments.

This sharp division between the mind and the body dates back to the seventeenth-century French philosopher, René Descartes. He believed that the body is a machine composed of matter that abides by the laws of science, but that humans are distinguished from all other animals by possessing an immortal soul. Descartes argued that the soul, or mind, cannot be perceived by the senses and therefore humans (mind) become distinguished from matter (body).

Descartes's dualism of mind and body has plagued our thought ever since. If the mind is ill, then the soul is ill too, according to Descartes, and none of us want a sick soul. This concept explains, to a certain extent, why we are so willing to accept and hope for a physical rather than a psychological diagnosis from the doctor. And it also explains, in part, the stigma that is attached to mental illness. Descartes made us think that if one's mind is troubled, then her or his soul is too.

We are all very well trained in making this split between our mind and body. Women, especially, are so accustomed to hearing that something is "all in your head" that they now make the diagnosis themselves, dismissing their own fatigue. Others tried to distinguish between mental and physical fatigue, as if "mental" fatigue was unacceptable and "physical" fatigue was legitimate. But even when they tried to distinguish between the two, many had difficulty doing so. Mabel, a twenty-nine-year-old married woman, said this:

> ". . . such a feeling of fatigue occurred two years ago when once again I was juggling school, a job, and a home. It's having my mind torn in a half a dozen directions that leads me to become run-down. I think the source of my fatigue is mental exhaustion, which leads me to feel physically tired as well."

Although Mabel identified her fatigue as caused by mental strain, the fatigue rippled through her whole being and was felt physically too. She expressed a very important concept I want you to remember: *Regardless of the source, fatigue is felt throughout the whole being.*

Descartes's mind/body dualism does not quite hold up when we talk about fatigue. As medical knowledge expands, doctors are discovering that other conditions, such as depression, anxiety, and pain, cannot be easily categorized into mind or body either. Medical research is showing that physical processes underlie mental events, and that thoughts, feelings, and perceptions can cause physical repercussions throughout the body.

In this chapter, I will further develop the concept that the mind and body form one continuous system. You will come to appreciate that neither the mind nor the body can be tired without affecting the other. I will explain how pressure at any point in the system can cause a ripple effect, spreading the waves of fatigue throughout. Regardless of whether the cause of fatigue is physical strain or mental strain, the end result is the same—you feel tired, your ability to function is impaired, and your sense of well-being is diminished.

THE FATIGUE SCHEME

The method that I have developed to conceptualize these ideas is called the Fatigue Scheme, as shown in Figure 5. It demonstrates pictorially how the body and mind are one continuous system, and that an energy drain at any level affects the rest of the system, sending a wave of fatigue throughout. In the Fatigue Scheme, the person is represented by five levels of organization.[1]

The drain, or energy utilization, can occur anywhere in our being. (I say "anywhere" because there is no real location for the "energy pool"; energy is stored and produced throughout the entire person.) No matter where the energy drain takes place, our mind is made aware of it and feels the sensations of fatigue.

Let us examine each of the levels in some detail and discover how energy depletion may occur.

THE FATIGUE SCHEME

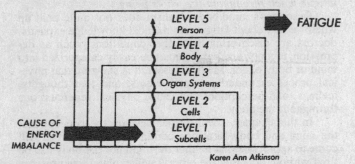

Figure 5: *An energy imbalance in any level is felt throughout the system, resulting in the sensation of fatigue when it reaches the highest level of organization, the person.*

Level 1, Subcells

This level includes all the chemical processes that occur inside the cell (the smallest working unit in the body). For example, hormones exert their influence and foodstuffs are converted into energy on this level. DNA, the genetic code of life, is also housed on this level. Level 1 is greatly affected by substances that we take in from the outside world.

Level 2, Cells

The cell is the smallest unit of structure of the body and is the site of all life processes. All of the tissues are made up of billions upon billions of cells—they are the basic building blocks of the body. However, cells are not all identical. Some are shaped differently than others, depending on their function. For instance, a muscle cell is long and spindle-shaped, while a blood cell is round; a nerve cell looks somewhat like a spider's web.

Because cells have different structures and functions, they are vulnerable to different kinds of injury and their energy can be drained in a multitude of ways. Fatigue can be caused by exercising muscle cells, depriving red blood cells of oxygen, or overworking brain cells by studying too long.

Level 3, Organ Systems

Cell parts make up cells, then thousands upon thousands of cells make up an organ, and several organs make up an organ system (such as the digestive system). Illness or prolonged strain in any one of the organs or organ systems can affect the entire body. A good example of this is a problem with the circulatory system. If the heart and blood vessels are not working properly, oxygen cannot be delivered to the tissues. If cells do not receive enough oxygen, they cannot function as they should. Diet, exercise, and drugs can all affect the amount of oxygen your tissues are getting.

Level 4, the Body

In order for us to be healthy, all of the body's systems—the circulatory system, the digestive system, the muscular system, the reproductive system, the nervous system, the endocrine system, and others—must operate in harmony. Each must pull its own weight and not cause any negative effects on the others. On Level 4, the body is represented as an integrated machine working in harmony. Its rhythm is orchestrated by the nervous system and endocrine system. A disruption in either is very likely to cause fatigue because the body cannot properly regulate itself, resulting in widespread disturbances.

Level 5, the Person

The fifth and final level of organization is the person, an individual with an identity, thoughts, feelings, hopes, dreams, and despairs. At this level, the mind (conscious and unconscious) is added. Many issues on this level can cause fatigue: boredom, dissatisfaction, conflict, grief, depression. All of these psychological responses consume energy, which is why they eventually lead to fatigue. This is also the level on which the sensation of fatigue is experienced. Fatigue is felt when energy imbalances on other levels are transmitted to the mind.

Why consider these levels of organization? By understanding how these levels affect one another, I hope you will come to appreciate how diverse causes can all lead to the general feeling of fatigue. Fatigue may result when a negative influence impinges on any level of the Fatigue Scheme; yet regardless of where the fatigue originates, it is always felt as a subjective sensation by the person.

PHYSICALLY INDUCED FATIGUE

Mary, a fifty-five-year-old married legal-library specialist, knows all about the sensation of fatigue. You would not know it from her accomplishments; she has a job with one of the blue-chip companies, she earned a college degree while working full-time, and just got married. The only daughter of an Italian immigrant, Mary has been coping with an inherited disease:

> "My entire life has been lived under a kind of fatigue, due to a blood disease—thalassemia minor or Mediterranean anemia. To counteract this, I am inclined to overcompensate by doing too much. *Rest* is the answer. I just make sure I stop everything and rest. The secret is to stop before getting too fatigued."

Mary's fatigue is caused by her mild anemia, which cannot be cured, only pampered. She inherited the anemia from one of her parents; thalassemia is caused by an abnormal gene that distorts the red blood cells and results in a failure to deliver an adequate supply of oxygen to the tissues throughout the body. Easy fatigability is the primary symptom.

Mary's problem is an example of fatigue tht originates on Level 1 of the Fatigue Scheme (see Figure 6). There is an error in her DNA, the genetic code inherited from her parent, which leads to fatigue that can be felt throughout her entire being because it affects the oxygen supply to all tissues.

Even though Mary's easy fatigability is the result of her anemia, which cannot be cured, she has learned several ways to alleviate her symptom:

"If the cause of fatigue is working too hard, we've got to find out what 'drives' us so much. Then one must simply *stop*. I found out that the world doesn't end if schedules are not met. I think I was my own worst enemy. Slowing down enabled me to not only recoup my energy, but to discover that the outside world did not expect as much as I was giving.

"Light exercise works marvelously. I usually get down on the floor and do leg raises, some push-ups, and then lots of stretching.

"A cocktail with a friend and a good long chat always works for me. Sharing the load relieves tired-ness.

"Getting over the idea that maids don't clean as well as I do has lifted quite a burden of fatigue off my back. Coming home after a hard day's work and

MARY'S FATIGUE SCHEME

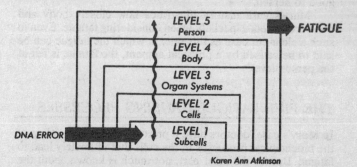

Karen Ann Atkinson

Figure 6: *An error in the DNA, a physical problem, results in anemia—which affects the entire person.*

finding a clean apartment is wonderful. Every other week is not too expensive, and can be supplemented by light cleaning in between."

And even though the basis for Mary's fatigue is physical, she has learned that mental attitudes have an effect. She said it is hard to separate her mind from her body:

"My therapist has a holistic approach to treatment, and we look at the entire picture of body and mind as we go on in therapy. Finding out what makes me tick has helped eliminate fatigue. Only then can one go on to make changes in one's life in the proper direction. Learning to care for oneself and treating oneself in a kind manner helps eliminate fatigue for me."

Mary has learned so many secrets about how to alleviate fatigue and maintain well-being. Exercise is terrific for increasing the blood flow and getting oxygen to tired tissues. Studies are beginning to show what Mary already knows: that confiding in someone relieves tiredness and stress. She has learned to delegate some of her work without feeling guilty and, perhaps most important, Mary has learned to be good to herself.

Mary's case history illustrates how closely body and mind are linked, especially when considering fatigue. Even in such a clear-cut case as this one, in which the fatigue can be said to be caused by a physical ailment, the fatigue is felt at the person level.

THE FIVE FATIGUE-CAUSING PROCESSES

In Mary's case, doctors have a pretty good understanding of the biochemical processes in the cells that ultimately lead to fatigue. But for the most part, not much is known about the physiology of fatigue from other causes. Much of our current knowledge comes from the study of the physical exertion of muscles. Even though fatigue is a symptom of literally hundreds of illnesses and conditions, very little research has concentrated on discovering the precise events that lead to the feeling of fatigue.

Nevertheless, we can make some general statements about the body processes that lead to a drained energy pool and subsequent fatigue. How exactly does this happen? There are five processes:[2]

1. Depletion of substances vital to energy production
2. Accumulation of waste products
3. Changes in the body's energy-producing machinery
4. Disruption in the body's ability to regulate itself
5. Failures in the body's communications system

Let us take a look at each one of these fatigue-causing processes in detail.

Vital Substances

An adequate supply of several vital substances is required by the body to make energy. One theory of fatigue states that the depletion of these substances—such as the proper fuel (food), vitamins, minerals, oxygen, water, hormones, enzymes, et cetera—leads to decreased energy production and a feeling of exhaustion.

You may think (especially if you have some extra fat on you) that running out of fuel will never be your problem. But it is not that simple. The body must be able to transport the fuel to the right spot at the right time. Often the body cannot transport new fuel to where it is needed fast enough from distant storehouses. So it is not always how much total food stores you have, but what they are, where they are, and in what form they are stored.

You can actually increase your potential energy pool by making sure your body has enough of the vital substances it needs. The most important activities that increase your energy potential are: eating the proper foods with adequate minerals and vitamins (not just eating), getting plenty of exercise (which ensures good delivery of substances), and making sure you get a proper night's rest (which allows time to restock the body's "warehouses").

Waste Products

Another theory states that fatigue is due to the accumulation of the waste products generated by energy production. The waste products may actually act as poisons, stopping the energy-making machinery. Or one of the chemical waste products may act directly on the brain, causing fatigue and sleep. A few studies hint that this chemical indeed might exist. Psychologist S. Howard Bartley, noted for his writing on fatigue, reported, "Blood of a fatigued individual injected into a rested person produces the overt manifestations of fatigue."[3] That is an exciting piece of research! However, to date, no one has identified the mysterious fatigue-producing substance.

The accumulation theory cannot completely explain fatigue, although waste products do inhibit the production of energy. The removal of these waste products is very important if you want to remain energetic and stave off fatigue. There are some things you can do to facilitate this. Physical exercise is the best method for increasing your capacity for getting rid of wastes. As you exercise, the blood supply to your head and the rest of your body is improved, which means faster cleanup.

Rest is mandatory for good waste removal. It normally cures the feeling of fatigue and refreshes the body. During rest or sleep the vital substances are being restocked while the body is being purged of sedating chemical waste products. In this way the body is being repaired from the wear and tear of the day's work. It is important for you to realize that the body needs a time of rest to clean out all the waste products of metabolism and carry out its reparative processes. Rest periods during the day can help achieve some renewal; this is why so many people are able to feel so refreshed after a "catnap." If you do not get enough rest every day to let reparative processes occur, you will surely be chronically fatigued.

Changes in the Energy Machinery

Exhaustive work can lead to actual structural changes in the body. For example, strenuous exercise can result in such obvious damage as broken bones, tendon or muscle pulls, or ruptured blood vessels. Subtle changes can also occur on the cellular level, affecting the body's ability to make energy. The chemical balance of such important constituents as sodium, water, potassium, or proteins in body cells may be altered, leading to handicapped cells. The protective covering around the cell, called a membrane, can also change with activity, resulting in the inability of those cells to do their job properly. If any of these changes occurs after prolonged exertion, recovery will take longer than usual because the damage will have been greater.

When we push ourselves in spite of fatigue, many of these structural damages may occur on a cellular level without our knowledge of them. If you pull a muscle, you would certainly stop walking on it; however, too many women continue to overwork in the face of fatigue. To maintain well-being, it is imperative you keep your energy-producing machinery, your body and mind, in good working order, which means resting them at appropriate intervals.

Disruption in Regulation

The body normally acts as a synchronized unit, with all the systems operating in harmony. When the systems that supply the body with vital substances and the systems that orchestrate the entire show do not operate harmoniously, the body starts to put limitations on the amount of energy it can produce—and fatigue creeps in.

The heart, lungs, and gastrointestinal systems are primarily responsible for delivering the vital substances throughout the body. The lungs bring oxygen into the body and expel carbon dioxide, the digestive system provides the body with its food, and the cardiovascular system transports all of the vital substances to the tissues. Illness or damage in any of these systems can interfere with the delivery of these substances. Heart and lung problems disturb the oxygen supply, while gastrointestinal problems can lead to nutritional deficiencies. You can see how difficulties in any of these organ systems can limit energy production. Diseases in these systems can cause fatigue in other ways; just fighting an illness consumes energy that could be used for other purposes.

As mentioned earlier, the nervous system and endocrine systems are responsible for regulating all the activities in the body. The nervous system sends impulses down its complicated network of nerves to all locations, telling muscles when to contract and sending messages of position, tension, and sensation back to the brain. Numerous factors, such as disease, drugs, chemicals, injuries, can interfere with this communication process.

The endocrine balance in the body can be altered either by disturbing the central regulation in the brain or by disturbing the production of hormones in the glands. Emotions play a part here, for they can dramatically affect the endocrine system. Perhaps you have experienced a disruption in your menstrual cycle at some time in your life due to a distressing event, or maybe you have felt the burst of adrenalin after a dreadful fright. The effect of emotions on the body and on fatigue is fascinating and very important; it is a topic I will cover in more detail later in this chapter.

Failure in Communication

The nervous system is the communications network in the body. It consists of the brain, cranial nerves, spinal cord, spinal nerves, and other specialized nerves. A generalized malfunction of this delicate network can lead to a major communications problem between the brain and the rest of the body. A disease called myasthenia gravis (MG) dramatically illustrates this point. It is characterized by great muscle weakness and increasing fatigability due to a failure of the nerve impulse to tell the muscles to move, or a failure in communications.

A flight attendant, whom I will call Susan, describes what it was like before anyone made the diagnosis of myasthenia gravis:

"He [a doctor] gave me an extra-careful checkup and passed me. He said I was in great shape. He said I was probably just tired—too much standing. Well, flying is all standing. You hardly ever sit down on a flight. So that made sense. But then my legs began to hurt. I wasn't just tired, I also hurt—at the end of a flight, or walking through the airports. Like O'Hare. Or, especially Dallas. You know how big it is. We were always having to walk from gate one to gate twenty-two. My legs would cramp. It was a real tight pain. I would have to sit down and rest for a couple of minutes. Then I'd be all right. But all the girls were always complaining about being tired, so I still didn't think too much about it."[4]

When she finally consulted another doctor, Susan was told that her tiredness and weakness were all in her head. For a few years, doctor after doctor repeatedly told her they could not find anything wrong. Finally, they were so convinced that Susan's fatigue was of psychological origin that she was hospitalized in a psychiatric ward. Luckily, she was seen by a very astute neurologist who made the diagnosis of myasthenia gravis. When she was treated with the appropriate drug, her symptoms improved greatly.

This dramatic story illustrates several points. First, you should take chronic fatigue seriously. Second, the diagnosis can be very difficult. Third, "psychological" fatigue is not easily differentiated from "physical" fatigue. Finally, it is important to determine the primary cause of chronic fatigue so it can be appropriately treated.

Iron supplements will not cure the fatigue of depression, and antidepressants and confiding in someone will not cure iron-deficiency anemia.

PSYCHOLOGICALLY INDUCED FATIGUE

In the cases of Mary and Susan, we have a pretty good idea of the underlying processes that lead to their fatigue: Mary had trouble delivering oxygen to her tissues, and Susan had trouble getting messages through to her muscles. Unfortunately, all cases of fatigue are not so clear; for instance, in fatigue caused by prolonged mental strain, we have little understanding of the underlying mechanisms. This is due primarily to two factors: The brain is harder to study than muscle tissue, and physically induced fatigue has received more attention from researchers than psychologically induced fatigue.

At this point, doctors and scientists cannot describe the biochemical mechanisms that lead to psychologically induced fatigue. But just because these biochemical changes cannot be described does not belie their existence. Biochemical mechanisms that lead to psychologically induced fatigue do exist; science is just not sophisticated enough to measure them. Psychologist S. Howard Bartley, writing about fatigue in 1965, maintained that the feeling of fatigue, no matter what the cause, represents some alteration in bodily processes: "Here it must be recognized that for every feeling, every sensory experience, every conscious attitude, there is a unique combination of body processes underlying it and accounting for it."[5]

It is very likely that the five fatigue processes discussed above will hold true for psychologically induced fatigue, as well as physically induced fatigue. For example, depression was once considered a psychological problem. But now researchers are discovering the biochemical mechanisms responsible for some of the mood changes. They have discovered that there is a depletion of specific brain chemicals in severely depressed people. This depletion of brain chemicals certainly fits one, if not more, of the five fatigue processes.

As knowledge expands, the line between the body and the mind will blur significantly. The fatigue that we experience as a result of physical strain on the body or mental strain on the mind can share the same underlying processes, feel the same, and have the same consequences in our life.

Louise knows about the fatigue from mental strain. She is a forty-two-year-old, twice-divorced, computer-systems analyst who primarily has difficulty in her relationships with men.

"Most of my family, relatives, and friends consider me a happy-go-lucky spirit with tons of determination and strength. To be perfectly honest, I can't imagine how I actually reached the age of forty-two. Although I'm quite happy at the moment, my life has been a seesaw of ups and downs.

"I was married the first time at nineteen. Just out of high school and working as a secretary. College was of no importance to me at that time; I just wanted to be married and have a family (the Cinderella syndrome—according to the book). The marriage lasted five years, was childless, and I found myself out on my own for the first time. This was frightening, to say the least. My income just about covered expenses, so I took on a part-time job.

"I really believed that I should not marry again; but, four years later I met, dated for two years, and married someone 'special.' He had a previous marriage, which produced two lovely children. After five years of trying to advance in my career with ———, perform the normal household responsibilities, entertain his children every other weekend, maintain and entertain on our boat weekends (without help or encouragement from my husband), I decided to throw in the towel for a second time. How do I spell relief? D-I-V-O-R-C-E!! Sorry, that's not an original.

"I met with a psychiatrist, then a psychologist, only to decide that in order to be free of endless sleepless nights and constant fatigue, I would fare much better alone. Facing my parents was the second most difficult item to deal with. I thought my dad would disown me, but he didn't."

Conflicts like the ones Louise grappled with are a major source of fatigue in women. Such conscious or unconscious struggles between two opposing desires or courses of action keep the brain working overtime, which uses more energy.

Psychiatrist George Engel is one of the few who have written on fatigue and mental strain. He writes:

> Conflict involves increased psychic work coupled with the frustration of little reward. Here the fatigue reflects the wish to be relieved of the necessity to continue the struggle, as well as a feeling of imminent exhaustion. It may disappear dramatically the moment the conflict is resolved.[6]

Doctors have known for a long time that in the fasting person at rest, the brain consumes about 75 percent of the glucose (sugar) being used by the body.[7] That is a remarkable amount of fuel for a three-pound brain to burn, but it demonstrates just how much work it is doing.

When we are plagued by a psychological issue—constantly worrying about something—the brain has much more work to do. If that issue or problem is not solved, the energy drain will continue unabated and chronic fatigue will become a way of life. In the Fatigue Scheme, this can be represented by the conflict creating an energy imbalance on Level 5, which leads to the feeling of fatigue on all levels.

LOUISE'S FATIGUE SCHEME

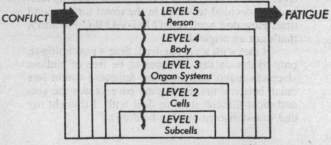

Karen Ann Atkinson

Figure 7: *Conflict, a psychological problem, results in increased psychic work, which leads to generalized fatigue that is felt throughout the entire person.*

Conflict is not the only psychological issue that consumes more energy. If you are, for example, emotionally dissatisfied, chronically angry or anxious, mourning a loss, or feeling depressed, then your mind has to work harder than normal. Fatigue is very often a dominant symptom in all forms of psychological dilemmas, and we will discuss many of them later in the book.

It may have crossed your mind that Louise was under a lot of stress. In fact, she used the word several times in her discussions with me. What exactly is stress and where does it fit into the Fatigue Scheme?

One of the first and foremost researchers on stress was endocrinologist Dr. Hans Selye. Dr. Selye described stress as the "nonspecific response of the body to any demand made upon it."[8] He distinguished stress—the body's reaction—from the stress-producing demands of life, which he called stressors. Research has shown that stressors may be either positive life experiences (marriage, job promotion, birth of a baby) or negative life experiences (divorce, getting fired, injury). It is the intensity of the demand for readjusting one's life or adapting to a new situation that counts, rather than just negative life experiences.

Does stress lead to fatigue? Absolutely, positively, yes! *Stress is the body's reaction to a demand. Fatigue is the result of the body's failure to meet that demand.* The demand, or stressor, can be anything in life.

Selye developed a model that explains how all living organisms react to stressors. He proposed that organisms respond with "certain reactions that are totally nonspecific and common to all types of exposure."[9] He eventually named these predictable reactions the "general-adaptation syndrome" (GAS) or the biological-stress syndrome. The GAS has three stages:

1. the alarm reaction
2. the stage of resistance
3. the stage of exhaustion[10]

When first exposed to a stressor, an organism will react with alarm and will consequently develop decreased resistance to infection and disease. If the organism survives the first stage, the body will begin to adjust to the stressor and build resistance. Then a period of adaptation and increased resistance will follow, the length of which depends upon the organism's innate ability to withstand stress and upon the energy pool available to fight the stress. Exhaustion sets in when the "adaptation energy," as Selye calls it, runs out.

The stress reaction, then, is simply a generalized body response that acts as a protective mechanism. It prepares the body to take action against a perceived or real threat. But keeping the body on such an alert takes energy. Over time the stress reaction depletes the body of energy and finally gives way to fatigue. Fatigue is the signal that the body needs rest in order to restock the energy pool. This stress reaction, and its attendant fatigue, can be represented quite adequately on the Fatigue Scheme (see Figure 8).

Selye found that an endless array of things could disrupt the body's equilibrium and trigger the stress reaction. The stressors on a person can range from a frostbitten toe to a disturbing emotion. The result is the same; the same set of chemical processes are activated in the body, regardless of where the stress was first felt.

STRESS AND THE FATIGUE SCHEME

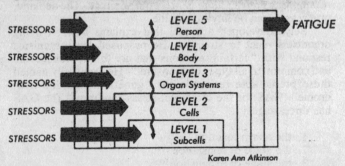

Karen Ann Atkinson

Figure 8: *Stressors can affect all levels of the Fatigue Scheme, triggering the stress reaction, which eventually leads to fatigue.*

We can say, then, that fatigue often follows the stress reaction. Is any particular stressor more fatiguing than any other? A stressor that keeps the stress reaction going for a longer period will cause fatigue more readily. In this day and age, psychological issues—emotions—are probably the most common stressors.

How much stress can we handle? Some people appear to cope with stress better than others. Those who deal with it poorly suffer more consequences. Selye believed that we are each born with an innate ability to cope with stress but that some people possess a more hardy constitution than others. He hypothesized that we each have a predetermined amount of energy available to us to expend over a lifetime. Once the wear, tear, and stress of life drains the energy pool, we enter the ultimate stage of exhaustion, or death. Selye wrote:

> We still do not know precisely just what is lost, except that it is not merely caloric energy, since food intake is normal during the stage of resistance. Hence, one would think that once adaptation has occurred, and energy is amply available, resistance should go on indefinitely. But just as any inanimate machine gradually wears out, even if it has enough fuel, so does the human machine sooner or later become the victim of constant wear and tear.[11]

I think this is a very important concept to understand. We can tolerate only so much wear and tear in a lifetime. And constant fatigue is a sign that you are a victim of constant wear and tear. This is why, as a physician, I feel strongly that chronic fatigue should be regarded as a symptom of too great a demand on the person. If we ignore fatigue and claim it is just a harmless feeling, then we are ignoring a warning from our bodies.

I am reminded of one of the women I interviewed. As she was talking to me, I thought about Selye's wear-and-tear theory. Although Sheila has lived a pretty good life, she has certainly had her trials and tribulations. In the past nine years, she has been through radical surgery and chemotherapy for cancer, mourned the deaths of four loved ones, and just recently lost her live-in boyfriend. After Sheila's cancer was discovered, her boyfriend Tom took up with another woman and subsequently moved out. Sheila told me she was just out of energy and does not know if she can survive this last blow:

> "In the course of four years I buried my father, my husband, my step-mother and my father-in-law, in that order, and I managed to hold myself together, but there have been times recently with all this business with Tom when I didn't know if I'd make it or not. It's been one of the roughest times of my life and I wish I could figure out why. I guess it's just a combination of everything, the illness and all the stress with that too, although I really had my guard down and didn't expect this latest development."

Sheila has had so much stress in the past few years that she is running out of energy. This last incident—her boyfriend deserting her—is almost too much for her to bear.

In the middle of this turmoil, Sheila found out she had a recurrence of her tumor. She asked me, "Doctor, isn't it true that stress is related to cancer? Could all this with my boyfriend have helped my cancer to return?" I told her yes. The stress could have lowered her resistance so that her body did not recognize the cancer had returned or so that it did not have the strength to fight it off.

Remember: In the first stage of the stress reaction, the alarm stage, the body's resistance to disease is down. Studies are showing that people who have more stress in their lives and who fail to cope well with the stress are more susceptible to almost any illness, from colds to cancer.

Individuals vary a great deal in the way they show the wear and tear of life. One person may develop heart disease, another may develop ulcers, while another may develop cancer. A number of factors, such as age, gender, genetic predisposition, diet, and drugs, determine how the stress reaction is manifested. We have control over many of these reactions. We can alter our diets to be more healthful, we can get more exercise, we can decrease our exposure to drugs, and we can learn to change our behavior toward stressful events. We can heed the warning of chronic fatigue.

Why listen to fatigue? I believe that chronic fatigue can be a step along the road to developing an illness. We know there is a relationship between stressful life events and subsequent illness. We also know there is a relationship between stressful life events and the development of chronic fatigue. It is, then, reasonable to assume that there is a relationship between chronic fatigue and subsequent illness.

In one study a group of people suffering from both chronic fatigue and a rheumatic disorder (e.g., arthritis) reported that the chronic fatigue started a year or two before the outward symptoms of the rheumatic disorder were felt. They also reported exposure to more severe and more frequent stressful events than people in the control group (normal people).[12]

The author concluded:

> This suggests that chronic fatigue should be regarded not just as a harmless subjective symptom but as an important indicator of failure to adapt to stressful events and a justification for prophylactic measures to prevent the development of certain diseases.[13]

I want to return to my warning that fatigue is a signal that your body needs rest. You should not ignore your fatigue, not only because it is distressing to live with it, but also because it could be the first sign of future illness.

You may have found that this has been a difficult chapter. We have covered a lot of territory and I have introduced some complex concepts. However, it is important for you to have a firm understanding of how one part of the body can affect the rest of it; how metabolic errors and emotions can both have the same effects on the body; and how various processes lead to the overall feeling of fatigue. I have used the Fatigue Scheme as a way of demonstrating to you that fatigue affects our whole being, regardless of where it starts. Remember: "Psychological factors always play a role in fatigue, regardless of its origin. Hence, the practical problem is to distinguish those instances in which physical factors are significantly involved from those in which they are not."[14]

Labeling the origin of fatigue as being primarily psychological or physical helps us. It is extremely important to figure out what is causing your fatigue and where pressure is being applied in the system, because the cures have to be directed at that level. For example, the treatment for Mary's anemia is quite different from the therapy required to resolve Louise's conflict. Our job now will be to identify your causes of fatigue and figure out what you can do to increase your energy reserve and decrease your energy drain.

Let me give you a good rule of thumb: Fatigue that is worse in the morning and gets better as the day wears on (or only during certain activities) is usually due to a psychological cause, whereas fatigue that grows as the day passes and persists despite changing activities tends to be caused by a physical problem. Furthermore, psychologically induced fatigue is not usually relieved by lying down or sleeping, whereas physically induced fatigue is often abolished or mitigated.

Fatigue is a signal that you need rest—*relief*. But relief from what? That may not be so obvious. In the next chapter, we will try to answer that question. We will spend the entire time developing your personal Fatigue Profile. We will discover the factors in your life that are adding to your fatigue. You have to identify the problems before you can solve them. I hope you will be able to identify psychological problems as well as physical problems, because as far as I am concerned, Descartes is dead and all causes of fatigue are equal.

WHAT TO DO

1. Set aside 10 percent of each waking day for yourself.

For most people, this calculates to be about an hour and a half out of every day. These ninety minutes should be strictly yours to do whatever you wish. Now, this should not include catching up on the laundry or running to the grocery store. If the time is not in your life now, then you must make it. You will find many ideas in the remainder of this book on how to make time. Do something you enjoy: Read a book, do some handiwork, take a walk, or use this time to get your daily exercise. Your ninety minutes should be relaxing.

2. At least once a day, take a rest period.

Try to find a quiet place, either lie on the floor or sit, but in either case, put your feet up (to help blood return to your head). Rest or doze for a half-hour. End your rest period by doing light calesthenics to get your blood circulating. Make sure your "rest" period is not a coffee break, filled with cigarette smoke, caffeine, and chatter.

3. Sleep one hour more each day.

Sleep is vital in alleviating fatigue and maintaining well-being. During sleep, hundreds of reparative processes are occurring, some of which occur only during sleep. Many women are chronically exhausted because they are forcing themselves to get by without enough sleep. In Chapter 9, I will cover sleep in detail; however, I want to establish this general guideline now. Most people cannot change the time of day they get up because of work schedules. Try going to bed one hour early.

4. Take at least a two-week vacation each year.

Include anyone who will help you relax: a friend, lover, or husband, but no children allowed! So often, women end up working just as hard on their "vacations" as they do the rest of the year because they are still busy taking care of everybody else's needs. Vacation should be a time of pleasure, relaxation, and rest for your body and soul. Do everything you must to take a vacation with only your special person along. And—a word to the wise—do not work your hectic pace up until the moment of your vacation. If you do, you will be sick your whole vacation, and just as it is time to go back to your routine, you will be feeling in a real "vacation" mood. To solve this dilemma, begin to rest up by slowing down your pace, lightening your schedule, and resting and sleeping more at least two weeks before your vacation.

5. *Put more pleasure into your life.*

Pleasure and enthusiasm raise the threshold for fatigue, whereas boredom and dissatisfaction lower it. If you are happy in life and taking time out to appreciate the people and things around you, you will have much more energy. Try planning events that put more music, dance, art, poetry, love, and humor into your life!

4

KNOW YOUR SELF

This is a self-assessment chapter. By taking fifteen exercises, you will find out something about your health, your life-style, your pressures, and your responses to life. By the time you complete this chapter, you should know a lot more about your fatigue and its causes. This will help you start your own program for increasing your storehouse of energy.

These fifteen exercises are scored. The score will indicate, generally, whether or not that particular area of concern is generating a lot of fatigue in your life. I will discuss the results and briefly indicate which scores place you in the Fatigue Zone. However, I want you to remember that these scores are not the final say on your fatigue and should be used only as general guidelines.

At the end of this chapter, all of the scores will be used to develop your individual Fatigue Profile. It will provide you with an overview of the results of all of your exercises and quickly help you pinpoint the areas in which you can go to work to increase your energy.

Try to answer the questions honestly. Just remember that self-assessment is the first step on the way to improvement. Think again of the new energetic you that you began dreaming of back in Chapter 1. You are on the road to becoming that new you, right now!

EXERCISE 1

GENERAL FATIGUE INDICATOR[1]

Which of the following describes how you feel most of the time?

1. Terrific
2. Very good
3. Energetic
4. Fairly well
5. Average
6. A little tired
7. Dragging
8. Exhausted
9. About to collapse

Your score on Exercise 1, **The General Fatigue Indicator**
Write the number you circled on the line below:

Score: _3_

If you circled a number between 6 and 9, you have some degree of chronic fatigue. Your goal should be to get this number, which represents the way you feel most of the time, in the range of 3 to 5.

EXERCISE 2

THE FATIGUE TEST[2]

1. Do you feel burning or heaviness in the head?
   Never   Sometimes   Frequently   Usually
2. Does your entire body feel tired?
   Never   Sometimes   Frequently   Usually
3. Do you feel as though you would like to lie down?
   Never   Sometimes   Frequently   Usually
4. Do your legs feel tired?
   Never   Sometimes   Frequently   Usually
5. Do your thoughts get confused or muddled?
   Never   Sometimes   Frequently   Usually
6. Are you drowsy?
   Never   Sometimes   Frequently   Usually
7. Do you yawn a lot?
   Never   Sometimes   Frequently   Usually
8. Are your eyes tired?
   Never   Sometimes   Frequently   Usually
9. Do you have trouble moving?
   Never   Sometimes   Frequently   Usually
10. Do you feel dizzy or have trouble standing?
    Never   Sometimes   Frequently   Usually
11. Do you have difficulty concentrating?
    Never   Sometimes   Frequently   Usually
12. Do you get tired of talking?
    Never   Sometimes   Frequently   Usually
13. Are you nervous?
    Never   Sometimes   Frequently   Usually
14. Do you forget things?
    Never   Sometimes   Frequently   Usually
15. Do you feel a lack of self-confidence?
    Never   Sometimes   Frequently   Usually
16. Do you have difficulty standing or sitting up straight?
    Never   Sometimes   Frequently   Usually
17. Do you have difficulty thinking clearly?
    Never   Sometimes   Frequently   Usually

71

18. Does your attention wander easily?
    Never   Sometimes   **Frequently**   Usually
19. Do you become anxious easily?
    Never   Sometimes   **Frequently**   Usually
20. Do you find that your patience is short?
    Never   Sometimes   **Frequently**   Usually
21. Do you have a headache?
    Never   **Sometimes**   Frequently   Usually
22. Do you feel stiff in the shoulders?
    Never   **Sometimes**   **Frequently**   Usually
23. Do you feel a pain in the abdomen?
    Never   Sometimes   Frequently   Usually
24. Do you have trouble breathing?
    Never   **Sometimes**   Frequently   Usually
25. Do you feel thirsty?
    Never   **Sometimes**   Frequently   Usually
26. Does your voice sound husky?
    Never   **Sometimes**   Frequently   Usually
27. Are you dizzy?
    Never   **Sometimes**   Frequently   Usually
28. Do your eyelids twitch?
    Never   **Sometimes**   Frequently   Usually
29. Do you have shaking in the arms or legs?
    Never   Sometimes   Frequently   Usually
30. Do you feel nauseated?
    Never   **Sometimes**   Frequently   Usually

Your score on Exercise 2, **The Fatigue Test**

Count the number of times that you circled "Never," "Sometimes," "Frequently," or "Usually." Enter the total of each in the following table, multiply by the number in the parentheses, then add all the numbers to calculate your final score. Number of times I circled:

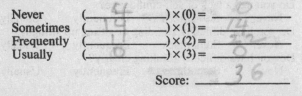

Never	(_____4_____) × (0) =	___0___
Sometimes	(_____14_____) × (1) =	___14___
Frequently	(_____11_____) × (2) =	___22___
Usually	(_____0_____) × (3) =	___0___
	Score:	___36___

If your total on the above test is between 0 and 30, you are fortunate to be experiencing very little fatigue. On the other hand, a total between 31 and 60 indicates that you are experiencing a moderate amount of fatigue. If your score was over 60, you are one of many women who are experiencing a great deal of fatigue.

The next six exercises are designed to help you learn more about your general health and your life-style. In these exercises, your nutrition; physical-exercise program; smoking, drinking, and drug-taking habits; and sleep pattern will be assessed.

NUTRITION[3]

1. Do you eat high-cholesterol foods, such as eggs or butter?

   Usually   Occasionally   Sometimes   Rarely

2. Do you use soft or liquid margarine?

   Usually   Occasionally   Sometimes   Rarely

3. Do you eat fatty meats, such as pork, bacon, steak, hamburger?

   Usually   Occasionally   Sometimes   Rarely

4. Do you eat whole-milk or cream products?

   Usually   Occasionally   Sometimes   Rarely

5. Do you eat sweets and refined sugar?

   Usually   Occasionally   Sometimes   Rarely

6. Do you use sugar substitutes?

   Usually   Occasionally   Sometimes   Rarely

7. Do you eat white (rather than whole-grain) bread?

   Usually   Occasionally   Sometimes   Rarely

8. Do you eat presweetened breakfast cereal?

   Usually   Occasionally   Sometimes   Rarely

9. Do you drink more than one "non-diet" soft drink per day?

   Usually   Occasionally   Sometimes   Rarely

10. Do you overeat?

    Usually   Occasionally   Sometimes   Rarely

11. Do you have indigestion?

    Usually   Occasionally   Sometimes   Rarely

12. Do you salt your food?

    Usually   Occasionally   Sometimes   Rarely

13. Do you drink tea?

    Usually   Occasionally   Sometimes   Rarely

14. Do you drink caffeinated coffee?

    Usually   Occasionally   Sometimes   Rarely

15. Is your diet low in fiber?

    Usually   Occasionally   Sometimes   Rarely

Your score on Exercise 3, **The Nutrition Test**

Count the number of times you circled each answer, write the numbers in the blanks below, and multiply each by the number in the parentheses. Add the subtotals to get your total score. Number of times I circled:

Usually (___1___) × (3) = ___3___
Occasionally (___2___) × (2) = ___4___
Sometimes (_____) × (1) = ___1___
Rarely (___0___) × (0) = ___0___

Add up the total of the four and write the answer below:

Score: ___8___

If your score was 0 to 15, your diet is low in fat, sugar, and other harmful dietary substances. Keep up the good work! If your score is between 15 and 30, you have made some good changes in your diet, although you still have room for improvement. With a score of 30 or above, you definitely need to improve your diet. Most likely, you are eating too much fat and sugar and you are not consuming enough vegetables and fiber. A high score on this test means that your diet is most likely contributing to your fatigue.

In the following exercise circle the choice that best describes your physical activity.

EXERCISE 4

PHYSICAL ACTIVITY

What is your weekly exercise?	Points
Little or none	5
Occasional exercise or sports participation	4
Individual program three times or more each week	3
Scheduled group exercise or sports program three or more times each week	2
More than thirty minutes aerobic exercise each day	1

Your score on Exercise 4, **The Physical Activity Test**
Record the number that you circled in the exercise test.

Score: _____

If your score is 2 or less, you already have an excellent exercise program in your life. If you scored 3, you should consider improving your exercise program. A score of 4 or 5 indicates that your lack of exercise is contributing to a low energy level.

EXERCISE 5

SMOKING

Have you ever or do you now smoke?

1. No, I have never smoked.   0
2. No, I have never smoked but I live with a smoker now.   1
3. Yes, but I quit over ten years ago.   2
4. Yes, but I quit less than ten years ago but more than one year ago.   4
5. Yes, but I quit within the last year.   6
6. Yes, I smoke less than a pack a day.   7
7. Yes, I smoke between one to two packs a day.   8
8. Yes, I smoke more than two packs a day.   9

Your score on Exercise 5, **The Smoking Test**

Score the Smoking Test by simply writing in the number that you circled in the space below:

Score: _____

The Smoking Test is easy to evaluate. A score of 6 or over means your body is still suffering from the ravages of smoking. You can accrue numerous health benefits, including reduction of your fatigue, if you and/or your partner stop smoking.

EXERCISE 6

ALCOHOL[4]

1. Are you ever defensive if a friend or relative mentions your drinking or the money it costs?
   Yes   No
2. Are you sometimes embarrassed or frightened by your behavior when you are under the influence of alcohol?
   Yes   No
3. Do you drink before bedtime, or to help you go to sleep?
   Yes   No
4. Do you ever have a drink to get going in the morning?
   Yes   No
5. Have you ever injured yourself as a result of drinking?
   Yes   No
6. Do you often wake up with a hangover?
   Yes   No
7. Do you often go to "happy hour" after work?
   Yes   No
8. Have you ever missed work because of a hangover?
   Yes   No
9. Has your work ever been affected because you were drinking the night before?
   Yes   No
10. Are there times that you feel that you must have a drink?
    Yes   No
11. Do you often have a drink before going to a party where drinks will be served?
    Yes   No
12. Do you ever decide to limit yourself to a certain number of drinks and then not keep your promise?
    Yes   No
13. Do you ever drink enough to get high when you are alone?
    Yes   No
14. Do you usually want a drink when you are angry, anxious, or frustrated?
    Yes   No

15. Do you ever need a "pick-me-up" drink before or after work, or before going out?

    Yes   No

16. Are there occasions when you feel disappointed or frustrated if alcohol is not served?

    Yes   No

17. When drinking in a group, do you ever try to have extra drinks without letting others know about it?

    Yes   No

18. Do you sometimes feel guilty or angry with yourself about your drinking?

    Yes   No

19. Are you drinking more than you did five years ago?

    Yes   No

20. Do you ever lie about how much you have had to drink?

    Yes   No

21. Do you tend to finish your first drink faster than most other people?

    Yes   No

22. Do you think it would be difficult to enjoy life if you never had another drink?

    Yes   No

23. At home, do you have drinks after dinner, as well as before?

    Yes   No

24. Do you ever use alcohol as a medicine, i.e., to make yourself happier, to kill pain, to help you sleep, to help you relax, to calm your nerves?

    Yes   No

25. Do you ever use alcohol to make yourself feel more feminine?

    Yes   No

Your score on Exercise 6, **The Alcohol Test**

Count the number of times that you circled "Yes" and write the answer below:

Score: _____

WOMEN AND FATIGUE

If you have answered "Yes" to any of the questions, you have some of the symptoms of a drinking problem. The use of alcohol can have a profound effect on your energy level and your overall health.

Almost all people in the United States take drugs of some kind. Many of them have significant side effects. In fact, fatigue is a major side effect of a large number of drugs. Often people lose track of the number of medicines that they take. So before you begin the next exercise, make a trip to your medicine cabinet (or wherever you store your medicine) and use the list below to refresh your memory of what you commonly use. Circle ALL the drugs you use; whether prescriptions, over-the-counter preparations, or illegal substances.

antacids or other
  stomach drugs
antibiotics
anticonvulsants
antidepressants
antihistamines
aspirin or acetaminophen
birth-control pills
blood-pressure pills
blood-thinners
cough and cold preparations
diabetic pills
diuretics (water pills)
heart medicines
hormones (estrogens, etc.)

insulin
minerals
muscle relaxants
painkillers (Rx)
sedatives
sleeping pills
steroids
stomach medicines
tranquilizers
vitamins
illegal drugs (marijuana,
    cocaine, heroin, etc.)
any other drugs

EXERCISE 7

DRUG USAGE[5]

1. Do those close to you often ask about your drug use?
   Yes   No
2. Have they noticed any changes in your moods or behavior?
   Yes   No
3. Are you defensive if a friend or relative mentions your drug use?
   Yes   No
4. Are you sometimes embarrassed or frightened by your behavior under the influence of drugs?
   Yes   No
5. Have you ever gone to see a new doctor because your regular physician would not prescribe the drug you wanted?
   Yes   No
6. When you are under pressure or feeling anxious, do you automatically take a tranquilizer?
   Yes   No
7. Do you take drugs more often or for purposes other than those recommended by your doctor?
   Yes   No
8. Do you take drugs regularly to help you sleep?
   Yes   No
9. Do you have to take a pill to get going in the morning?
   Yes   No
10. Do you think you have a drug problem?
    Yes   No

Your score on Exercise 7, **Drug Usage**
   Count the number of times that you answered "yes" to the questions above and write the answer below:

Score: _____

If you answered "Yes" to any of these questions, there is a good chance you have a drug or medication problem. I hope that it caused you to think carefully about your use of drugs and medications. Many medications can add to your fatigue, either directly, through side effects, or indirectly, by disturbing your sleep.

EXERCISE 8

SLEEP

1. Do you get up feeling tired in the morning?
   Yes   No

2. Do you have difficulty falling asleep?
   Yes   No

3. Do you wake up often during the night?
   Yes   No

4. Do you wake up very early in the morning and have difficulty getting back to sleep?
   Yes   No

5. Do you have physical symptoms, discomfort, or pain that awaken you during the night?
   Yes   No

6. Do you use pills, alcohol, or other drugs to get to sleep?
   Yes   No

7. Does your job involve work on shifts other than daytime?
   Yes   No

8. Do you sleep at different times on weekends than during the week?
   Yes   No

9. Do you ever feel an uncontrollable urge to sleep during the day?
   Yes   No

10. Do you find that you sleep poorly after consuming alcohol?
    Yes   No

Your score on Exercise 8, Sleep

Count the number of times that you circled "Yes" on the sleep exercise and write the answer below:

Score: _3_____

If you answered "Yes" to two or more of the questions, disturbed sleep may be contributing to your fatigue.

WOMEN AND FATIGUE

The next exercises cover a variety of topics that deal with your personal life: such as conflicts you feel, stress, your job, homemaking, and other struggles with which you may be dealing. All of these facets of life impinge on your energy level—your well-being—and are extremely important in looking for the psychological causes of fatigue.

To answer the next set of questions, circle the response that best indicates the extent to which the statement is a concern in your life.

EXERCISE 9

YOUR CONFLICTS[6]

1. Your partner's being unavailable or not home enough.
   Not at all   Somewhat   Considerably   Extremely
2. Poor communications.
   Not at all   Somewhat   Considerably   Extremely
3. Not getting enough appreciation or attention.
   Not at all   Somewhat   Considerably   Extremely
4. Conflicts about the children.
   Not at all   Somewhat   Considerably   Extremely
5. Lack of companionship.
   Not at all   Somewhat   Considerably   Extremely
6. Not getting along with others, personality clashes.
   Not at all   Somewhat   Considerably   Extremely
7. Conflict over who does housework.
   Not at all   Somewhat   Considerably   Extremely
8. Not getting enough emotional support—his not backing you up.
   Not at all   Somewhat   Considerably   Extremely
9. Finding it difficult to talk about sexual matters with your partner.
   Not at all   Somewhat   Considerably   Extremely
10. Feeling dissatisfied with the emotional aspect of your sexual relationship.
    Not at all   Somewhat   Considerably   Extremely
11. Conflict between your sexual actions and your real feelings.
    Not at all   Somewhat   Considerably   Extremely
12. Feelings of discomfort with your sexuality.
    Not at all   Somewhat   Considerably   Extremely
13. The financial strain of having children.
    Not at all   Somewhat   Considerably   Extremely
14. Worrying about children's physical well-being—health problems, accidents, sex, drugs, and so forth.
    Not at all   Somewhat   Considerably   Extremely
15. The heavy demands and responsibilities of having children.
    Not at all   Somewhat   Considerably   Extremely

16. Not being sure if you are doing the right thing for your children.
Not at all   Somewhat   Considerably   Extremely
17. Your children not showing appreciation or love.
Not at all   Somewhat   Considerably   Extremely
18. Not having enough control over your children.
Not at all   Somewhat   Considerably   Extremely
19. Your having too many arguments and conflicts with your children.
Not at all   Somewhat   Considerably   Extremely
20. Your children do not help you enough.
Not at all   Somewhat   Considerably   Extremely
21. Problems with child care or schooling.
Not at all   Somewhat   Considerably   Extremely
22. General feeling of discomfort with yourself.
Not at all   Somewhat   Considerably   Extremely
23. Feeling that others are better or more competent than you are.
Not at all   Somewhat   Considerably   Extremely
24. Feeling of guilt for not getting more done.
Not at all   Somewhat   Considerably   Extremely
25. Finding yourself being "driven to do it all".
Not at all   Somewhat   Considerably   Extremely
26. Difficulty in saying No to the demands of others.
Not at all   Somewhat   Considerably   Extremely
27. Feeling that you give, give, give while others always seem to take, take, take.
Not at all   Somewhat   Considerably   Extremely
28. Finding that you take on the burdens of others.
Not at all   Somewhat   Considerably   Extremely
29. The feeling of being torn between work and home.
Not at all   Somewhat   Considerably   Extremely
30. Difficulty in seeing that your own needs are met.
Not at all   Somewhat   Considerably   Extremely

Your score on Exercise 9, **Your Conflicts**

Count the number of times you circled each answer, write the numbers in the blanks, and multiply each by the number in the parentheses. Add the subtotals to get your total score. Number of times I circled:

None at all	(_____ *15* _____)	× (0) =	_____ *0*
Somewhat	(_____ *5* _____)	× (1) =	_____ *5*
Considerably	(_____ *4* _____)	× (2) =	_____ *8*
Extremely	(_____ *4* _____)	× (3) =	_____ *12*

Now add up the total of the four and write the answer below.

Score: _____ *31*

If your score was 0 to 30, you are fortunate enough to have a life that is relatively free of concern. A score of 31 to 60 indicates that there are areas in which you could improve. Above 60, you are experiencing a high amount of frustration and stress, which is draining you of a considerable amount of energy.

EXERCISE 10

HOMEMAKING CONCERNS[7]

1. Having too much free time.
   Not at all Somewhat Considerably Extremely
2. Not having your own money.
   Not at all Somewhat Considerably Extremely
3. The lack of adult company.
   Not at all Somewhat Considerably Extremely
4. Having to structure or plan your own time.
   Not at all Somewhat Considerably Extremely
5. Disliking housework.
   Not at all Somewhat Considerably Extremely
6. A lack of challenge.
   Not at all Somewhat Considerably Extremely
7. Having to justify not having a "job" outside the home.
   Not at all Somewhat Considerably Extremely
8. Lack of appreciation from others for all the work you do.
   Not at all Somewhat Considerably Extremely
9. Not contributing to the family income by earning money.
   Not at all Somewhat Considerably Extremely
10. Boredom and monotony.
    Not at all Somewhat Considerably Extremely

Your score on Exercise 10, **Homemaking Concerns**

Count the number of times you circled each answer, write the numbers in the blanks below, and multiply each by the number in the parentheses. Add the subtotals to get your total score. Number of times I circled:

Not at all   (_____) × (0) = _____
Somewhat   (_____) × (1) = _____
Considerably   (_____) × (2) = _____
Extremely   (_____) × (3) = _____

Add up the total of the four and write the answer below.

Score: _____

If your score was 0 to 10, you are fortunate enough to have a role that is relatively free of stress and one which you enjoy. A score of 10 to 20 indicates that you are reasonably free of frustration, although there is some room for growth and development. Above 20, your feelings about your job as a homemaker are causing you significant concern and may be contributing to your fatigue.

As in the previous exercise, circle the word that best describes if the given factor is a *concern* to you in your *present* job.

EXERCISE 11

JOB STRESS[8]

1. Having too much to do.
    Not at all   Somewhat   Considerably   Extremely
2. Job insecurity.
    Not at all   Somewhat   Considerably   Extremely
3. The job's causing conflicts with other responsibilities.
    Not at all   Somewhat   Considerably   Extremely
4. Not liking the boss.
    Not at all   Somewhat   Considerably   Extremely
5. Not being given the advancement you want or deserve.
    Not at all   Somewhat   Considerably   Extremely
6. The job's not fitting your skills or interests.
    Not at all   Somewhat   Considerably   Extremely
7. The job's being too regimented—too much supervision.
    Not at all   Somewhat   Considerably   Extremely
8. Bad physical working conditions.
    Not at all   Somewhat   Considerably   Extremely
9. Lack of recognition or appreciation.
    Not at all   Somewhat   Considerably   Extremely
10. The job's dullness, monotony, lack of variety.
    Not at all   Somewhat   Considerably   Extremely
11. Being dissatisfied with income.
    Not at all   Somewhat   Considerably   Extremely
12. Problems due to your being a woman.
    Not at all   Somewhat   Considerably   Extremely
13. Having to do things that shouldn't be part of your job.
    Not at all   Somewhat   Considerably   Extremely
14. Lack of opportunity for career growth.
    Not at all   Somewhat   Considerably   Extremely
15. Unnecessary busy work.
    Not at all   Somewhat   Considerably   Extremely

16. Lack of challenge.

       Not at all   Somewhat   Considerably   Extremely

17. The people you work with.

       Not at all   Somewhat   Considerably   Extremely

18. The job's taking too much out of you—it's too draining.

       Not at all   Somewhat   Considerably   Extremely

19. The hours you work.

       Not at all   Somewhat   Considerably   Extremely

20. The number of hours that you have to spend away from your family.

       Not at all   Somewhat   Considerably   Extremely

Your score on Exercise 11, **Job Stress**

Count the number of times you circled each answer, write the numbers in the blanks below, and multiply each by the number in the parentheses. Add the subtotals to get your total score. Number of times I circled:

Not at all   (_____) × (0) = _____

Somewhat   (_____) × (1) = _____

Considerably   (_____) × (2) = _____

Extremely   (_____) × (3) = _____

Add up the total of the four and write the answer below.

Score: _____

If your score was 0 to 20, you are fortunate enough to have a job that is relatively free of stress. A score of 20 to 40 indicates that you are reasonably free of frustration. Above 40, you are experiencing a high amount of frustration and stress from your job.

WOMEN AND FATIGUE

We all suffer losses at some time in our life. Losses include people, personal attributes (such as job, youth, or beauty), or ideals (such as dreams). People often forget to take losses into account when they try to explain their fatigue. When we do lose somebody or something we experience a period of grieving, whether we know it or not. And such grieving drains us of considerable energy. In the questions below, circle the terms that describe the losses that you have incurred over the last two years.

EXERCISE 12

LOSSES

Death of a spouse
Death of a child
Divorce
Separation from spouse or partner
Death of a close family member
Victim of violence or a violent crime
Major personal illness or injury
Mastectomy, hysterectomy (or removal of any other body part)
Loss of a pregnancy (abortion or miscarriage)
Death of a close friend
Loss of job
Last child leaving home
Nonfulfillment of a dream (childless, never married)
Menopause
Retirement from job
Moving to a new location
Any other _____

Your score on Exercise 12, Losses
Count the number of items you marked and write the answer below.

Score: _____

If you have experienced two or more losses within the last two years, mourning is probably a big contributor to your fatigue.

EXERCISE 13

YOUR MOOD

1. Do you experience difficulty in concentration?
   Yes   No
2. Have you lost interest in your usual activities?
   Yes   No
3. Do you feel disappointed with yourself?
   Yes   No
4. Have you experienced any change in your sexual drive?
   Yes   No
5. Have you experienced any change in your appetite?
   Yes   No
6. Do you ever think of harming yourself or of death?
   Yes   No
7. Have you noticed any change in your physical movements; are they either slowed down or speeded up?
   Yes   No
8. Do you feel as though you just do not have the energy to perform your usual activities?
   Yes   No
9. Have you experienced any change in your sleep?
   Yes   No
10. Do you feel guilty?
    Yes   No

Your score on Exercise 13, **Your Mood**

Count the number of times you circled "Yes" and write the number below.

Score: _____ 5

If you marked "Yes" up to three times, you are generally in a good state of mind. A score of four indicates that you are probably feeling depressed. If you felt that five to ten of the statements applied to you, then you have some degree of depression. The higher your score, the more severe your depression.

WOMEN AND FATIGUE

The last two exercises are designed to discover the physical causes of fatigue—physical symptoms of illness and physical factors on your job. In Exercise 14, circle any symptoms that you presently have. Mind you, we all have aches and pains, we all occasionally have headaches or constipation. I want you to circle those that either worry you or that you think are consistently out of the ordinary.

EXERCISE 14

THE REVIEW OF SYMPTOMS (ROS)

abdominal pain
aches
anemia
apathy
appetite change
arm or leg pain
back pain
bed-wetting
black stools
bleeding gums
bleeding problems
blind spots in vision
blood in urine
blurring of vision
bowel-movement change
breast lump(s)
breast pain
bruising
bulging eyes
burping
calf pain
cataracts
change in birthmarks
change in body size
change in glove or shoe size
change in hair distribution
change in skin color
chest pain
constipation
convulsions
cough
coughing up blood
cramps
dentures
depression

diarrhea
difficulty starting urine
difficulty swallowing
discharge from ear
discharge from nose
discharge from vagina
dizziness
double vision
dribbling urine
enlarged lymph nodes
excessive drinking of fluids
excessive eating
excessive urination
facial pain
fainting
fatigue
fevers
fibroid tumors
frequent urination
gas
goiter
hair change
headache
head trauma (blow)
hearing change
heartburn
heart murmur
heat or cold intolerance
hemorrhoids
hernia
hoarseness
infection in ear
infections
infertility
insomnia

95

irritability
itching
joint deformities
joint heat
joint redness
joint sprains
joint stiffness
joint swelling
kidney stones
laxative needs
leg cramps
limited motion of joints
limping
loss of vision
malaise
memory loss
menopause
menstrual irregularity
menstrual pain
mole changes
mouth sores
muscle cramps
muscle pain
muscle paralysis
muscle wasting
muscle weakness
nail change
nausea
neck pain
nervousness
nightmares
night sweats
nipple discharge
nosebleeds
numbness
obstruction in nose or sinus
pain
pain in ears or eyes
pain on urination
palpitations

paralysis
phobias
pins-and-needles feeling
postnasal drip
rashes
ringing in ears
sexual difficulties
shakes (tremors)
shortness of breath
shortness of breath
  on exertion
shortness of breath on lying
  down or sleeping
sinus discharge
sinus pain
skin changes
skin changes over breast
sleeping problems
sore throat
sore tongue
speech difficulties
spotting (vaginal)
sputum production
sweating
swelling
taste problems
teeth problems
thirsty
transfusions
tuberculosis skin test positive
turning yellow (jaundice)
unusual menstrual bleeding
upright sleeping position
urgency of urination
urination at night
urine color change
vomiting
vomiting blood
vomiting hair
wheezing

Your score for Exercise 14, **The Review of Symptoms**

Count the number of symptoms that you circled and write the number below.

Score: _____

If you circled three or more, you have a physical condition that is probably consuming a lot of your strength and you should see your doctor. Of course, someone could have just one or two symptoms, such as stomach pain and vomiting blood, which would indicate a serious problem that needs attention. Or someone could have four symptoms, none of which suggest anything serious. There is no magic cutoff point for how many symptoms spell trouble, but three symptoms can usually give you a good clue if a disease is present and which one it may be.

PHYSICAL JOB FACTORS

1. Does your job require that you stand in one position for sustained periods of time?
   Yes   No
2. Does your job involve twisting or stooping?
   Yes   No
3. Do you stand on a hard surface?
   Yes   No
4. Does your job involve sustained sitting?
   Yes   No
5. Does your job involve the lifting of heavy objects?
   Yes   No
6. Do you have to reach or twist to do your job?
   Yes   No
7. Are you required to use repetitive physical motions?
   Yes   No
8. Do you use machines or tools in your work that subject your body or appendages to vibrations?
   Yes   No
9. Does your job require concentrated visual acuity?
   Yes   No
10. Do you handle chemicals or toxic materials in your job?
    Yes   No
11. Is your work area dirty or crowded?
    Yes   No
12. Is your work area noisy?
    Yes   No
13. Is your work area too hot or too cold?
    Yes   No
14. Are you subjected to poorly fitting tools or safety devices?
    Yes   No
15. Is your work area arranged so that devices or papers with which you work cannot be reached with minimum movements?
    Yes   No

Your score on Exercise 15, **Physical Job Factors**

Count the number of times that you circled "Yes" and write the answer below:

Score: _____

If you answered "Yes" more than four times, your job is probably excessively tiring. Although there are many more factors on a job that could be causing fatigue, the biggest offenders were covered here.

You have worked hard to analyze a variety of elements in your life that could contribute to your fatigue. We will now use the results of your past work to develop your Fatigue Profile, which will help you look at the consolidated results of all the exercises and give you an overall view of what is causing your fatigue. First, go back to the exercises indicated on the chart on the next page and fill in the table with the scores from each one.

SCORE TABLE

	Exercise	Your Score
1.	General Fatigue Indicator	3
2.	Fatigue Test	26
3.	Nutrition	8
4.	Physical Activity	3
5.	Smoking	0
6.	Alcohol	0
7.	Drug Usage	1
8.	Sleep	3
9.	Your Conflicts	31
10.	Homemaking Concerns	5
11.	Job Stress	0
12.	Losses	0
13.	Your Mood	5
14.	The Review of Symptoms (ROS)	17
15.	Physical Job Factors	

Now, I want you to develop your Fatigue Profile. The following graphs are designed to give you a quick picture of the areas that may be contributing to your fatigue. To develop the Profile, take your score from each of the exercises as you recorded in the table above and mark the score of each exercise with an X on the appropriate line in the Fatigue Profile.

For instance, if your score on the General Fatigue Indicator was 7, mark an X on the General Fatigue Indicator line as shown below:

Example:

Exercise 1. General Fatigue Indicator

```
        0                3              6   (7)     9
------------------    =======    *****X *****
                                        Fatigue Zone
```

Your Fatigue Profile

Exercise 1. General Fatigue Indicator

```
       0            3            6            9
       --------------------======= *************
                                    Fatigue Zone
```

Exercise 2. Fatigue Test

```
       0           30           60           90
       --------------------======= *************
                                    Fatigue Zone
```

Exercise 3. Nutrition

```
       0           15           30           45
       --------------------======= *************
                                    Fatigue Zone
```

Exercise 4. Physical Activity

```
       1                        4            5
       ----------------------------------- *************
                                    Fatigue Zone
```

Exercise 5. Smoking

```
       0            3            6            9
       --------------------======= *************
                                    Fatigue Zone
```

Exercise 6. Alcohol

```
                                  0           25
       -------------------------------- *************
                                    Fatigue Zone
```

Exercise 7. Drug Usage

```
                                  0           10
       -------------------------------- *************
                                    Fatigue Zone
```

Exercise 8. Sleep

```
                        0      2            10
       -----------------------|---- *************
                                    Fatigue Zone
                                    101
```

WOMEN AND FATIGUE

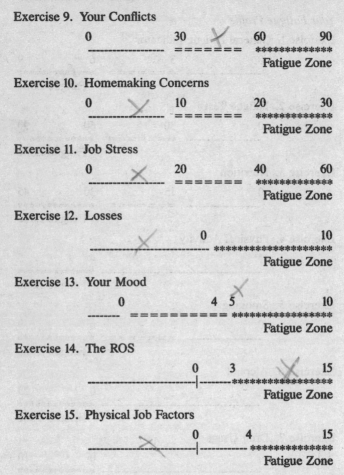

Exercise 9. Your Conflicts

```
0            30    ✗    60          90
----------- ======= ***************
                          Fatigue Zone
```

Exercise 10. Homemaking Concerns

```
0    ✗    10         20          30
----------- ======= ***************
                          Fatigue Zone
```

Exercise 11. Job Stress

```
0    ✗       20         40          60
----------- ======= ***************
                          Fatigue Zone
```

Exercise 12. Losses

```
        ✗       0                    10
--------------------- ********************
                          Fatigue Zone
```

Exercise 13. Your Mood

```
0              4 5  ✗               10
------- ========== *****************
                          Fatigue Zone
```

Exercise 14. The ROS

```
            0    3        ✗        15
------------------------|---------*****************
                          Fatigue Zone
```

Exercise 15. Physical Job Factors

```
        ✗    0         4          15
------------------------|----------- **************
                          Fatigue Zone
```

You have come to the end of the exercises. By now, I bet you feel as if you have been exercising! But be encouraged—your work here is extremely important. Identifying the causes of your fatigue is the first step to eliminating them.

WHAT TO DO

1. Use your Fatigue Profile as your guide to identifying the areas in your life that are causing your fatigue.

This chapter was designed to help you get a better understanding of your own personal fatigue. By answering a lot of detailed questions, you are now probably much more aware of conditions under which you feel tired. This chapter also forms a data base that will help you analyze your fatigue further as you read through the additional chapters in the book. For the most part, each exercise in the Fatigue Profile has been designed to reflect one chapter of the book. (In a few cases, more than one test is associated with a given chapter; for example, alcohol and drugs are both considered in Chapter 8.)

As you read, refer back to the work you have done here and look for patterns or trends that run throughout your answers and recur in your thinking. This will help you pinpoint the crucial area in your life that needs the most attention. I have divided the causes of fatigue into three sections: life-style causes, psychological causes, and physical causes. Do you have weak areas in all three categories, or do all of your Fatigue Zones fall within the same category? Study your Fatigue Profile.

2. Retake these exercises to assess your progress.

As you start making changes in your life, return to this chapter and repeat some of the exercises. If you continue to answer the questions the same way and your Fatigue Profile stays the same, you need to work more diligently to bring about the necessary change. If you are succeeding, the outline of your Fatigue Profile should change over time—it should shift to the left. Also, use your changing responses and changing Fatigue Profile as a subject of conversation between you and your loved ones or your doctor as a means of gaining their assistance in supporting your efforts and bringing about changes in your life.

3. Follow through on your findings.

I hope, at this point, you have a good idea of what is

contributing to your fatigue. The next step is to examine each cause of fatigue individually and discover what can be done about it. Some of the suggestions for changes will take time and effort; others can be brought about quite quickly. Whatever the case may be, continue to work on those areas you have identified as energy drainers. And do not expect miracles! Change takes time. Have a little patience with yourself. Make it a lifelong goal to look for ways inside and outside this book to boost your energy!

Part Two
CHANGE YOUR LIFE-STYLE

5

EAT FOR ENERGY

Americans have been called the most overfed, underexercised people in the world; one in three persons in America is overweight. Unfortunately, this statement is much more true for women than it is for men. One out of every five women is considered to be significantly overweight. And this statistic does not include the millions of women who are slightly overweight and are constantly struggling to lose that extra ten to fifteen pounds.

Then, there are millions of women who may be envied for their slimness and apparent lack of a weight problem, but people know little about the price these women pay to stay fashionably slender. Many women who appear to be free of a weight problem are locked into a compulsive eating style, such as semistarvation, or binges and purges. All told, it is estimated that more than half the female population between the ages of fifteen and fifty suffer with some form of an eating problem.[1]

Many of these women do not realize the extent of the price they are paying—that the fatigue and other ill health from which they may be suffering is largely a result of their eating and dietary habits. Although American women rarely connect fatigue with eating, either the lack of it or too much of the wrong kind can be an important cause of fatigue.

Recently, I saw the results of a survey in a women's magazine that reported that 80 percent of women said they had been on a diet within the previous year. I am sure that the majority of those women never reached their goal; they probably ended the diet in frustration and discouragement. I think fatigue caused by diets is one of the major reasons women find it so hard to stick to them. They lose their stamina and willpower as their energy flags, and finally they give in to the body's urgent clamoring for food.

I want you to read this chapter with your own eating habits clearly in mind. Go back to your Fatigue Profile in Chapter 4 and see how you scored on Exercise 3, Nutrition. Are you presently overweight or do you regularly overeat? How did you answer the questions about sugar consumption? Do you eat refined sugar, sweet foods, and soft drinks on a daily basis? Is your diet high in fat? A high-fat diet would include meats such as pork, organ meats, hamburger, and steak; dairy products made out of whole milk and cream products; and a lot of junk and fried food. And finally, are you taking large doses of vitamin supplements? If you answered these questions with a "yes," your diet may well be a major contributor to your fatigue.

In this chapter we are going to look at the link between food and fatigue. I will explain why the typical American diet is fatiguing, how the diet techniques you are using may be sapping you of energy, and how you should select a diet plan.

EATING AND FATIGUE

Most people know intuitively that eating a large meal—especially a pasta feast—makes them groggy and sleepy. The very act of eating, in and of itself, often appears to bring about a state of transient fatigue. This seems reasonable, for the body must do some work to process fuel. But there is much more to it than this.

Studies are beginning to reveal the marvelously complex effects that food has on us. Eating can either induce sleep or produce wakefulness, depending on which foods are eaten, by producing chemical changes in the brain. The food actually triggers the release of the chemical messages.

We can think of the brain as having two pathways, each

one stimulated by the interaction of a group of chemicals. One pathway—the adrenalin pathway—acts to energize us, wake us up, and put the body on alert. Opposing this pathway is another—the indoleamine pathway—that works to calm us down, sedate us, and put us to sleep.

Certain foods activate one or the other pathway. One expert summed up the effects as follows:

> Researchers have shown that a meal composed primarily of *high-protein* foods, such as fish, fowl, eggs, meat, dairy products, and beans, stimulates the adrenalin pathway and gives you up to five hours worth of long-lasting energy. In contrast, a meal consisting principally of *high-carbohydrate* foods, such as pasta, salad, fruit, and rich desserts, gives you a surge of energy for up to an hour, but then actually encourages you, by influencing the indoleamine pathway, to go to sleep.[2]

Use this knowledge to help you select food and plan your meals. If you have a very busy morning or afternoon, stay away from a large high-carbohydrate meal. If you have an especially important meeting or engagement after lunch, watch out for the combination of the effects of a high-carbohydrate meal and the afternoon slump! Have your daily allotment of protein at lunch and save your carbohydrate meal for supper, to help you relax in the evening. On the other hand, if you do have an important evening engagement and want to be at your best, choose a high-protein dinner to help "rev" you up. Pay attention to the size, timing, and content of your meals!

DIETARY COMPONENTS AND FATIGUE

Food not only has the ability to affect chemicals in the brain, it is our source of fuel and essential minerals and vitamins. Deficiencies or excesses of any of the essential dietary components have the potential to create fatigue—especially chronic fatigue. Let us now take a look at the basic food groups and the essential dietary components. A healthful diet includes adequate calories in the form of carbohydrates, as well as adequate amounts of protein, fat, minerals, and vitamins.

Carbohydrates

Carbohydrates are the most abundant chemical compounds on earth and constitute one of the three classes of nutrients. They include sugars, glycogen, starches, and cellulose (fiber). Carbohydrates are preferred by the body as the basic source of energy, its fuel. This is because the body's energy-making machinery is designed to burn primarily glucose (sugar), not fat or protein.

Carbohydrates are absorbed from the digestive tract in the form of either glucose, galactose, or fructose. These three simple sugars can be used directly by the body to make energy or they can be stored after being changed into glycogen. The stored glycogen is available for conversion back to glucose whenever there is need for reserve energy.

Occasionally, the body can run out of glucose and

CARBOHYDRATES AND THE FATIGUE SCHEME

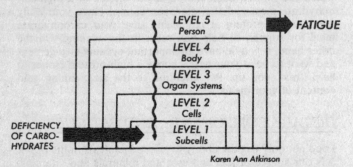

Karen Ann Atkinson

Figure 9: *A deficiency of carbohydrates leaves the body's energy-producing machinery relatively empty, causing weakness and fatigue.*

110

glycogen, for instance when you are fasting or dieting. Then what does it use for fuel to make its energy? The body will burn protein and fat when it is deprived of carbohydrates, but that still leaves the glucose-burning metabolic pathway relatively empty and causes the body to become weakened and clamoring for carbohydrates.

We can visualize this on the Fatigue Scheme, shown in Figure 9. A deficiency of carbohydrates will starve the energy-producing machinery in cells throughout the entire body, which causes fatigue. We can experience this fatigue between meals if we go too long without eating or as a side effect of a diet.

Most of the popular diets that have hit the best-seller list are low-carbohydrate diets. On a low-carbohydrate diet, you will feel fatigued and crave candy, pies, cakes, breads, et cetera. Although you can live off your own fat and protein, and lose weight on a low-carbohydrate diet, you pay the price of eating away at some important organs and suffering from weakness and lethargy.

A nonfatiguing diet must be one that is low in calories and adequate in carbohydrates, so it forces the body to burn a little fat each day and spares you from burning protein. The regular glucose-burning metabolic pathway must be satisfied in order for you to keep your energy. Any other kind of diet may whittle away at your fat some, but it will also whittle away at your muscles, liver, spleen, and willpower. You cannot succeed on a diet if you are exhausted by it!

The form of carbohydrate, simple (sugars) versus complex (starches), is also very important when considering food fatigue. Many people think sugars (including brown sugar, honey, syrups) give one quick energy. Well, they do—but they also give you a quick letdown because sugars are so rapidly absorbed into the bloodstream and into the cells that they are quickly depleted. The resulting hypoglycemia makes you feel weak, light-headed, irritable, fatigued, and hungry. Then hunger may drive you to a candy bar or soda pop once again to raise your blood-glucose level—starting the cycle all over.

By eating complex carbohydrates (whole-wheat breads, grains, cereals, potatoes), you can avoid these vacillating blood-sugar levels, because complex carbohydrates get broken down slowly in the digestive system and, hence, are absorbed into the bloodstream over a longer time period. The slow, steady absorption maintains a more constant blood-sugar level and avoids the symptoms of hunger, weakness, and fatigue.

Many people think of starches as fattening foods; I often hear women who are contemplating beginning a diet say, "Well, I'll have to cut out my bread and potatoes." This is exactly opposite to what you should do for a successful, healthful diet. Starches are no more fattening than sugar or protein on a weight-for-weight basis. But watch out for fat. Fat is over two times as fattening as the starches, sugars, or protein. Fat, as found in meats and dairy products, should be cut out of your diet.

Carbohydrates should make up 60 percent of a healthful diet. Simple and refined sugars should be avoided in all forms, including white sugar, brown sugar, honey, cakes, pies, cookies, soda pop, et cetera. Complex carbohydrates are the best source of calories. These are found in fresh vegetables, fresh fruits, whole-wheat bread, whole grains, cereals, potatoes, corn, beans, rice, and pasta. The closer the food is to the "harvest" the better; in other words, try to select foods that are unprocessed.

Fat

Fat is the most energy-rich form of food available from either animal or plant sources. When we metabolize fat in the body, it yields twice as much energy on a gram-per-gram basis as do carbohydrates or protein. This is the same as saying fats are higher in calories than the other two, given the same weight.

Even though the body prefers carbohydrates as fuel, it cannot store large amounts of them. *So, when we consume more calories than the body needs, they are stored as fat, no matter what the source: carbohydrates, protein, or fat.*

Because excess calories from any source are converted into fat in the body, we need to eat very little fat in our diets, yet the typical American diet is very high in fat as a consequence of eating meats, whole milk, butter, cream, ice cream, and other animal products. It is also rich in eggs, which are high in cholesterol. Approximately 35 percent to 40 percent of the calories in the typical middle-class diet come from fat, another 15 percent from protein, and the remainder from carbohydrate. At this level of consumption, however, Americans are dying from heart disease, strokes, and cancer.

These diseases do not develop overnight. It takes years for the fat and cholesterol to harden the arteries and clog the passageways throughout the body. As that silent process takes place in your body (and it is going on this very moment), one of the earliest symptoms you might experience is fatigue. Excessive fat in the body causes fatigue in a variety of ways. Let us see how that happens.

Fatigue can result from the depletion or lack of a vital substance, such as oxygen which is transported to all tissues in the body by red blood cells. These are extremely small cells (about 5 million red blood cells will fit in the lead tip of a pencil), so they can squeeze into very tight passages.

As the blood vessels get farther and farther away from the heart, they get smaller and smaller in diameter. Finally, they become capillaries and are so narrow that only one red blood cell can pass through at a time. The red blood cells have to move through in single file, and to do so, they must be able to contort their shape. Red blood cells with normal shapes can slip and slide and wiggle their way through. At this point, they release the oxygen they are carrying to the tissues that lie just on the other side of the thin capillary wall.

Fat can significantly interfere with the delivery of oxygen to these tissues, and thus cause fatigue. Animal studies have shown that after meals high in fat content, changes occur in the blood that make it hard for red blood cells to deliver their precious cargo of oxygen.[3] Fat in the blood causes the red blood cells to become sticky and clump together. The blood consequently becomes thicker and moves very slowly through the smaller vessels. In the tiniest branches, the capillaries, the blood may actually stop. Hence the blood cannot deliver an adequate supply of oxygen to some tissues. Dramatic pictures of this sludging of blood have been taken in animals. Although the same experiment

113

NORMAL BLOOD

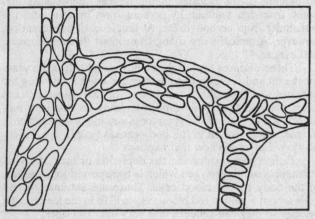

Karen Ann Atkinson

Figure 10: *The red blood cells in normal blood move easily through vessels without clumping.*

cannot be done on people, it has been seen in test tubes, and many researchers believe that the same process occurs in our blood after a high-fat meal.

Fat not only causes immediate fatigue after a fatty meal. Over the course of a lifetime this fat builds up in the blood vessels through which it travels, like grease building up in your kitchen sink, until it finally plugs the drain. This process of fat buildup, or atherosclerosis, starts very early in Americans and continues for years. We all have some degree of hardening of the arteries right now.

Over time, the linings of the arteries become thickened by deposits of fat, cholesterol, calcium, and other materials. As these deposits harden, the vessels become more rigid. This makes it much more difficult for the blood to move through the arteries; the heart has to work harder to push the

HIGH-FAT BLOOD

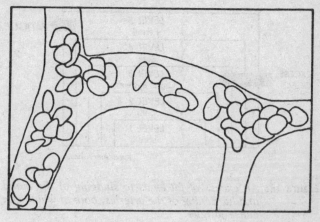

Karen Ann Atkinson

Figure 11: *The red blood cells in blood with high fat levels are sticky and clump together, which causes them to move slowly and clog smaller vessels.*

blood around the body. All of this spells easier fatigability and developing disease. From the early stages of sludging of the blood to the later stages of hardening of the vessels, fat does most of its damage at the organ level of organization. We can represent the effects of fat on the Fatigue Scheme, as seen in Figure 12.

As atherosclerosis progresses, organs may become damaged. If a complete blockage occurs in an artery, the tissue beyond the clot usually dies (unless blood comes from another nearby vessel). In a heart attack, the heart muscle dies; and in a stroke, part of the brain dies. At this stage of the disease, fatigue is just one symptom among many more serious ones.

An excess of fat in the diet can, obviously, lead to obesity as well. Obesity is considered a health risk. It has

FAT AND THE FATIGUE SCHEME

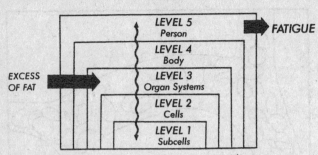

Karen Ann Atkinson

Figure 12: *An excess of fat leads to sludging of the blood and hardening of the arteries, both of which can cause fatigue.*

been associated with an increased risk of cardiovascular diseases, diabetes, osteoarthritis, varicose veins, clots, hernias, and gallstones. Just moving a heavy body around takes work and can quickly exhaust you.

We have such a powerful weapon for preventing disease and treating it. And yet, even though research has shown that the American diet is far too rich in fats and cholesterol, doctors have been lax in telling their patients to change their eating habits. One individual who had been admonishing both doctors and the public to change on this score was Nathan Pritikin, author of *The Pritikin Diet*. He said, "The major cause of death in the United States is food poisoning. It is not the kind of food poisoning that you usually think about. Our food poisoning comes from the normal foods in our diet."[4] The poisons that Nathan Pritikin was talking about are fat and cholesterol.

Fat, then, is something you can and should do without in your diet. Try to wean it out. This is one of the most important actions you can take to increase your energy pool, decrease fatigue and weight, prevent disease, and prolong your life. Your fat intake should not exceed 20 percent of total calories and your cholesterol intake should not be greater than 100 milligrams per day.

Proteins

Proteins are the building blocks of life. They make up the major part of all plant and animal tissues. They are found almost everywhere in our body; for example, proteins comprise the skin, hair, muscles, spleen, liver, bones, and teeth. They are essential for growth of new tissue or the repair of injured tissue. Proteins are also very important parts of many of the compounds in our bodies that control metabolic processes. And if necessary, although not ideal, protein can also be burned by the body as a source of heat and energy.

If the body is deficient in carbohydrate, it will begin to burn fat and protein as sources of heat and energy. Protein will yield the same amount of energy as carbohydrate. The price for doing this, however, can be great. Protein can be taken away from organs, such as the muscles, liver, and spleen. Furthermore, waste products from burning protein—ammonia and urea—are toxic to cells, especially cells in the kidneys. High-protein diets (which prevent robbing protein from the organs) are harmful for this reason. They put stress on the kidneys.

Proteins are actually constructed out of smaller subunits called amino acids. There are twenty or more amino acids in nature. All of them are necessary for proper growth and functioning of the body; however, since nine of these amino acids must be supplied by the diet, these nine are called the essential amino acids. The remaining eleven or so are called nonessential amino acids because they can be synthesized by the body from fragments of old broken-down proteins. Old proteins are recycled into an amino-acid "pool," from which new amino acids and proteins are made.

Because the body has the ability to break down old proteins and resynthesize what it needs, we actually do not need to eat much protein every day. Yet Americans have been raised to think they need a diet rich in protein. Americans are eating at least twice if not three times the protein they need. The minimum recommended daily allowance calls for 40 to

117

50 grams, although some experts are now saying even that is too high. Only 20 percent of your calories should come from protein.

Minerals

Minerals are elements of neither plant nor animal origin that are found throughout nature and in our food. They make up a great percentage of the hard parts of the body, such as the teeth, nails, and bones. Minerals also play a major role in a number of important regulatory functions throughout the body.

They are lost daily from the body and, hence, we must replace them in order to avoid a mineral deficiency. At this time, twenty minerals are known to be needed in the diet. These twenty include major electrolytes, such as potassium and sodium, and trace elements (needed in minute quantities), such as cobalt and nickel. The best source of these minerals is unprocessed, fresh food, especially leafy green vegetables.

MINERALS ESSENTIAL FOR LIFE

sodium	cobalt
potassium	copper
calcium	fluorine
chloride	manganese
phosphorus	molybdenum
magnesium	nickel
iron	selenium
zinc	silicon
iodine	vanadium
chromium	tin

You may remember from Chapter 3 that a disruption in regulation is one of the five processes that leads to fatigue. Because minerals play such an important role in regulatory functions throughout the body, a deficiency of one of any of these minerals is quite likely to cause fatigue. Several conditions known to be directly the result of a mineral deficiency have fatigue as a primary symptom.

Iron deficiency is of particular concern. Even with our high standard of living, American women are not getting enough iron in their diets. It has been estimated that at least 20 percent of women of childbearing age[5] and nearly 60 percent of pregnant women are iron-deficient.[6]

Fatigue is often a complaint of iron-deficient women, even when an obvious anemia cannot be demonstrated. That is because you can be iron-deficient without showing iron-deficiency anemia in your blood. (Anemia is a decrease in the number of red blood cells circulating in the blood.) And doctors often overlook this important distinction. Iron deficiency comes long before iron-deficiency anemia. And yet, a test for anemia is the first one many doctors order. They rarely will order an iron-level test if anemia is not found. However, if doctors were to check iron levels, they might discover that a mineral deficiency is responsible for a lot of fatigue.

A deficiency in several of the other minerals can also lead to anemia. Whenever blood cells are made by the body, zinc is in demand. Without the proper amount of zinc, this process can be disturbed. A copper deficiency or manganese deficiency can interfere with the proper utilization of iron. Cobalt is part of Vitamin B_{12} which is needed for the development of normal blood cells. You may have heard of pernicious anemia before; it is a deficiency in Vitamin B_{12}.

Iodine is a mineral that you probably relate to salt. Iodized salt is impregnated with iodine. This is done to make sure there is an adequate amount of iodine in our diets. We need iodine for the proper development and functioning of the thyroid gland. A deficiency of iodine causes goiter (an enlargement of the thyroid gland) and hypothyroidism. Fatigue is one of the cardinal symptoms of hypothyroidism.

Sodium, potassium, calcium, and magnesium are all considered major minerals. These are extremely important in regulating many body functions. A deficiency in any one of them leads to widespread changes throughout the body. For instance, low levels of sodium, potassium, or chloride can cause muscle weakness and lassitude. Magnesium deficiency can create weakness, muscle tremors, and heart-rhythm abnormalities. Fatigue often accompanies deficiencies of any of these major minerals.

Vitamins

A vitamin is any dietary component necessary for growth and good health that cannot be burned as energy in the body. Most vitamins have important functions as regulators of the metabolic processes. In general, the body cannot make vitamins; they must be derived from outside plant and animal food sources.

It is very important for you to realize that either a deficiency or an excess of vitamins may result in fatigue. The key here is moderation. An excess of vitamins can be just as harmful as a deficiency of vitamins. Do not believe the magical claims in the magazines and health-food stores about the curative powers of vitamins. Vitamins are not magic. You might even think of them as a drug; just because two aspirin help a headache does not mean that a whole bottle is better. The whole bottle might make your headache go away, but it can kill you as well. Too much of anything is poison.

In light of the campaigns to get people to take vitamins and the belief of some people that large doses of vitamins can cure almost anything, doctors have become just as concerned—if not more so—about people overdosing on vitamins as they are about their being deficient. This is especially true for the so-called fat-soluble vitamins: vitamins A, D, E, and K. These vitamins are absorbed by fat, stored in the body, and accumulate over time.

The body has the ability to get rid of excessive amounts of the water-soluble vitamins such as C and B complex in the urine, but it cannot dispose of the fat-soluble vitamins, A, D, E, and K that way. Too much vitamin A can lead to headaches, irritability, dizziness, diarrhea, loss of hair, and fatigue. Vitamin D excess leads to calcification of the tissues and can damage the kidneys. Vitamin K toxicity causes gastrointestinal disturbances and anemia. Vitamin E in large amounts can cause weakness and fatigue.

Often, in an attempt to treat the symptom of fatigue, women will begin to self-medicate with large doses of vitamins. Unfortunately, companies tend to take advantage of the public's belief in the magical powers of vitamins. One study in the medical literature reported,

> The J. B. Williams Company has long exploited women's possible need for diet supplementation. The company has paid a number of fines for false and misleading advertising in connection with its product Geritol®, which claims to be a "pick-me-up" for people with "tired blood." Such promotion capitalizes on the most widespread health misbelief in the United States—that extra vitamins provide more pep and energy.[7]

As I write, one of the tabloids has come out with a huge headline that screamed, MIRACLE VITAMIN BEATS TIREDNESS. It turns out the vitamin referred to was B complex—not a miracle vitamin, just an ordinary one. I will tell you firmly that vitamin pills do not provide pep and energy (although three-fourths of Americans still believe this). There is no way to put "pep and energy" into a capsule or a pill. The only thing a vitamin supplement will cure is a vitamin deficiency.

Mild vitamin deficiencies are definitely a problem for some people, but there are not good statistics to show how many fit this category. Some experts say Americans are getting all the vitamins they need, even from processed foods, while others claim that as many as 85 percent are deficient. Quite frankly, it is hard to make a diagnosis of a mild vitamin deficiency because our methods of measuring vitamins in the body are time consuming, costly, and not very accurate.

Nevertheless, some vitamin deficiencies are commonly associated with fatigue. Check your diet to make sure you are getting enough folate (folic acid) and Vitamin B_{12}. Deficiencies of both these vitamins can lead to anemia. Also, check your intake of biotin and pantothenic acid. Fatigue is reported to be a primary symptom of deficiencies of these vitamins.

If you should have a vitamin deficiency that is corrected by taking a vitamin pill, your body may restore some of its energy. If, however, you already have the appropriate amount of vitamin in your body, the extra vitamin pill will not affect your energy level. Vitamin supplements are potentially hazardous to your health and large doses can cause serious imbalances in your body. Do not become a victim of the vitamin salespeople!

Should You Take a Supplement?

Mineral and vitamin deficiencies can clearly lead to fatigue. And fatigue is a particular problem for women. That might lead one to think that women may suffer from more mineral and vitamin deficiencies than men. Some studies now suggest that approximately half of all American women are deficient in some essential mineral or vitamin (the same is not true for men). Why? Nutrition expert Dr. Myron Winick has identified four primary reasons women are so susceptible to nutritional deficiencies today.[8]

First, women's unique biological role in bringing life into the world creates extra nutritional needs. The monthly menstrual cycle causes a significant blood loss. Iron, other minerals, and vitamins are used when the body works to replenish that monthly loss. Furthermore, during pregnancy and lactation the demand for certain nutrients increases dramatically. Nutrient deficiencies will occur unless dietary adjustments compensate for the change.

Second, because many women equate slimness with beauty, women seem to be constantly dieting. Dieting does not necessarily lead to nutritional deficiencies. However, the styles women often use to diet (purging, fasting, low-carbohydrate diets) frequently do lead to certain deficiencies.

Third, many women use oral-contraceptive pills, without realizing that many of these pills interfere with the absorption and metabolism of certain vitamins.

Finally, women are now consuming much more alcohol than in the past. Alcohol reduces the absorption of several vitamins and minerals, and also increases the excretion of some of them.

These four factors—the biology of the female, dieting, oral-contraceptive use, and alcohol consumption—predispose a woman to develop mineral and vitamin deficiencies. Well—should you take a mineral-and-vitamin supplement?

I confess, this is a difficult question to answer. There is lively debate in the medical community about this, let alone in the public sector. If you are confused about all the advice you get from television, radio, and in the print media about vitamins, I do not blame you. I get so frustrated when I see the misleading advertisements and when the "experts" get on television simply to push another food fad on an accepting public. I cannot begin to tell you how much information out there is simply not true. Because science does not have all the answers, there will always be room for the quacks and hucksters to take advantage of people.

I can only tell you that debates over the correct recommended daily allowance for vitamins and minerals as well as other nutritional issues will continue for some time. For instance, we just found out that the recommended level of calcium in the diet was set too low. Perhaps in the future, we will find out that other values are incorrect.

Nevertheless, enough is known about mineral and vitamin requirements to make some reliable statements about supplements. I strongly believe that everyone should attempt to satisfy mineral and vitamin requirements by eating balanced meals. It is really very simple to achieve this by concentrating on eating complex carbohydrates and unprocessed fresh fruits and vegetables. Make sure you are eating the proper foods to assure an adequate intake of minerals and vitamins.

According to the results of a Food and Drug Administration study, "86 percent of the public believed that 'anyone who eats balanced meals can get enough vitamins in his regular food'; yet the majority of the respondents still used or had used supplements because they didn't think *they* ate balanced meals."[9] If you are one of these people, you should make every effort to change your diet to include more unprocessed foods.

Food should be our primary source of these vital substances, yet I cannot say across the board that vitamin supplements have no place. If you are convinced that your diet is not balanced and you refuse to change, then a multiple-vitamin pill once a day (which provides *only* the recommended daily allowances and no more) is allowable. Also, if you are dieting, a multiple-vitamin pill once a day is a good idea.

Do not take any large doses (large is anything over 100 percent of the recommended daily allowance) of any vitamins or minerals, unless your medical doctor has diagnosed a specific condition (such as iron-deficiency anemia). Vitamin supplements could well be contributing to your fatigue, not alleviating it. If you are taking megadoses of vitamins or minerals, you should stop.

Let me give you a rule of thumb: Use extreme caution when dealing with supplements of minerals or vitamins; they are poisons in large doses, just like anything else. If anyone makes the claim that a vitamin supplement will cure several conditions, especially as diverse as from colds to cancer, watch out. The only condition a mineral or vitamin supplement will cure is a deficiency of that very same mineral or vitamin.

DIETING AND FATIGUE

Unfortunately for many women, food is more than fuel for the body. It often becomes a way of feeding one's emotional as well as physical needs. Consequently many women get locked into destructive eating habits, which in turn lead to metabolic imbalances and nutritional deficiencies. Furthermore, because of our culture's obsession with female slimness, most women are dieting, at least occasionally. All of this spells chronic fatigue.

The most common eating disorder among women is compulsive overeating. This is just a fancy name for eating more than one wants or eating uncontrollably between meals. Most women who have this problem do not seem able to stop eating even when they want to stop. As you might imagine, they tend to be on the heavy side.

Consequently they usually go on diets, either by trying the latest fad diet or by fasting and taking diet pills. For the most part, these efforts at dieting fail and are followed by a period of increased eating—a binge. Over a course of years, these women alternate between overeating and dieting, which causes their weights to fluctuate considerably.

Fatigue often accompanies compulsive overeating. It is created either by the foods eaten during a binge (usually fatty foods and sweets) or by the absence of carbohydrates while dieting. Remember: When a person does not diet properly, the body starts craving carbohydrates for energy. This craving often helps precipitate a binge on junk food and sweets that occurs after breaking a diet.

The key to successful weight loss without fatigue lies in the selection of the reducing diet. The best way to lose weight is to decrease calories, but maintain a balanced selection of healthful foods. You should increase the amount of complex carbohydrates and decrease the amount of fat in your meals.

However, many popular diets will tell you the opposite. They promise quick results, but are based on severely unbalanced diets that emphasize eating mostly fat or protein. I am not saying that these diets will not work; they will. One can lose weight on a severely imbalanced diet, but weight loss is usually maintained only as long as the diet is continued. That is because the intitial weight loss on these diets is mostly in the form of water. Once the diet is stopped, weight is regained because the body reclaims the water it lost. And of course, the diets fail to keep weight off in the long run because they do not change eating habits.

Although the names all differ, most of the diets that have hit the best-seller list in the last several years are such low-carbohydrate diets (for example, *The Complete Scarsdale Medical Diet, Dr. Atkins' Diet Revolution,* and *The Doctor's Quick Weight Loss Diet*). They usually advise consuming unlimited calories in the form of fat and protein. It is hard to stay on many of these diets. Furthermore, they can be expensive and tiring, and some of them are downright dangerous.

Carbohydrates are considered the culprits in these diets; but remember, without carbohydrates the body is without its favorite fuel. Fatigue, then, can be a major symptom of all low-carbohydrate diets. These diets also lead to many vitamin and mineral deficiencies because they are nutritionally inadequate. Low sodium levels and dehydration can occur, in addition to deficiencies in vital substances such as fiber, calcium, riboflavin, folic acid, and Vitamin C. Both dehydration and low sodium cause weakness and lethargy, and folic-acid deficiency causes anemia. So many aspects of a low-carbohydrate diet are fatiguing it is a wonder anyone can walk around while on the diet, let alone function up to par.

Another style of dieting is fasting, or starving by choice. I think you can understand why fatigue and weakness would be a problem with this type of diet. The body is quickly depleted of its storehouse of nutrients. Mineral and vitamin deficiencies occur, as well as depletion of water, glucose, and glycogen. Once the glycogen (stored sugar) reserves are utilized, then the body starts burning protein—from the muscles and the liver and the spleen—and fat to make energy. This situation usually leads to significant hypoglycemia—low blood sugar—with the attendant symptoms of weakness, light-headedness, irritability, hunger, and fatigue. For unknown reasons, the hypoglycemia that develops in starving women is more severe than in starving men. It can be as low as 40 milligrams per deciliter compared with normal fasting blood sugars of around 100 milligrams per deciliter.

The body tries to adapt to these starvation conditions by decreasing the metabolic rate. This is analogous to turning down the thermostat on your furnace to save oil. It is the body's attempt to conserve energy. But, as a result, the slowed metabolism also slows down weight loss. A decrease in metabolic rate can also occur in other energy-depriving diets, such as the ones I discussed above, and this is just the opposite of what you want to happen.

There is, however, a way to diet and increase your metabolic rate that will lead to more rapid weight loss—exercise. We will look at this in detail in the next chapter.

Fasting or starvation is the hallmark of the eating disorder anorexia nervosa. This is a serious eating disorder usually found in young white women from middle- and upper-class backgrounds. Each of these women has a profoundly distorted body image and exercises rigid control over her caloric intake. Despite the weight loss that ensues from this calorie restriction, these women usually deny being thin or feeling hunger or fatigue. Anorexia can progress to a serious condition that may require hospitalization or lead to death.

Any woman suspected of having anorexia nervosa should be seen by a doctor and referred to receive long-term counseling.

Another eating disorder that may be related to anorexia is bulimia. This problem is more widespread than once thought and appears to be on the increase. Bulimic women have a morbid fear of becoming obese, yet they tend to maintain an average weight. By the appearance of many of these women, you would be surprised to find out that they have an eating problem.

Bulimics typically consume large amounts of food and then make themselves vomit. This usually occurs on a daily basis. You may think such eating behavior would be easy to spot, but it is not. Secrecy is usually the rule—the binges and purges are carried out privately.

The repetitive cycles of binges and purges can drastically upset the body's chemical balance. This is often made much worse by the use of laxatives. Many bulimic women will use large quantities of laxatives in an attempt to keep weight down. Vital substances in the body, such as potassium, can be lost during these purges and subsequently lead to deficiencies and metabolic disturbances. Fatigue and weakness are predominant symptoms. Sometimes the chemical imbalances are so serious that hospitalization is needed to correct them and, of course, to help treat the underlying psychological problem.

Many women with anorexia or bulimia are, sadly, never cured of their eating disorder and suffer from a lifetime obsessive relationship with food. In a number of cases, these women will go on to develop obesity. Other women find that obesity has been a lifelong problem for them, either because of eating too much or because of a metabolic disorder that predisposes them to weight gain.

Obesity is a condition marked by an abnormal amount of body fat. The term is properly used when a person's weight is 20 percent over the average for her age and height. Obesity is a result of an imbalance between food intake and energy expenditure. The imbalance can be caused either by eating too much food (exogenous obesity) or by an abnormality of metabolism in the body (endogenous obesity), but the under-

127

lying reasons for these conditions are very hard to discern.

Fatigue is often associated with obesity for several reasons. Ingesting excessive amounts of food, especially fat, will lead to fatigue. Many of the metabolic conditions that make a person susceptible to obesity, such as hypothyroidism, have the symptom of fatigue. Furthermore, fatigue is compounded by the excess weight that must be moved about.

Eating disorders and the poor nutrition that accompanies them are a major source of fatigue in women. Whether you are eating a normal high-fat American diet, trying to lose weight on a low-carbohydrate diet, fasting, or struggling with one of these eating disorders, chances are you are being drained of precious energy.

The typical American style of eating and dieting causes fatigue, fatness, disease, and premature death. You can combat fatigue and a weight problem, as well as take some of the strongest preventive health measures possible, by changing your diet. Make good nutrition a top priority; it is the best way to ensure a healthy, long life full of energy and vitality.

WHAT TO DO

1. Select meals for their ability to perk you up or slow you down.

Foods can trigger the release of chemical messengers in the brain that either energize or sedate us. Pay close attention to how you feel after a meal high in carbohydrates. Although carbohydrates should be the mainstay of calories in your overall diet, try to balance individual meals so that each works in your favor. Avoid a large high-carbohydrate meal, especially at lunchtime when important activities follow or at dinner if you have to be especially alert afterward. On the other hand, use a large high-carbohydrate meal in the evening to help relax you.

2. Change your diet to a nonfatiguing and healthful one with the intent of making it a lifelong habit.

A nonfatiguing, healthful diet is one that provides you with adequate calories and nutrients yet is devoid of harmful foods, such as fat and cholesterol. All Americans should be urged to change to a very low-fat, low-cholesterol, high-carbohydrate diet. In selecting your foods, remember these major points:

- Carbohydrates are the primary source of energy. The body utilizes carbohydrates first as fuel and prefers burning glucose over proteins or fats. If you deny the body of carbohydrates, you will feel fatigued and hungry with cravings.

EAT MORE: complex carbohydrates, such as fresh vegetables, fruits, whole-wheat bread, whole grains, cereals, potatoes, corn, beans, rice, pasta.

EAT LESS: simple sugars, such as white sugar, brown sugar, honey, syrups, and any sweets with these ingredients.

- Extremely little fat is needed in the diet; too much fat only leads to an impaired ability of the blood to deliver oxygen, which causes fatigue— and to atherosclerosis, which is the primary cause of cardiovascular diseases.

EAT MORE: poultry, fish and nonfat dairy products.

EAT LESS: fatty foods, such as red meat, whole milk, cold cuts, whole-milk dairy products, butter, margarine, lard, oils.

- Cholesterol has been identified as one of the substances that aids in the development of atherosclerosis. Your cholesterol intake should be cut down to about 100 milligrams each day.

EAT MORE: noncholesterol foods.

EAT LESS: eggs, meat, organ meats, shellfish.

- A deficiency or excess of many of the essential minerals and vitamins can cause fatigue. Make sure you are consuming a well-balanced diet, paying extra attention to getting iron (if you are premenopausal) and calcium. The only supplement worth considering is a multiple-vitamin pill that has all the recommended daily allowances in one dose. Taking individual pills for each mineral and vitamin can lead to imbalances in the body. Do not take megadoses of any vitamin, individually or in combination. Megadoses of vitamins are dangerous to your health.

3. Undertake dieting properly!

Give up, for all time, the idea that you will quickly lose weight. There is nothing that is more likely to make you fail than to expect miracle diet cures overnight. Tomorrow's fad diet is not going to work any better than yesterday's fad diet. The only way to get weight down and keep it under control is to change your eating habits, and that takes time! You have to change your taste buds and your metabolism—these do not change rapidly. Set some long-range goals.

The best diet for weight loss (and to maintain health) is a high-carbohydrate, low-fat diet that is low in calories. The best diet plan I have seen is the *Pritikin Diet*. It has been called a "radical" departure from the normal American fare, and because it is, many critics say Americans will not go for it, yet they agree it is probably the healthiest way to eat. I have been so convinced by all the data I have read and heard that my husband and I changed our diet two years ago to Pritikin, which primarily calls for increasing the amount of complex carbohydrate and decreasing the fat in the diet.

Making these changes can be difficult at first, only because we are all creatures of habit. I suggest using a cookbook to guide you (we used Nathan Pritikin's *The Pritikin Promise*, New York: Simon and Schuster). We have altered our cooking and eating habits, our taste buds have changed, our food bill has gone down and so have our weights. We "diet" all the time for health reasons, not weight reasons, but we have never felt better or been more energetic!

4. If you have an eating problem, try to figure out why you eat.

Most women with eating problems are eating for an emotional reason. In some way, eating and the associated extra weight serve a positive function. The task is to figure out what need is being satisfied when you eat without really being hungry.

Try to keep a record of when you eat and how you feel. What are you feeling when you go to the refrigerator: frustrated, unloved, angry? Once you are able to separate your need for food from your need for emotional fulfillment, you will gain control over your eating.

If you have a serious eating problem you have not been able to solve on your own, get help. Consider talking with a counselor or joining a weight-loss group to give you support and guidance. Women tend to be more successful in losing weight and changing their habits when they are in a women's support group.

6
EXERCISE FOR
FITNESS

If I told you that a wonder drug had just been discovered that reduces your fatigue, increases your energy, speeds up your metabolism, helps you lose weight, improves your mood, slows your aging, decreases your risk of illness, and prolongs your life, would you take it? You bet you would. All of America would be gobbling it down, and people would be willing to spend huge sums of money on it. Well—sorry, there is no such pill. But there is exercise, which will bring about all those wonderful changes for a much cheaper price than you would pay for the pills.

If all those positive effects were compacted into one little pill, it really would be a miracle drug. And yet most women do not think of exercise as the miracle for which they have been wishing; rather, they groan and think of the difficulty of exercising. It is work, something else on the list that should get done but usually does not.

Obviously, exercise is not a new subject to women. The women's magazines continue to be chock-full of articles on it. However, as a doctor, I find a flaw with many of these articles. Exercise, for the most part, is being marketed as the new way to become sexier (to get a new body), rather than a disciplined way to become truly physically fit—healthy. Many women exercise today, but relatively few are fit.

Physical fitness is inseparably linked to one's energy level. If I were asked, what is the one thing a woman could do to combat chronic fatigue, I would give the boring, yet predictable answer: exercise. It is safe to say that a woman who does not exercise regularly has some degree of chronic fatigue. The flip side of that statement is, any woman who is physically fit does not suffer from chronic fatigue.

EXERCISE INCREASES ENERGY

Why is exercise the great energy booster? Exercise is the activity that leads to physical fitness. Fitness implies an ability of the person to carry on—to do work—for a sustained period without fatigue setting in. This entails a certain level of performance on the part of the heart, lungs, and muscles. The more fit you are, the more you can endure—mentally and physically—without feeling tired. Exercise substantially raises the threshold at which fatigue will occur and is the only way to increase one's endurance.

At first glance, that may seem like a contradiction because exercising does take energy. Women patients have said to me: "But, Doctor, I am so tired already. If I exercise, I will not have any energy left." Although it is true that exercise does consume fuel, in the long run it produces far more energy than it utilizes. Many women have discovered the wonderful fatigue-fighting effects of exercising. When I asked one twenty-nine-year-old woman what she would do to combat fatigue, she replied:

> "Although you'd think it to be the opposite, I would exercise, such as do Jazzercise. This often diminishes my feelings of tiredness by improving my mental health and giving me more energy and invigoration to do other things."

Exercise creates energy in several ways. For instance, it alters the energy pool by increasing the size of the reservoir, strengthening the structure of the basin, plugging any leaks in the pool, delivering more fresh "water" faster, and cleaning out the poisons in the pool. Let us look at these energy-pool concepts in terms of actual body changes.

Exercise Builds More Energy-producing Machinery

Exercise stimulates the body to build more of the "machinery" that generates energy. It also strengthens the structures that are already there. Anatomical changes occur throughout the body; for example, the heart becomes larger and stronger, so it pumps better with less effort; the lungs work better, so the transport of oxygen is more efficient; the number of muscle fibers increases in all muscles in the body, so more power is generated; new blood vessels grow through the tissues, so delivery is improved; the nerves conduct messages better and faster; and the very energy-producing chemicals inside cells are geared up.

All of these changes act in harmony to allow us to go for longer periods of time before feeling fatigued. This new machinery allows for the production of more energy—increasing the capacity to do work, both mental and physical.

Women are at a great disadvantage in this area, which is one of the primary reasons why women are susceptible to more fatigue and experience more fatigue than men. First, because women have smaller bodies than men, they have smaller hearts, less lung capacity, and less muscle mass. Women are starting out with a smaller energy "factory," which means that they cannot perform as much work and will tire more quickly than men.

More important, however, women fail to develop the energy-making machinery they do have. Obviously, this tragedy is one of the by-products of the traditional image of femininity. Women have always been called the "weaker" sex, but social institutions have kept women far weaker than they need to be. Exercise and fitness has not been considered feminine. Consequently most women have never been physically fit at any point in their lives—their hearts, lungs, and muscles are all "flabby" and are producing at levels far below that of which they are capable. Chronic fatigue is just one of the prices that women pay for this underdeveloped state.

One medical study found that the complaints most often heard from women tend to be ones of long duration but not severe, such as fatigue, menstrual problems, colds, allergies, headache, low backache, digestive disorders, and upper-respiratory problems.[1] Compared to unfit women, those who were physically fit generally had fewer of these complaints, indicated very little disability, and—they had the least amount of fatigue. Those women who were out of shape had the most fatigue, backaches, menstrual problems, difficulties with labor and delivery, postdelivery complaints, colds, digestive problems, and allergies.

This study was conducted in a group of women who were found to have no physical disorders. The lack of physical fitness alone could account for their chronic fatigue. However, doctors seldom make a diagnosis of "not physically fit" as a cause of women's medical problems because of their social biases about what it is to be female. As a result, women are not given serious advice and treatment plans to improve their fitness as a cure for fatigue or other chronic problems.

Exercise Fights the Fatigue-causing Processes

Remember the five processes that lead to fatigue? They are the (1) depletion of substances vital to energy production, (2) accumulation of waste products, (3) changes in the body's energy-producing machinery, (4) disruption in the body's ability to regulate itself, and (5) failures in the body's communications system.

The very act of exercising fights all of these fatigue processes. Vigorous activity stimulates the heart to pump blood through the body faster, which whisks vital substances to the working muscles and other organs and sweeps away waste products that cause fatigue. Exercise also helps the body regulate itself; it assists in keeping all the working parts well "oiled" and operating in unison. On the other hand, disuse and inactivity lead to rusty, creaky parts that are hard to get back in harmony—like the tin man in *The Wizard of Oz*.

Exercise also wakes up the entire nervous system. It opens up all the channels of communication. This is extremely important in combating fatigue, because fatigue is a state that is much like sleep. There is a general reduction of activity in the nervous system and hence a slowdown in the rest of the body's organ systems. Exercise creates an electrifying force that travels throughout the network of nerves and mobilizes the entire body.

Exercise Speeds Up the Metabolic Rate

The amount of energy you have is directly related to your metabolic rate. Some people seem to go through life blessed with boundless energy, while others seem to drag through life always in need of it. A fast metabolic rate ensures an ample supply of energy and little fatigue, while a slow metabolic rate often spells perpetual lethargy.

Although these energy differences are part of our natural constitutions, you can speed up your metabolic rate—by exercising regularly. This is particularly important for women to understand. Generally, females have lower resting metabolic rates than males—which is another reason why women suffer from more fatigue than men. These metabolic differences between the sexes apparently occurred as a result of evolution.

Men evolved faster metabolic rates so that they could quickly turn calories into energy used for hunting, fighting, and protecting their families. On the other hand, females evolved slower metabolisms so calories would not get turned into energy so easily; rather, they would be saved in the form of fat. In the case of famine, a slower metabolism—and more fat—offered a greater chance for the offspring to survive if the mother could live through it and continue to nurse her young. The species had a better chance of survival.

In this day and age, women pay some prices for having evolved slower metabolisms. Exhaustion sets in faster, stored calories are more difficult to mobilize and burn when energy is needed, there is a greater susceptibility to obesity, and it is harder to lose weight. Women were meant to do well under the conditions of starvation (dieting)! Many women stumble on this biological truth when they try to shed their extra pounds.

Dieters who do not exercise often find that after they have been on a successful diet for a few weeks, they stop losing weight. If they cut their calories down further, their weight loss seems to slow down even more and, of course, so do they. This has been called "the plateau effect." At this point, dieters usually become so discouraged and are so fatigued that they give up dieting and go back to their usual eating habits.

Researchers have found out why this plateau effect occurs in dieters who do not exercise. The body reacts to the dieting as if it were starving and responds by slowing down the metabolic rate. It is the body's way of saving fuel and energy during a famine. For women who already start out with a relatively slow metabolic rate, dieting acts to lower it further—resulting in disabling fatigue (and less weight loss). The only way to keep the metabolic rate up and still keep the caloric intake down is to engage in vigorous activity. Exercise increases the metabolic rate, not only during the activity but for as long as eight hours after. The body is forced to start producing energy and consuming calories again.

Whether you are fighting only fatigue or fatigue and the battle of the bulge, you must increase your metabolic rate—and the only way to do that is to exercise.

Exercise Improves Mood

Fatigue is a feeling that is composed of both psychological and physical sensations. Recent medical research has shown that exercise exerts its effects at both of these levels—it is beneficial to the mind as well as the body. Not surprisingly, exercise has a remarkable ability to alleviate and combat fatigue on the mental as well as the physical level. The old saying "A healthy body *is* a healthy mind" is proving to be true.

Exercise is clearly associated with improvements in mood. Elevating the mood is an excellent way to abolish fatigue. The precise mechanism of how this is brought about is not exactly known, but the link is a very strong one. We know that whenever people feel down, they tend to feel fatigued; on the other hand, when people are in good spirits, they have more energy. As you will learn in Chapter 14, sometimes fatigue and depression are indistinguishable. Treating a mood problem is often a cure for fatigue—exercise takes aim at both!

Exercise is thought to exert its beneficial mental effects by altering brain chemistry. Vigorous activity apparently releases chemicals that produce feelings of pleasure and relaxation—they act as natural tranquilizers. In some studies, exercise was better than drugs at reducing anxiety and stress. Increasing pleasure and relaxation raises the threshold for fatigue, and reducing anxiety and stress stops an energy drain. All of these effects lead to an increased energy pool.

Exercise is also a very powerful weapon against depression, which is often the cause of chronic fatigue. The effect is especially helpful in those people who are particularly distressed or physically unfit at the start. Exercise works in the brain to increase norepinephrine, the chemical neurotransmitter that is depleted in depression. This antidepressant drug effect seems to explain why running appears to be at least as effective as psychotherapy in reducing depression.[2]

Exercise Slows Aging, Prevents Disease, and Prolongs Life

Strength and energy naturally decline with advancing age. Part of aging gracefully may be accepting more fatigue in life. However, research is now showing that many of the physical and mental signs of aging that were thought to be inevitable can be retarded. Many of the "aging" changes that take place in the heart, nerves, blood, bones, and metabolism are actually the result of physical inactivity. Aging and its attendant fatigue can be staved off with regular exercise.

Besides slowing down the aging process, exercise has now been shown to reduce the risk of developing several of the major killers, such as heart attack, stroke, hypertension, and osteoporosis. It has long been suspected that exercise prevented disease and prolonged life, but it was not until the summer of 1984 that the first two studies clearly linking exercise with prolongation of life came out. Researchers reported a direct relationship between the level of physical activity and the length of life.[3] In the group who exercised, fewer deaths occurred from a wide variety of diseases. Those with cardiovascular disease, the leading cause of death in this country, got the most benefit out of exercise. People who did not exercise were found to have twice the death rates at the same age as those who expended 2,000 calories or more a week in physical activity. Constancy of the habit of exercise was found to be very important. The study concluded, "regular sustained exercise during nine or more months of the year may be necessary to maintain cardiovascular health."[4] This study points out the importance of changing one's lifestyle so that exercise becomes a lifetime habit.

Let us review how exercise increases energy and fights fatigue; it

- builds energy-producing machinery
- improves delivery of vital substances
- facilitates removal of waste products
- helps the body regulate itself
- opens the channels of communication throughout the nervous system
- increases the metabolic rate
- improves mood and relieves anxiety
- retards the aging process
- helps prevent disease, especially heart disease
- prolongs life

Exercise is one of the best activities in which you can engage to alleviate your fatigue. Exercise increases your sense of well-being through increasing your energy pool and refreshing your body and mind. Once you begin a program of exercise, you will feel a new surge of energy.

You may be convinced of all the benefits you will reap from exercise yet feel a bit overwhelmed by the challenge of making the change in your life. However, there is a road back from sedentary living to an active, vigorous life. Your new motto should be "Fitness Is Feminine and Fatigue-fighting."

ON THE ROAD TO FITNESS AND LESS FATIGUE

You should start thinking of exercise as that miracle pill I spoke about at the beginning of this chapter. I admit, exercise is one of those horse capsules that is hard to swallow, at least in the beginning. But remember, it is a pill you should take every day; you will feel worse the next day if you miss a "dose." Think to yourself, "I haven't taken my pill yet today." If you do not take the pill, you will probably drag through life being perpetually tired and overweight. Furthermore, you will probably feel bad about yourself and die sooner than you might have.

Why is exercise such a hard pill for most women to swallow? To find the answer, I think you have to peer into your dim past. If you really examine your innermost attitudes, you will probably find that you received the clear message while growing up that physical activity was not feminine. Oh, it was (sort of) all right to be a tomboy as a girl child, but when we reached puberty we were told to stop dangling from the tree limbs and start acting like young ladies.

The phrase is "act like a lady," and I think the word *act* was quite appropriate. We were taught how to act out a role that included inactivity and passivity. As a doctor, I shiver to think how women's upbringing contributes to their poor physical and mental health. It is not natural for a human being, male or female, to be physically inactive; and yet I see so many women who were taught to be inactive.

Now many women have to be retaught to be active. It is difficult to start exercising, because it goes against that deeply rooted image of femininity that says sports and physical exercise are for males, not females. Although we may laugh and say, "Oh, nonsense" and have new ideals, it is very hard to get those old notions and emotions out of our system.

Exercise is the only road to physical fitness; no real pill or easy-way-out method will provide the equivalent benefits. You should think of physical fitness as simply a healthy state of mind and body that allows you to carry out the activities of life. An unfit body cannot perform up to its full capacity; it tires easily, deteriorates faster, and is more susceptible to disease. Exercise builds the cardiovascular, respiratory, and muscle systems to their full capacity. We need to exercise for fitness in order to build our energy pool, not to meet superficial goals of looking "sexier."

Unfortunately, many women think that the only way to physical fitness is through jogging, long-distance swimming, or other torturous activities. Women, especially older ones, may immediately feel overwhelmed and defeated, thinking, "I will never be able to do that." Consequently they refuse to initiate any activity. I do not blame them.

Jogging is not the only exercise in the world. There are many other physical activities that will lead to fitness. The idea is to get involved in any activity that does three things: moves the joints, uses the big muscles in your body (legs, arms, back), and stresses your heart and lungs (aerobic activity). Walking, bicycling, rowing, dancing, ice skating, and roller skating all fit the requirements. Exercise does not, by definition, have to be monotonous and boring. Pick an activity that is fun.

Some people prefer to exercise in a group; others like to be by themselves. I find that I prefer to exercise alone. That is my quiet time, away from everybody and everything, and I do not want to have to engage with someone else. Others have expressed the same feelings. When I asked one woman how she had learned to deal with fatigue in her life, she replied ". . . long walks help me put life's happenings into perspective." It sounds like a peaceful time, something that most of us women could use a bit more of in our hectic lives.

Some people find that if they exercise with a friend or in a group it gives them incentive; a partner can help get you out on the days you are feeling blue and lacking motivation. A fifty-six-year-old married woman who just put exercise in her life told me:

> "I started taking two classes a week in the morning. I may be real tired and not feel like doing anything, but it makes you feel better. And I can't do it on my own even though I have a tape on the VCR machine. I can't do it as well as with the class. There's something about that interaction with other people."

Obviously, if you take up a recreation like dancing or tennis, you will need a partner. But for other activities you will not. You will have to learn your own style.

The idea behind all this is for you to begin to develop a lifelong habit, to develop an interest in an activity or sport that will give you the exercise you need to derive the health benefit while keeping boredom to a minimum. This will take time because it is hard to change old habits. Inactivity is a very old, ingrained habit.

Do not expect great changes overnight; that is the surest way for you to be disappointed. Rather, look ahead to a year from now. If you do not take this approach, chances are that a year from now you are going to be in the same position as you are now. If you start with realistic expectations, you will be delighted at the results next year. Be patient.

You must take the attitude that exercise should receive your highest priority in your daily list of activities. This is not a selfish attitude. If you exercise, you will find you have much more to give to your family and your work. It may take a few minutes away from them every day, but it will return far more. By keeping yourself energetic, healthy, and happy, you will be giving them more than they would ever get in thirty minutes with the "old" you. Make the time, let something else go by the wayside if you have to. Give yourself the gift of exercise.

WHAT TO DO

1. Make a lifelong habit of exercising for good health.

Exercise is one of the most important ingredients of any program to banish fatigue. It increases the size of your energy pool in a myriad of ways and as a result, your capacity to perform in all spheres—mental and physical—is expanded. Not only do we need exercise, we need the "miracle pill" every day—physical activity must be woven into the fabric of our lives. It is a necessity for all women of all ages. Even if you have been inactive for years and years, it is never too late to start.

You eventually want to reach the goal of exercising for at least thirty minutes nonstop every day. The activity should be an aerobic exercise—any continuous, muscular activity that increases the heart and breathing rates. You need to elevate your heart rate from 60 percent to 75 percent of your maximum rate and sustain that rate for the thirty-minute period. The activity should be vigorous enough to elevate your pulse in the right range given your age. I suggest that you consult some of the good books on the market about aerobic exercises for more details about how to plan your program.

Soon after you stop exercising regularly, your body will return to its former low level of strength and tone. Exercise must become part of your daily health routine, just like brushing your teeth. You may be thinking, "This is all well and good but I don't have thirty minutes a day to devote to exercise. I just can't find the time." Find it, make it, steal it—those thirty minutes will be some of the most important in your entire day.

2. Get a physical exam before you start exercising.

Although you may feel in picture-perfect health, if you are over thirty-five or out of shape, you should have a complete physical before you start exercising. The doctor's examination can help detect any physical problems that could limit you to certain types of exercise and it can also help determine the type of program that will fit your particular needs. Not every exercise is for everyone.

Try to locate a doctor who specializes in sports medicine or a clinic that offers fitness evaluations. You are more likely to get an accurate determination of your present level of physical fitness and what kinds of activities you should begin with.

3. Choose the right activity and the right partner(s).

When you pick an activity, keep two things in mind: your level of fitness and what you can enjoy. If you are bored, you will not continue your program.

Get creative. If you are working, have children, and seem to have no time left to yourself, try working physical activity into the time you spend with the children. Take them roller skating or ice skating, and do not sit on the sidelines. If you do not know how—learn. Another way to sneak in exercise is to put a stationary bicycle near the telephone and pedal while you talk, or put one in front of the television set. When you go on a trip, carry your own bags and suitcases. Take the steps instead of elevators and escalators. In short, take the more physically difficult route when you can.

Check with your local community groups, churches, synagogues, YMCAs, or YWCAs to see if any of them have exercise programs. Many of them do. Call your regional Blue Cross/Blue Shield Association and your state or regional American Heart Association for exercise programs in your area and ask for brochures on exercise. Both of these organizations distribute excellent health brochures on diet and exercise. Listen for local public-service announcements on the radio and television to see what is available in your area. Make a habit of clipping the newspapers and women's magazines for exercise ideas. Join a spa if you can afford it.

The right partner can be an encouragement as you go about your plan. If you choose to get some exercise with another person, make sure it is someone who is at your level. The quickest way to defeat is to start a strenuous activity with someone who is in better shape than you are. That is guaranteed disaster. It is hard enough to get out there and do something without being constantly reminded of how out of shape you are. Instead of being a positive experience, the exercise becomes another negative input on a long list of things that already make you feel bad. Remember: The goal of your program is to improve your health, not put you in competition.

If you have no partner, are afraid to go out alone, or the weather is too bad, and you have absolutely no idea what to do for exercise, buy an exercise record or videotape (depending, of course, on what type of equipment you have at home). So many are available today at a variety of fitness levels, you should be able to find something to suit you. Also check your local television listings to see what kind of exercise programs are offered. These shows are great for providing incentive and instruction. Tune in regularly!

4. Proceed slowly.

Do not expect much when you start out—be kind to yourself. Set a reasonable long-term goal and be realistic about your expectations. Avoid the trap of tantalizing quick cures, promising overnight diets, and miracle pills. Do not set out with a short-term goal, such as crash dieting and starting an exercise routine to lose weight for the holidays or that party coming up. How many times has that approach failed before?

Revamp your thinking; start thinking about slowly, slowly putting activity into your daily routine and that a year or two from now your life will be different. Remember: A year will go by anyway. If you do not do it this way, chances are you will look and feel the same one year from now as you do right this moment. Go slowly and, little by little, you will feel less tired, more fit, and pleased with yourself.

Do not compare yourself to others either. Other people's problems or conditions do not matter; what matters is your activity, given your particular condition. Keep in mind that it will take time to reach your fitness goals. Some experts say that to achieve fitness, it takes a month of regular exercising for every year of inactivity. Are you counting? Do not be discouraged. Be patient. If you take the approach of trying to make a long-term change, it will be very easy. All you have to do is make tiny, little changes every day.

5. Listen to your body.

While you exercise, pay attention to your body's signals. If you get in touch, your body really will tell you a lot. Do you have backaches, shoulder aches, or aching calves? That may be a sign that those areas need more exercise than others. On the other hand, if you experience hurtful pain, stop exercising. Pain does not mean the exercise is working; it means the activity is unsafe or too strenuous for you. Movements that often cause this kind of pain are bouncing, arching the back or neck, swinging arms or legs, exercising too fast (such as lifting weights rapidly, where the momentum takes you through the lift), overflexing, and locking the joints—keep these out of your exercise routine.

If you feel dizzy, nauseated, or breathless, stop exercising. Try it for a shorter period of time the next day. If the feeling persists, see a doctor. You should see one immediately if exercise ever brings on pain in your jaw, shoulder, arm, chest, or upper abdomen. This could be a symptom of a compromised heart and you should not wait to see if it goes away on its own. Once you start exercising, listen to your body's messages.

6. Learn how to push your "GO" button.

This is the hardest step. Even if you mean well and want to start exercising, sometimes it is very difficult to muster up the energy to break the vicious cycle of inactivity. How do you get going? Do things to motivate yourself to exercise. Pick a pleasant activity; choose clothes you like; buy a colorful sweatsuit; find pleasant surroundings. Make your exercise program elicit pleasant images in your mind.

Try to start with very small steps. For instance, today write down what you would like to do and tell yourself, "Maybe I'll do it tomorrow and maybe I won't." Set your mind to getting out the next day. If you cannot drag yourself out to do anything, dress in some sneakers and exercise garments every day as if you were going to exercise. Walk around the house in them. Slowly add a few stretches to this routine. Then very gradually increase your activity as the days or weeks go by.

Be patient with yourself and reward yourself for what you do; do not punish yourself for what you do not do. And if you ever give up or miss a day, a week, or a month, do not berate yourself. That is okay. It does not mean you cannot start again. You can—immediately.

7. Support the notion that "Fitness Is Feminine."

We become better people, more capable of carrying out the important tasks in life—working, loving, giving—if we are physically fit. Carry this message in your mind and share it with your loved ones, friends, and acquaintances. Whenever you can, encourage women's and girls' participation in sports and exercise. It is imperative that as a group women begin to support other women and change the old notion that being feminine is synonymous with being weak and unfit. What that translates into is, being feminine means being unhealthy. Many women's medical problem—chronic fatigue—stems from simply being out of shape. We have to change the message the next generation gets through what we say and especially what we do. We have to change the old notion to a new one—that Fitness Is Feminine!

_____ 7 _____

QUIT FOR GOOD

In some fashion, every woman has prospered from the women's movement, regardless of whether or not she agrees with its general goals. Even though there are many barriers yet to be overcome, women can now at least dream of opportunities that previously were closed to them because of gender. But, progress has its price. As they gained the right to vote and work for wages, women also gained the right to smoke cigarettes, abuse alcohol, and engage in other harmful habits. I am reminded of one of my favorite quotes by Albert Camus:

> Freedom is nothing but a chance to better ourselves, but most of us use the word to justify our desires to be worse without penalty.

Well, there are penalties—great penalties—for choosing to smoke cigarettes and abuse alcohol. It turns out that many of the things we put in our mouths—the food we eat, the cigarettes we smoke, the beverages we drink, or the medications we take—can all sap us of our energy. The woman who smokes, drinks alcohol, and takes the birth-control pill may be walking around tired because all three directly cause fatigue.

In this chapter, we will look at the particular problem of smoking—one that is having an increasingly deadly effect on women's health and vitality. We will look at how smoking drains your energy pool, why it is so difficult for women to stop smoking, and talk about ways to beat those difficulties.

I used to smoke. So keep in mind that whatever I tell you in this chapter I say not only as a doctor, but also as a woman who has gone through quitting. It is hard—but it can be done. And it is worth the effort! I cannot begin to tell you how much more energy I have now. Life is so much nicer without cigarettes.

There are some 4,000 substances in cigarette smoke. Although we are a long way from knowing how all of them affect the body, some, such as nicotine, are known to be extremely harmful. Nicotine is a poison that acts very rapidly. The lethal dose for a human is only 50 milligrams, about the amount in two cigarettes. Because most of the nicotine is burned, smoking two cigarettes is not deadly. However, the body rapidly absorbs the nicotine from inhaled smoke and in about 7.5 seconds the nicotine starts to exert its effects on the brain.

Nicotine has a variety of effects; it can act as a stimulant or a depressant. It usually stimulates the brain initially, but then later exerts a depressant action. Either one of these actions can cause fatigue; the brain uses energy excessively when it is overly stimulated, whereas depression of brain function leads directly to the feeling of fatigue.

Nicotine affects other parts of the body in addition to the brain. It affects organs such as the heart, the stomach, the intestines, the muscles, and the nerves. For instance, by stimulating the nerves, nicotine can increase respiration, heart rate, and blood pressure; increase acid secretion in the stomach and activate the intestines; cause the skin to become cold and clammy; and induce shakiness, water retention, and nausea.

With all of this increased activity in the body, the heart has to beat faster to deliver blood, consuming a great deal of energy. But there is more to it. In order to beat faster, the heart must work harder and therefore needs more oxygen. This is where cigarette smoke delivers a double whammy to the body. Another constituent, the toxic gas carbon monoxide, actually decreases the ability of the blood to carry oxygen. So, at the same time the body needs more oxygen, it gets less.

Oxygen is carried by hemoglobin in red blood cells. But so is carbon monoxide. As a matter of fact, carbon monoxide binds to hemoglobin two hundred times faster than oxygen! So any carbon monoxide in the air we breathe or the smoke we inhale will quickly attach itself to hemoglobin, beating out oxygen. This is exactly what happens when people accidentally die or commit suicide by breathing carbon monoxide from the exhaust of an automobile. They just get a bigger dose than a smoker. In essence, every time you take a puff you are asphyxiating yourself. It is no wonder fatigue is one of the major effects of cigarette smoking.

Where does this process fit in the Fatigue Scheme? Anything that affects the delivery of oxygen to the tissues can cause profound fatigue. Remember Mary in Chapter 3? She inherited a type of anemia from one of her parents that made it difficult for her red blood cells to carry oxygen. Her fatigue was from a very basic disturbance inside the cells. Cigarette smoking can be thought of in the same way; it

SMOKING AND THE FATIGUE SCHEME

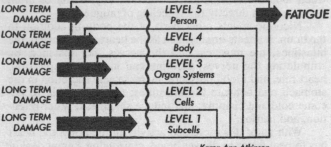

Karen Ann Atkinson

Figure 13: *The toxins in cigarette smoke all exert their harmful effects in concert, which leads to widespread changes throughout the body resulting in fatigue.*

creates a "functional" anemia. The carbon monoxide, just one of the many toxins from the smoke, handicaps the red blood cell's ability to carry oxygen. The result is the same: The tissues are deprived of vital oxygen and fatigue occurs.

There are at least twenty ingredients in cigarette smoke that are *known* to be toxins. All of these toxins exert their effects at the same time and cause widespread changes throughout the body. Many of these changes contribute to the development of fatigue, which is a very common symptom in smokers.

What are the other hazards of smoking? I think a knowledge of the hazards will help you prepare for quitting, or will help nonsmokers to support the attempts of smokers to quit. While I was smoking, it helped me greatly to go through the list of smoking-related illnesses in my head. I could not go on denying my medical knowledge about smoking (nor could I ignore my tiredness and cough). I had to quit; I am so happy I did. Let us go through the list I developed from the Surgeon General's report on women and smoking:[1]

- Working women who smoke report more days lost from work than nonsmoking working women.
- Acute conditions, such as influenza, are 20 percent greater in smokers than in nonsmokers.
- Smoking may affect a woman's response to selected drugs.
- Women under sixty-five who smoke report more limited activities.
- The lungs of women smokers function more poorly than the lungs of either ex-smokers or nonsmokers. The condition of the lungs is directly related to the number of cigarettes smoked.
- Smokers have more respiratory symptoms, such as cough, sputum production, wheezing, and shortness of breath.
- Chronic bronchitis is more frequent in women smokers, increasing with the number of cigarettes smoked daily.

- The severity of emphysema found on autopsy is related to the number of cigarettes smoked during a lifetime.
- Cigarette smoking may interact with a physical or chemical agent to which women are exposed on the job, leading to a greater health risk. For example, women smokers who are exposed to cotton dust have a higher risk of developing bronchitis and abnormal lungs. Also, women smokers who are exposed to asbestos have more lung cancer.
- Peptic ulcer disease is more common in women who smoke.
- Coronary heart disease is more frequent in women who smoke.
- Smoking is a risk factor in the development of hardening of the arteries.
- Severe hypertension is more likely to develop in women who smoke.
- The risk of stroke (subarachnoid hemorrhage) is increased by cigarette smoking; the risk is even greater if a woman simultaneously uses the birth-control pill.
- Cigarette smoking is causally associated with cancer of the lung, larynx, lip, tongue, gums, buccal mucosa, hard and soft palate, salivary glands, floor of the mouth, oropharynx, esophagus, kidney, and urinary bladder.
- Smoking may impair a woman's fertility.
- The more a woman smokes during pregnancy, the greater her risk of spontaneous abortion, fetal death, and death of the baby at birth.
- Maternal cigarette smoking may account for up to 14 percent of all premature deliveries in the United States.
- Babies born to women smokers generally weigh less than babies of nonsmokers.
- Maternal smoking during pregnancy increases the risk of an infant developing "sudden infant death syndrome."

- Children of smoking parents have more respiratory infections and hospitalizations in their first year.
- Women who smoke during pregnancy may harm their child's long-term growth, intellectual development, and behavior.
- Smoking lowers the age at which menopause begins.

And that is not a complete list; I was selective. Obviously, if the risk becomes reality and you do develop any of these chronic diseases, such as emphysema, bronchitis, or heart disease, you will experience fatigue as part of the illness. There is a good chance that you would feel the fatigue years before the disease produces any obvious symptoms. At that stage, the long-term damage brought on by smoking will affect you at all levels of organization and thus drain you of energy.

If you smoke, you have less energy and pep than you could have. You may not think you are chronically fatigued from smoking; but when you quit, the energy drain—of

CHRONIC DISEASE AND THE FATIGUE SCHEME

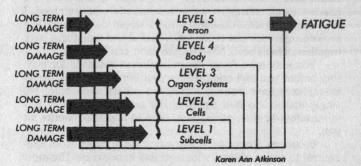

Karen Ann Atkinson

Figure 14: *The long-term damage caused by smoking will, in and of itself, begin to drain energy and exacerbate fatigue.*

153

which you may not have been aware—will stop. You will probably have to suffer a brief withdrawal period, but in the long run, you will be surprised at how much more energy you have.

When a person stops smoking, she immediately begins to accumulate health benefits. Experiments have shown that the body goes to work immediately to repair damaged lung and other body tissues. You can immediately lower your risk of heart disease and cancer by giving up the smoking habit.

You can quit. I am not saying you are going to quit the first time you try. And that is okay. Too often, people expect to quit on the first go-around. Then if they cannot quit, they consider their efforts a lost cause, shrug their shoulders, and view themselves as hopeless.

Research has shown that ex-smokers usually tried to quit several times before they finally succeeded. I stopped smoking three times with at least a year between attempts before this last (and final) time. I am reminded of the line "It's easy to quit smoking, I've done it a million times." That is what it felt like to me. I would buy one pack at a time, smoke a few cigarettes, and then get extremely angry with myself. (Getting down on myself only made me want another.) In this fit of anger, I would take all the remaining cigarettes, break them, and throw them away. Then a few hours later, the craving would start. Sometimes, when my will crumbled, I was so desperate, you know what I would do? I would dig broken cigarettes out of the wastebasket and tape them back together! That shows how bad the habit can be.

You may have to try several different methods for quitting before you find one that fits your personal needs. Many ex-smokers have done it alone, but others need help. No single method to quit smoking has been shown to be any more effective than others; you have to find what works for you.

Programs from which you can choose range from self-control to group efforts, with a variety in between. The most important factor in all programs is your commitment to stop. You know why you should quit; I have given you a number of good reasons, and you probably have a list of your own. But do not let your fear of failure stand in the way of trying. Keep thinking of all the energy you will have and how much better your health will be after you stop.

Quitting smoking seems to be more difficult for women than it is for men. Studies have shown that no matter what type of program is used, women fail more often than men. I tell you this not to discourage you, but so that you can learn from other women's failures and successes.

It seems that women do better than men in some programs, and more poorly in others. Women tend to be more successful at quitting if they are in a group situation, particularly an all-female group. There, women can receive support and understanding, and have a chance to share their feelings in a sympathetic environment.

Women also seem to do better when they have a partner with whom to quit, such as their husbands. A helpful and considerate spouse can go a long way to provide support to a woman's efforts. It is important to plan for this and make other people around you aware of your intentions. Otherwise your effort to quit can be sabotaged by your spouse, relatives, or friends.

Encouragement from an organized group, friends, or a spouse is extremely important to women. Women tend to do poorly when they try to quit alone or are put in situations where they do not receive individual attention. Lectures and other educational approaches do not work as well on women as on men. Neither does treatment with drugs. Each woman must decide what is the best situation for her, but being aware of the general needs of women might help you think through yours a little more clearly.

Researchers have offered up a variety of reasons to explain why women have such a rough time. Studies have indicated that women are under more life stress than men, show more symptoms of emotional distress, and report more apprehension and tension. I do not doubt any of this.

Interestingly, there is one group of women who have more difficulty quitting smoking in treatment groups (it is hard to test women who quit on their own because it is hard to identify them). Homemakers have the highest failure rate. The Surgeon General's report explains, "These women explained that cigarettes served as companions and they reported the difficulties of being without adult company all day and of being deprived of outside activities as obstacles to giving up smoking."[2]

The biggest obstacle to women seems to be their negative emotions. Many women smoke to quell bad feelings, whereas men often say that they smoke because they enjoy it. Women appear to use smoking as a psychological coping mechanism. This would explain women's difficulty with stopping. The stresses and the burdens will not go away overnight, so a new coping mechanism must be found. So one big question to ask yourself is how you are going to cope with bad feelings when you are trying to quit.

This tends to be the time you will break your commitment and say, "Oh, what the heck. I feel so bad anyway, who cares?" And that is the point. You may be feeling so bad about yourself that you truly do not care about your physical health. It may appear to you that the effect of cigarettes on your long-term health may be trivial compared to the psychological stress you may be feeling right now. You may feel that you might not even live long enough to get lung cancer if things continue the way they are, so why not smoke a cigarette?

You must begin to think about different ways of coping when you feel that low. What little things make you feel good, or special, or pretty, or feminine? When I was trying to quit and found myself in one of those terrible low spots, I would make a cup of hot tea (not coffee—it made me crave a cigarette), take a long hot bubble bath, and then put on bath powder. Find something to compensate for the cigarette when you are anxious and tense. Think about the problem and make a list of a few ideas for activities to substitute for smoking before you try to quit. Then when you need it, pull out the list and put some of it into action.

You are most likely to relapse and go for the cigarette when you are under stress, or feel anxious or low. If you do give in and smoke a cigarette, do not view it as proof of failure, proof that you "cannot do it." Having one cigarette while struggling to stop is far better than continuing to smoke a pack or more a day, feeling it is useless to even try to quit. Any decrease in the amount you smoke is an improvement, and you should be pleased with yourself. Try to look at taking a cigarette during quitting as part of the process; psychologically prepare yourself for the idea that you might slip. Just because you stumble does not mean you have to give up trying altogether. You can quit again, immediately— as many times as it takes.

Another obstacle that women often need to overcome while quitting smoking is the fear of weight gain. Once again, the stereotypical image of the sexually attractive woman worms its way in. Women are constantly trying to do everything possible to lose weight and keep it off. I have been told by many women that they would stop smoking if they could keep their weight down without smoking. It is true that smokers tend to be thinner than nonsmokers, although we do not understand how smoking contributes to this.

Some of the answer could rest with nicotine. Nicotine is a stimulant, and stimulants can suppress appetite. However, I think a large part of it is psychological; cigarettes satisfy a craving for oral gratification. (What could be closer to sucking on the bottle than sucking in on a cigarette?) Food is often used as a means of emotionally "feeding oneself"; cigarettes can serve the same purpose. Once someone stops smoking, the cigarette is often replaced with food as a means of fulfilling oral needs.

Think about the times you smoke and the times you eat. Keep track of when you really crave a cigarette. What are you feeling and what is the situation? By examining your answers, you will learn when you take cigarettes for psychological reasons and you can prepare yourself mentally to combat those times when you are trying to quit.

Watch out for food substitution and accept the notion that you may have a small weight gain when you quit. You will probably gain only a few pounds. These few pounds will not hurt your health; but if you keep smoking, the cigarettes surely will! And give up the idea that if you just had that figure of your dreams, your life would be fine. Chances are that a new body will not fix any of your old problems.

When I stopped smoking I found that hard candy, diet beverages, and herbal teas really helped get me through moments of craving. The best replacement I found, though, was exercise. When I really went nuts for a cigarette, I dragged myself outside and went for a walk.

It is amazing what fresh air and vigorous walking will do. Somehow the fresh air in my lungs did away with the urge to smoke. I found this was even more true in the winter. I quit in December, just as winter set in. I have never seen it reported before, but I found breathing cold air was particularly useful in beating the cravings. If you have tried quitting before and failed, try it during the winter months the next time (if you live in a winter-belt area) and plan on using long walks in the cold as a way to deal with tension and cravings. Remember, the more exercise you get, the better you will be able to cope with withdrawal symptoms and the more calories you will burn.

Withdrawal symptoms can be another obstacle to quitting. Many people are dismayed to find out that they feel miserable for the first few days and finally give in to treating the symptoms with a cigarette. Be prepared to feel uncomfortable the first few days—expect it. Smoking is a physical addiction and, therefore, withdrawal will cause symptoms, some unpleasant. These can include headaches, nervousness, abnormal bowel movements, irritability, and, yes, fatigue.

Be prepared to feel more fatigue at first. That may seem contradictory, but remember that nicotine can act as a stimulant. When you first deprive your body of the substance to which it has been accustomed, it may react with a cry for more stimulant. At first you may feel as if you cannot get going in the morning, or you may feel a bit sluggish all day. Work your way through this time. Do not give in to this fatigue by getting a boost from lighting up. Give your body a chance to kick the habit and increase your energy pool.

Once you quit smoking, changes will begin to occur in your body almost immediately. Within twelve hours, your body will begin a big cleanup process in your lungs, and begin to heal the damage throughout your body. After about forty-eight hours, your blood could be carrying as much as 8 percent more oxygen. You will feel better by the third day, although you may still feel the craving because nicotine and carbon-monoxide levels will be low.

Remember that the withdrawal symptoms will pass. You will soon begin to notice many changes. Not only will you have more energy and be less fatigued, you will be able to breathe more easily. Your cough will begin to clear and your sputum production will decrease. Your senses of taste and smell will improve. Your head will clear and your stomach will not be so queasy. You will begin to feel good about yourself because you will have kicked the habit.

You know what got me to kick the habit? Something very small, yet very powerful. I had been struggling for months with myself, feeling guilty about smoking. I was gearing up in my head to get ready to quit—I kept going over that list of harmful effects; sometimes I would sit and write it down. I would buy one pack, finish it, quit, struggle for a day or two, and finally give in during some low point or stressful period. Then I planned on quitting on my birthday in October. That did not work. The weeks wore on. Then early in December, my husband said to me late one night in bed, "I hate kissing you, you taste terrible." That was it. I quit. And now my husband says I taste wonderful.

WHAT TO DO

1. Decide to quit smoking.

The most important step in quitting is to make a commitment. It does not matter how long it takes you to stop, as long as you are in the process of trying. I went for months, struggling with quitting in my mind. Start thinking about it. Make a list of reasons why you would like to quit. Include on it everything from physical diseases, to smelling and tasting better, to the money you will save.

2. Decide how to quit smoking.

There are a variety of programs from which you can choose. Remember that women tend to be more successful at quitting when they participate in an all-women's group, because they receive support from one another. Check your yellow pages for programs or call your local cancer society or local heart association. Both should be able to tell you what kinds of stop-smoking programs are available in your area. Also, consider your local YWCA, church, or temple. Many of these organizations run programs.

Perhaps you would rather try going cold turkey alone; consider finding a partner with whom to stop—your spouse or maybe a friend at work. Women find that it is particularly helpful to have someone to talk to during the stressful times.

3. Learn what to expect when you quit.

Read about the subject of smoking so that you will be ready for withdrawal symptoms. Many health organizations have good brochures on the subject. Call your cancer society, heart association, or Blue Cross/Blue Shield regional office. If you know what to expect, it will be easier to beat it.

Decide how you will cope with nervousness and tension before you stop. Make a list of things that you enjoy, activities that can help you when you are under stress or feeling blue. When those times come, refer to the list for a suggestion and give it a try.

Do not forget about EXERCISE.

4. Prepare for a relapse.

Praise yourself for any amount that you are able to cut down. Do not be hard on yourself. Quitting is a process, and at times that process may have to include slipping back and smoking a cigarette or two. A relapse does not mean that you are defeated. Stopping smoking is very difficult, and you should be proud of yourself for any successes. If you slip, forgive yourself and quit smoking again.

When you do succeed, you will feel very proud of yourself—as you should. I must share with you what I found on the résumé of a woman who answered my fatigue questionnaire. Under a section entitled "Accomplishments," she had written:

> "My most important accomplishment was in March of 1980 when I quit smoking. This not only improved my chances for having a quality life but convinced me that anything in this world is possible."

8

ABSTAIN FOR SPIRIT

As I talked to women around the country, I found that very few of them are aware of the energy toll that they are paying due to the effects of drugs or alcohol. Almost all women use medications of some type, and it seems that most consume at least some alcohol. Alcohol and many medicines, whether over-the-counter or prescription, are major causes of fatigue.

In this chapter, I will discuss some of the problems that cause women to seek solace in the medicinal effects of alcohol or in the swallowing of pills. Although alcohol is a drug, I have decided to cover it as a special case in the first part of this chapter. In the second part, I will discuss the use of legitimate drugs. I have chosen to concentrate on the use and abuse of prescription and over-the-counter rather than illicit drugs because I believe that ordinary medications have the biggest effect on women's energy today. So, when I use the word *drug,* I am generally referring to a medication, not an illegal substance. Nevertheless, remember that the so-called recreational drugs take their tolls too.

ALCOHOL

Many people still think of alcohol as a beverage or a food. I also used to look upon it that way. However, after seeing alcohol destroy the lives of countless patients and learning about the subtle effects it had on people, I have come to appreciate that alcohol is a powerful drug. It should be used cautiously.

Alcohol can have a particularly devastating effect on women. Alcohol drains women of more energy than they ever imagined. Even women who do not abuse alcohol can suffer from its effects. Beware—one drink can pull the plug in your energy pool!

There was a time when women were not allowed to use alcohol at all. Ancient Roman law ordered the death penalty for any woman who drank it. Women were judged by a standard of morality that lumped drinking, promiscuity, adultery, and immorality all together.

Although the laws have changed, the attitudes and beliefs of ancient Rome are still somewhat with us. Women today receive double messages about drinking. On the one hand, drinking is considered to be sophisticated and liberated; on the other, drinking and all its consequences are still judged more harshly in women than in men. Drinking is not "ladylike."

Even though this attitude still persists to some extent, more and more women are drinking. Today, more than 60 percent of women in the U.S. drink, the highest number ever. The percentage is higher in younger women; 85 percent of college-age women drink. Although women are no longer put to death for drinking, there are serious prices to be paid.

Some of the prices are readily visible, such as drunken-driving accidents and alcoholism. Other consequences—such as problems with family and friends, job difficulties, and emotional and physical ailments—are not always so apparent. Sometimes alcohol can create new problems or make existing difficulties worse, without the moderate drinker knowing it.

Kathy, a forty-eight-year-old divorced counselor with three children, told me how alcohol affected her life. Kathy decided to go back to school to get a college degree when her youngest child started kindergarten. Since her teenage years, she had wanted to go to college, but had fallen into an early marriage that immediately produced a child. Her third child was the result of an unexpected pregnancy that made Kathy feel particularly trapped and frustrated.

Her marriage had gone sour years before, but Kathy was afraid to divorce, because she feared the economic consequences. She dreamed of being free and finding a good job to take care of herself and the children; college was the road to that dream.

As her youngsters went off to school, so did Kathy. She was always working. She did all the chores in the house, made the meals for the entire family, attended classes, and did homework. She did not dare let any of her tasks slip at home, because her husband did not particularly favor her going back to school. Their battles became frequent and grew in intensity until violence entered the picture.

After months, Kathy finally went to the doctor, complaining of chronic fatigue. "I'm always tired. I'm tired when I get up in the morning, I fall into bed exhausted at night," she said. "I want to do things and I like pretty much what I'm doing. Now I have the chance I have always wanted, but I can't seem to drag myself out of bed to do anything. I can hardly smile at my baby anymore."

When you think of Kathy's situation, there are a million reasons why she should have been chronically tired. She was in a bad marriage, she was feeling unappreciated as a homemaker, she was terribly overworked, and she was also in conflict about her role as a woman. She was feeling particularly guilty about wanting to do something for herself. All of these factors contributed to her fatigue.

But there was something else. The doctor asked her what she did to relax and she casually replied, "I have a glass of red wine in the evening to wind down." The truth of the matter was that the glass of wine was a very big glass indeed.

Kathy was drinking a half-bottle of wine several nights each week. The arguments with her husband usually occurred when she was drinking. And the next day, she was always irritable, short-tempered, and terribly tired. She never thought of these symptoms as resulting from a hangover. To her, hangover meant headache. But once the doctor pointed out the connection between her drinking and her symptoms and behavior, it started to make sense. She had never considered that alcohol could be the source of some of her fatigue and other difficulties.

Kathy was a problem drinker.[1] The National Institute on Alcohol Abuse and Alcoholism (NIAAA) reports that "6 percent of drinking women are problem drinkers, although not necessarily alcoholic, and another 21 percent may be potential problem drinkers."[2] This means that women account for somewhere between one quarter to one half of the 10 million problem drinkers in the United States. That is a lot of women.

Unfortunately, alcohol abuse in women is getting worse. One out of every three new members of Alcoholics Anonymous is a woman, an all-time high. More women in their twenties and thirties have alcohol-related problems than women in any other age group. Almost two out of three women now being treated for alcoholism are under the age of thirty-five.

Why? Why are so many women having difficulty controlling their alcohol use? First, society has taken a more permissive view of women who drink alcohol. Today, drinking alcohol by women is not only acceptable, it is often a rite of passage for teenage girls, just as it has always been for boys.

Second, the circumstances of many women's lives are conducive to using alcohol as a coping device. It seems that women drink for different reasons than do men. From what little research we have on women and alcohol (most research has been done on men), it seems that problem drinking among women "may stem from conflicts over acceptance or rejection of the traditional feminine role, traumatic life crises, peer pressure to drink, and drinking to escape from problems."[3]

The struggles women are grappling with in most of these situations all seem to be related to their position in society; the stresses, frustrations, and sense of inadequacy that position engenders.

It has been documented throughout mental health literature that groups in our society who are devalued or who lack control over their lives are particularly prone to depression and other emotional problems. Studies show that women, a group designated and treated as inferior throughout history, suffer significantly more emotional illness than do men. Seen in this light, alcohol abuse may represent one among many mechanisms women use to cope with a psychological condition linked to their subordinate status in society.[4]

Many women today are struggling with the notion of what femininity means to them. Caught between the old concept of passivity and compliance and the new concept of autonomy and assertiveness, many women are having problems resolving the clash. This role conflict seems to play a large part in why women are drinking so much. Many women report that drinking makes them feel more feminine and enables them to play out the traditional role more easily. Alcohol, of course, only obscures the problem temporarily.

Alcohol is a drug, and one of its major side effects is drowsiness. Many people think alcohol is a stimulant, because initially it causes gregariousness, aggressiveness, and excitability. But that is only because alcohol makes some of the control mechanisms in the brain falter. The initial "high" from alcohol is rapidly followed by dulled thinking, slowed-down reflexes, uncoordinated movements, and drowsiness.

Alcohol is a depressant. It dampens the neurons in the central nervous system, which leads to decreased mental and physical abilities. That is why alcohol is sometimes effective in decreasing anxiety; it is relaxing because it is sedating. For many people, this sedating effect does not vanish overnight. Fatigue is often the residual result the day after a few drinks in the evening.

I have had numerous women tell me that they just do not function at their top level if they have as little as one or two beers or glasses of wine the night before. You do not have to drink heavily to suffer from the fatiguing effect of alcohol. One of these women told me:

> "Strangely enough, the effect of alcohol on me is felt not the day I take it, but the day after. The effect is more psychological rather than physical. I lose my sense of self-confidence. I tend to use all

sorts of defense mechanisms when I talk to people—that show my insecurity.

"Also, I become hard on myself—I get critical of myself and these little critical messages run through my head. It seems like the alcohol changes me; it's like a Dr. Jekyll and Mr. Hyde.

"And I find that just two beers will do it—with four, I have extreme psychological effects the next day. I also feel fatigued and irritable—I try to overcome those feelings with exercise. So unless I really, really feel confident about myself, I tend to avoid the alcohol."

Studies suggest that women are more susceptible to the effects of alcohol than men. As one expert said to me, "Women get sicker quicker."

First, because women are physically smaller than men, they will get more intoxicated on a given amount of alcohol.

Second, even if a woman is the same size as a man, she will become more intoxicated imbibing the same amount of alcohol. This is because of the difference in their respective body makeups. Usually a woman has more fat and less fluid than a man, thus the alcohol becomes more concentrated in her body. Ounce for ounce, a woman will feel the effects more.

Third, a woman's menstrual cycle and the birth-control pill can affect how a woman reacts to alcohol. Generally, a woman is more likely to get intoxicated while drinking just before her menstrual period. Fluctuating hormones apparently decrease the liver's ability to metabolize alcohol.

And fourth, women are more likely than men to develop liver cirrhosis and other life-threatening organ diseases. The reason for this is not yet known.

Women also tend to become alcoholics faster than men. This can be accounted for by the physical differences mentioned above, by the way women drink, and by dual addiction (to both alcohol and other drugs). Women as a group tend to drink alone, usually in the privacy of their homes. Because no one is around (such as a bartender to say "no more"), women may drink until they pass out. Consequently, they get exposed to higher alcohol blood levels over a period of time. Also, it is far more common for women to be dependent on both drugs (tranquilizers, sedatives, hypnotics) and alcohol than men. Drugs combined with alcohol can result in a variety of serious, even fatal consequences.

The majority of people who drink alcohol do so to relax and to enjoy themselves socially. And for most, alcohol never seems to become a problem. Yet even social drinking can have a marked effect upon its participants, because even moderate amounts of alcohol create the depressive effect. And, as we discussed, the depressive qualities of alcohol cause fatigue. A small amount of alcohol can temporarily decrease the efficiency of the mind and body.

In most cases, those effects are short-lived, but for others, that line between social drinking and problem drinking becomes blurred. If you drink alcohol to get to sleep, to get going, as a pick-me-up, to cope with frustration or anxiety or sadness or loneliness, or to feel more feminine, you are using alcohol to medicate your emotions. Using alcohol for its drug qualities means you may be having difficulty controlling your drinking. Go back and check your Fatigue Profile; how did you do on Exercise 6? Did you answer "yes" to any of the questions?

Women, in particular, need to be careful about the use of alcohol. Alcohol can decrease your effectiveness in carrying out your responsibilities and cover up your ability to deal with the real problems in your life. The fatigue that comes from alcohol consumption can be, like many of alcohol's other effects, a silent monster that saps your energy and well-being. You will have more spirit and energy if you abstain—abstain for spirit.

WHAT TO DO

1. Learn about alcohol.

Remember that alcohol is a powerful addictive drug. In order for you to use the drug safely, you must know how it affects you. Keep track of your drinking until you become fully aware of your habits and responses to alcohol. Be sensitive to how your susceptibility to alcohol varies during your menstrual cycle.

Pay close attention to your energy level. If you experience fatigue the day after a drink or two, then you should avoid alcohol when you wish to be in top mental and physical shape. Drink only when you are willing to pay the price of fatigue.

2. Set a good example.

Each woman is responsible for making her own decision about her drinking habits. Decisions not to drink should be respected. Learn to say no if that is what you desire. Do not hesitate to refuse alcohol, even in the face of considerable peer pressure. There is some evidence to suggest that women drink more in the company of men, so women who do not drink can help serve as role models and lend their support to other women in resisting the pressures to drink.

3. Do not use alcohol as a medication.

If you begin to use alcohol as a medication, it may quickly become a habit. All of us experience frustration, anxiety, stress, and emotional turmoil. Drinking may seem like a good antidote for whatever is bothering you. But there are other ways to cope with those feelings. Try to delineate exactly what is eating at you. Talk about it with a friend. Write about it in private. Take a walk and try to find an action that will change your circumstances. Exercise instead of drinking. Give yourself a test—see if you can go one week without a single drink.

4. Get help if you need it.

If this chapter has made you feel uncomfortable, perhaps because of your drinking habits, it is understandable. Drinking when compelled to do so is a very painful, lonely experience. You should know, however, that relief is available. You can stop drinking, even though it may seem impossible to you right now.

When one is a compulsive drinker, life without alcohol seems intolerable. But there is a place, somewhere on the other side of a few weeks, where life is better. Many wonderful people are ready to help you get there. All you have to do is say "Help."

- call your local crisis center and hotlines, or
- call your local council on alcoholism, or
- call your community mental health center, or
- call your local chapter of Alcoholics Anonymous, or
- call Women for Sobriety

The numbers should be in your telephone directory. You do not have to give your name. Just ask, "Do you have a program to help women with a drinking problem?"

DRUGS

As I studied fatigue, I came to realize more than ever, that a tremendous amount of the fatigue experienced by women is caused by the medicines they take. Many times the tired feeling is a small price to pay for the wonderful results that can be achieved through modern drug therapy. But in other cases, fatigue is too great a price to be paid.

New medicines are giving us the means to treat or control previously disabling or life-threatening illnesses. From chemotherapy for control of cancer to antidepressants that help severely depressed patients, pharmacological treatment is achieving dramatic results. There have been tremendous strides in the development of medicines in the last fifty years. Every day we read of a new treatment method. The pace of these developments has, however, led to other problems.

First, it is difficult for physicians, let alone the general public, to keep up-to-date on all of the developments. Doctors are faced with the demanding task of choosing the right treatment for each patient's particular condition. Second, it is often difficult to judge the overall effect of these complex chemical substances on the human body. It is hard to measure the potential impact of side effects. The Food and Drug Administration, of course, has a sophisticated approval process through which all drugs must pass before they can be used to treat the general public. This process mitigates much of the risk in using new drugs. But even though the risks of certain side effects are known for a particular drug, the degree of severity varies a great deal from patient to patient. The doctor must monitor each individual carefully.

Of course, the side effect with which we are concerned here is fatigue. A considerable number of drugs list fatigue, drowsiness, sedation, lethargy, et cetera, as potential side effects. For example, physicians have reported fatigue in patients using beta-blockers, a class of drugs used in the treatment of angina and high blood pressure. Of course, not all patients who take beta-blockers experience fatigue, but those who do must make a choice of whether the benefits outweigh the fatigue. In most cases, they seem to adjust to their fatigue and plan their life accordingly.

Plan their life accordingly—that seems to be the answer for many people who need to take medicine to control a chronic illness. And, of course, there are millions of women in this country who are doing just that. I suggest, however, that you do not automatically accept fatigue as a side effect of your treatment.

First, tell your doctor about your symptom. As we have discussed before, some doctors may not be sensitive about the complaint of fatigue or know what to do about it; but you should persist in seeking solutions (in Chapter 15, I will discuss how to talk to your doctor).

Second, work with your doctor to find alternatives. Perhaps your dosage can be reduced and still provide you with the appropriate therapeutic benefits. Often, the time that you take the medicine can be changed (for instance, take your pills before going to bed) so that the peak of the fatigue side effect would occur while you sleep. For instance, some people on antidepressants can take the whole dose before going to bed, instead of spacing the doses around the clock. On this schedule, little fatigue is experienced during the day, and the tiredness they feel from their dose before bedtime helps them to sleep.

The effect of drugs varies by individual. Sometimes another drug in the same class that does not cause fatigue in you can be used. We all have personal reactions to drugs.

(And, I might note, women sometimes react differently from men.)

Third, if you have fully explored the alternatives and you must take the medication, then you must compensate in other ways. If you can identify one period during the day when you are more tired, work around it. As we discussed in Chapter 2, accept this kind of fatigue and learn to organize your life around your lowest period by taking naps or avoiding demanding tasks then.

You can also boost your energy pool by eating the proper foods, getting exercise, staying away from alcohol and tobacco as much as you can, and getting plenty of rest. All of these activities will diminish the fatiguing effects of the drug.

Although fatigue is a well known side effect of some drugs, people (including a lot of doctors) rarely think of drug use as a cause of chronic tiredness. Furthermore, the drugs that most frequently cause sedation are, for the most part, prescribed for women. These are called psychotropic drugs—drugs that affect the mood—and include tranquilizers, hypnotics, sedatives, and antidepressants. According to some estimates, over one half of all the women in the United States have used psychotropic drugs for a medical reason. Of all the prescriptions written for these drugs, 73 percent are written for women![5] This means that women use over two times as many mood-altering drugs as men.

Because of sex-role stereotypes, doctors expect more psychological problems in women and prescribe drugs accordingly for vague complaints. What may be a problem of living often gets "medicalized" and masked with a drug. Women frequently become dependent on these drugs, even at therapeutic levels, which only intensifies the problems in their lives.

So often women find themselves leaving their doctor's office with a prescription in hand. And in the short run, the drug may seem to help. After all, people take drugs because they provide some kind of immediate relief or pleasure. Often women are taking drugs that do nothing to solve their underlying problem but may be simply dulling the pain of life. In the long run, the drugs often create more problems.

Instead of investigating the real source of the symptom,

many doctors simply prescribe antianxiety medications, hypnotics, sedatives, or antidepressants to "treat" a symptom presumably arising from some "inherent" weakness in the individual. The side effects from these drugs can often worsen the very condition from which the patient originally sought relief.

Fatigue is such a condition. Apparently, housewives, the unemployed, and the retired are the most likely to seek help from physicians for the symptom of fatigue.[6] Such symptoms may be the result of the life situation in which these people find themselves. Tragically, the fatigue is often compounded. Studies have reported that "physicians are prepared to prescribe mood-modifying drugs to housewives in the belief that they do not need to be alert for their jobs, but they are reluctant to do so for students."[7]

Doctors are not prescribing these medicines only for housewives; they are being given to women in all walks of life. It seems as if every week I hear about another famous woman entering a rehabilitation center for treatment of a problem with drugs or alcohol or both: Betty Ford, Elizabeth Taylor, Liza Minnelli, Mary Tyler Moore. We hear all the gory details of their lives, but we do not hear about the other women, the millions of obscure women struggling with their lot in life who have resorted to pills to ease the pain.

What is happening? Why have so many women turned to pills (and alcohol) to cope with life? One researcher who studied women who used tranquilizers reported this:

> While reasons for initial use varied widely, continued use was most often discussed in terms of its [Valium's] ability to allow subjects to maintain themselves in a role or roles they found difficult or intolerable without the drug. The most common role strains and conflicts mentioned by females centered around their traditional roles as wife, mother, and houseworker. One woman said she took diazepam (Valium) so that she could cope with a demanding social role as hostess. A woman with four teenagers reported that she took diazepam to protect her family from her irritability. Another

woman took diazepam as an escape from an unsatisfying family situation. Many women reported initial tranquilizer use following the birth of children and the attendant physical and emotional strain. Women who continued tranquilizer use over a prolonged period expressed clearly conflicting attitudes regarding their maternal role. Almost all the women described situations of extreme role strain, inability to comply with traditional role expectations, and the feeling that they lacked the right to express their dissatisfaction and preferences.[8]

Although you occasionally read that the increase in drug use has come about because of role-overload stress in mothers who work outside the home, quite the opposite is true. It turns out that studies are showing that women who are in the dual roles of both worker and homemaker have less illness and take fewer tranquilizers and sleeping medications than women who are traditional homemakers.

Housewives—women in traditional roles—seem to be experiencing some of the most serious psychological problems. Housewives are subject to many stress-related diseases and often use drugs or alcohol as coping mechanisms. In study after study, women who experienced strains in their roles as housewives had the most difficulty coping and used the greatest variety of substances.[9]

If our grandmothers struggled with a sense of low self-esteem, they kept it to themselves and just considered it a woman's lot in life. Today, low self-esteem is viewed as a problem and, sadly, many women now turn to the many drugs available to try to ease the pain that goes with it.

Unfortunately, many doctors interpret women's symptoms that result from these stressful life situations as the result of "innate female emotional instability." Women may be taking medications to cope with their life circumstances; however, one cannot lose sight of the fact that doctors are prescribing these medications for women. Physicians are contributing to the women's drug problem by inappropriately prescribing these drugs and issuing repeat prescriptions without reassessing the patient's situation. Much of doctors' behavior has been shown to be a result of their attitudes toward women. One study reported:

> The little literature available on physicians' attitudes toward female patients shows that physicians believe female patients to be more mentally disturbed, to have more social problems, and to be less stoic than men during illness. Physicians are also more likely to consider that women, more than men, provide unreliable information.[10]

Consequently women's symptoms are taken less seriously by doctors and often automatically attributed to psychological or psychosomatic illness. As a result, women are overusing or abusing tranquilizers, sedatives, and hypnotics because of the widespread indiscriminate prescribing habits of patronizing doctors. The real problems of these women are not identified and remain unsolved, while their symptoms are simply dulled.

It would be so much more helpful if they were told that their emotional reactions to circumstances (such as divorce, wife abuse, frustration with their roles, poverty, discrimination, et cetera) are normal; that anyone in their situation would feel the same way (including men); and that the task is to change life's circumstances. Tough, yes, but it can be done. Psychotropic drugs do not change such situations, they only dull some symptoms and create a few more. Fatigue is one of the most common.

In addition to psychotropic drugs, a variety of other medications can have the side effect of fatigue. In the following list, I have indicated various classes of drugs that are known to be associated with fatigue and have given a few examples of the more popular drugs in each. Many drugs are used for a variety of conditions and so may fit in more than one of the categories. It is impossible to develop a complete list of drugs that may cause fatigue as a side effect; there are hundreds.

Although I have not discussed illegal drugs used for recreational purposes, I should note that a number of those also cause fatigue. Any drug that causes a depressive effect on the brain should be suspect. Be careful of substances that may be considered mild, such as marijuana. Also remember that each person reacts differently to drugs. One person may experience a given side effect, while the next will not.

Fatigue has been reported as a side effect of the following classes of drugs.

Analgesics and Salicylates

An analgesic is a painkiller. Analgesics include drugs from ordinary aspirin (a salicylate) to more powerful, non-narcotic medicines, such as Talwin. You should be aware of drowsiness or other fatigue-related effects, especially if you are on large dosages.

Anticonvulsants

Anticonvulsants are generally used in the control of seizures. Any drug that is used to alter brain function has the potential to cause fatigue. These drugs include Dilantin, Phenobarbitol, and Tegretol.

Antidepressants

These are drugs that have been growing in popularity in recent years because they are so effective in the treatment of depression. These include Elavil, Norpramin, Parnate, Sinequan, Lithium, and Triavil. Antidepressants should be administered under the close supervision of a physician.

Antihistamines

Antihistamines are commonly used in the control of the symptoms of colds, flu, allergies, and motion sickness. Most are sold in over-the-counter forms. Because of the possibility of drowsiness, almost all antihistamines come with information warning the user to avoid driving a car or using machinery when using the medicine.

Antihypertensives

Antihypertensive medications are used to lower the blood pressure. Many different types of drugs are used to do this; some of them are fatigue-causing, while others are not. The antihypertensive drugs most commonly associated with fatigue are Inderal (see beta-blockers below), clonidine, methyldopa, and reserpine.

Antipsychotics

These drugs are usually employed in the treatment of patients with serious psychological illness. Antipsychotic drugs may also be considered major tranquilizers and are extremely helpful in preventing and controlling episodes of severe emotional upset. Included in this category are Compazine, Haldol, Mellarill, Stelazine, and Thorazine.

Beta-blockers

These are drugs that are typically used in the treatment of angina, hypertension, and other symptoms of cardiovascular disease, as well as migraine headaches. They work by blocking part of the messengers of the sympathetic nervous system. Examples of beta-blockers are Inderal and Tenormin.

Birth-control Pills

By now, every woman knows about birth-control pills; and most know about the wide range of side effects. Fatigue is one of them. It is not known for sure whether the estrogens or the progesterones in the Pill are responsible.

Cough and Cold Preparations with Narcotics

By law, only prescription cough and cold preparations can contain narcotics, such as codeine. Effects can include lightheadedness, dizziness, or sedation. One should avoid operating machinery or driving a car while using medicines containing even mild narcotics. If your doctor has prescribed a cough medicine, make sure you know what is in it.

Hypnotics

Hypnotics are a broad class of drug typically used to induce sleep. These sleep aids include sedatives, analgesics, intoxicants, and anesthetics. Examples of hypnotics are Dalmane, Doriden, Halcion, Nembutal Sodium, and Restoril.

Muscle Relaxants

These include a variety of substances used for the relief of muscle spasms associated with acute, painful conditions of muscles, such as severe backache. This class includes such drugs as Soma, Robaxin, and Valium.

Narcotics

Narcotics are effective in the control of pain but are addictive. Sedation is one of the most common side effects of narcotics. Narcotics should be used only under the strict supervision of a physician. Examples of legal narcotics include Darvon, codeine, and Demerol.

Sedatives

A sedative is generally used to designate any substance that has a relaxing, soothing, or tranquilizing effect on the body. The term "sedative" is applied to a variety of substances and includes the following categories:

Barbiturates

Barbiturates are often used to treat anxiety, tension, and insomnia. Such drugs as Amytal, Butisol, Nembutal, and Seconal are in this class. In addition to incurring the risk of drowsiness, confusion, and loss of memory, patients can easily become psychologically and physically addicted to barbiturates.

Nonbarbiturates

Nonbarbiturate sedatives are often used for a variety of reasons. For example, Phenergan can be used to treat allergic reactions or to calm apprehension, or Remsed can be used to control nausea and motion sickness. This class can also include drugs considered to be major tranquilizers (Equanil) or hypnotics (Dalmane and Noctec).

Major Tranquilizers

Major tranquilizers, such as Equanil, Miltown, Prolixin, and Serentil, are often used in a variety of disease states to reduce severe tension and anxiety. Some drugs in this class are also in the antipsychotic class, depending upon their usage.

177

Minor Tranquilizers

Tranquilizers are most often used to relieve anxiety and tension and to relax muscles. Tranquilizers include such drugs as Valium, Librium, and Xanex. These are some of the most frequently prescribed drugs in America.

I hope that I have been able to increase your awareness of your use of drugs in your life. This chapter, along with the exercises in Chapter 4, were designed to help you recognize when your medicines are a help and when they are a hindrance. How many medications did you circle in the list preceding Exercise 7? Were you in the Fatigue Zone at all with Exercise 7, Drug Usage? It is important for you to remember: When in doubt, ask questions, get the answers, be cautious. As with alcohol, make sure that you are using your medicines for the right purpose. If you are experiencing fatigue as a side effect of a drug, make sure that the benefits outweigh the cost of reduced energy.

WHAT TO DO

1. Determine what fatigue-causing drugs you use.

Many women use more than one drug that has drowsiness or fatigue as a side effect. For example, someone could be taking birth-control pills, Valium, and antihistamines. Make a list of all the drugs you use. For each one, answer the following questions:

- What is the name of the drug?
- What is it being used to treat?
- What kind of drug is it (e.g., tranquilizer, etc.)?
- Is this drug one of the drugs that commonly causes fatigue?
- Are there any other side effects?
- What is the proper way to take the drug? (When do you take it, how often, with what, and for what length of time?)

- Does this drug interact with any other drugs (such as birth-control pills)?
- Is it safe to take this drug and drink alcohol?

If you have difficulty answering any of these questions, you can receive information from the following sources:

- your doctor
- your nurse
- your pharmacist
- a book entitled the *Physicians' Desk Reference* (It is a yearly publication that contains information about all prescription drugs.)

Decide if you really need to take the over-the-counter medications. Obviously, you have two choices if you want to get rid of drug-induced fatigue: Either stop the drug or try lowering the dose.

2. Have your doctor help you with prescription drugs.

Keep track of how you feel throughout the day, discover when you are the most alert and when you are the most drowsy. Based on this information your doctor might be able to prescribe a substitute drug, decrease your dose, or alter the times you take your dose, thus moving your tired period to a less critical time of day. If you must take a drug that causes fatigue, do not just give in to the tiredness, learn how to manage it.

3. Learn other ways to cope with stress.

Stress is part of life; it is always present in one form or another. You can cope with stress either in productive ways, such as exercising or doing something creative, or in nonproductive ways, such as taking drugs, which drastically decreases your ability to function. The key to dealing with stress successfully is to make it work to your advantage. When you find yourself under stress, discover ways to turn it into something that will benefit you.

- Take time-outs, do something for yourself.
- Talk to someone you are close to, tell them how you really feel.
- Do something with your hands; knit a sweater, sew a dress, crochet an afghan, do needlepoint, start a garden.
- Exercise; take a walk, go swimming, go dancing, play tennis, play badminton, play horseshoes, play croquet.
- Get involved in local groups that are working to change situations affecting women.
- Take courses at a local community college in an area in which you think you would like to improve.
- Learn new job skills by taking adult-education courses, job-training programs, or college courses. [11]

4. Get help if you are depending on drugs to cope with life.

Beware of using drugs for nonmedical reasons. Be careful of using any drug—nicotine, alcohol, over-the-counter drugs, prescription medications, and illicit drugs—for escape. All have the potential to create serious side effects, as well as provide temporary relief. Try to get in touch with why you are really using a drug. Because the drugs are taken on the orders of their doctor and "medicines" are acceptable therapeutic agents, many women fail to realize they could be dependent on drugs. Remember: Just because a doctor has prescribed a medication for you does not mean that it is the best way to treat your particular symptom. Do not be afraid to challenge a doctor's assumptions.

Too often, chronic drug taking only makes life worse and makes a woman feel more guilty and worthless than she already feels. Make a change for the better. I know it sounds impossible, but it can be done with help from others.

Problems are solved one at a time. The first one that should be solved is the overuse of drugs to blunt feelings, the bad feelings you would rather not be aware of. Once the haze is gone, you can begin to become the person you would like to be. Life without pills may seem intolerable right now, but with some personal counseling and support you will learn that it is so much better without them. And once you make the commitment to help yourself, it will not take long to see how much better you can feel. If you need help with the drugs you are using:

- call your local crisis center and hotlines
- call your local council on alcohol and drug abuse
- call your community mental health center
- see a doctor, private counselor, minister, or rabbi

The numbers should be in your telephone directory under Drug Abuse, Alcohol and Drug Abuse, or Mental Health. You do not have to identify yourself. Just ask, "Do you have a program to help women with a drug (medication) problem?"

_____ 9 _____

SLEEP FOR VITALITY

"Tired night's sweet restorer, balmy sleep."

—Edward Young, *Night Thoughts*
(1742–1745)

Sleep is the great restorer of our energy pool. We count on a good night's rest to give us vigor and enthusiasm for the next day's tasks. After we have finished a day of stimulating active work and play, we look forward to bedtime, to spending a few minutes with a good book and eventually drifting off to sweet dreams.

However, for the millions of people who have trouble sleeping, this view of sleep is but an elusive dream. Without their daily rest, they cannot replenish their energy supply and their fatigue mounts. It is estimated that up to 15 percent of the American population has difficulty getting the right quantity or quality of sleep.

In one specific study, which surveyed about four thousand people covering all age groups and both genders, 44 percent of the respondents reported that their sleep was restless. Another indicator of the size of the sleep problem is the wide variety and quantity of over-the-counter sleep aids and prescription sleep pills that are used each year. About 11 percent of American adults use sedative or hypnotic drugs to help them sleep.

Sleep is vital to our energy, our well-being, and our outlook on life. Without sleep, we soon cease to function properly. Sleep is a natural part of our lives, but as we shall see, it is somewhat fragile and easily disturbed. In this chapter, I will explore some of the mysteries of sleep and its complex cycles. I will give you a brief description of the mechanism of sleep. Then we will look at some of the things that can disturb its intricate mechanism. Finally, we will discuss some of the things you can do to make sure that you get enough of the most restful sleep.

THE MECHANISM OF SLEEP

Although we spend about one third of our life sleeping, most of us know very little about what happens to our bodies while we slumber. We tend to take sleep for granted until something disturbs it. When that disturbance occurs, whether it be for one night or a longer period of time, it can severely disrupt our lives. Even after one night of poor or limited sleep, the effects of sleep deprivation are strongly felt; we perform poorly at our work, we become irritable, we become moody, we lack concentration, we feel lethargic—tired.

My husband laughed when he saw me reviewing a study that concluded that people feel fatigue after they are deprived of sleep. "Well, isn't that studying the obvious?" he said. "My grandparents taught me that when I was a child." He was right in one sense, that we have always known that sleep deprivation causes fatigue. Yet researchers have spent years trying to understand the mechanism of sleep and its exact relationship to a person's energy level.

If we understand that process, we may be able to adjust certain aspects of our daily habits to help us sleep better. I certainly found that to be true. As I have been studying sleep in relationship to fatigue, I have learned that relatively simple changes in my schedule and my personal routine can have a big effect on the quality and amount of rest I receive. I will share with you some of those changes in this chapter.

Sleep is a vital part of our daily rhythm; we need some prolonged rest every twenty-four hours. There seem to be two primary functions of sleep. First, it helps restore energy levels. In one scientific study, a group of people was deprived of sleep while researchers kept track of the subjects' behavior patterns and a variety of chemical indicators in their bodies.

After about one hundred hours (over four days) of being awake, the researchers reported that the "people began to hallucinate and show slightly psychotic behavior. They would see fire bursting from the walls and suspect their friends of conspiring to kill them. They also showed changes in motor performance and in energy-transfer systems."[1]

At about the same time that behavior changes were noted, analysis of the subjects' blood showed that energy-carrying chemicals were beginning to run down. Initially, the body handled the challenge of no sleep by using an emergency energy-making system, but that too broke down around four days into the experiment.

When the subjects of the experiment were finally allowed to go to sleep, their psychological symptoms and chemical imbalances disappeared.

Experiments of this type indicate that the body uses sleep time to renew its energy coffers with energy units. It appears that some part of the rejuvenating process can happen *only* during sleep.

The second important function of sleep is that it helps the body to regulate and synchronize itself. Once the body gets accustomed to a certain rhythm of daytime work and nighttime sleep, hundreds of other biological rhythms fall into phase. Temperature, pulse rate, and respiration change with the sleep/wake cycle. So do the levels of very important brain chemicals and hormones.

Experiments have shown that temperature and a variety of other vital body signs fluctuate in a twenty-four- to twenty-five-hour period. We see a lot of variation from person to person, though. For example, people vary in their need for sleep. We all know people who consistently need ten hours of sleep and yet still seem to drag through their daily tasks. Others can get by on as little as four hours of sleep a night and are extremely active during the day. Most people sleep on the average of seven to eight hours a night. If sleep is disrupted, there is a double whammy: Our daily rhythms are disturbed and we are deprived of the restorative rest we need.

THE CYCLES OF SLEEP

Although we may not be conscious of them, each night we go through cycles while we are sleeping. As we drift off to sleep, our sleep gradually deepens until we are in a deep, deep slumber. Then we return through a period of lessening depth to a state that is relatively light. This cycle normally takes about ninety minutes. If nothing disturbs us, we begin the cyle again, going down to a deep slumber and, later, back up to light sleep again. Each night we go through three to five of these cycles.

As we go through the night, the depth of each cycle decreases. As morning approaches, the sleep becomes lighter, body temperature rises, the pulse and respiration begin to speed up, and certain hormones begin to surge. The body is getting ready for the activities of the day.

CYCLES WITHIN SLEEP

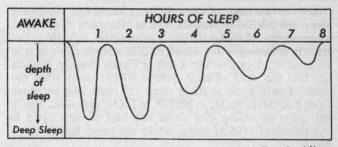

Karen Ann Atkinson

Figure 15: *A night's sleep consists of three to five cycles, each one going from a light sleep down to a deep slumber, and back up again.*

If anything disrupts any portion of one of these sleep periods, our rest can be disturbed profoundly. For instance, if you are suddenly awakened out of the deep portion of one of the cycles, you probably will be groggy, lethargic, and irritable. On the other hand, if you are awakened out of the lighter portion of sleeping, you may feel relatively wide awake even though you did not get a complete night's rest.

Did you ever wonder why the alarm clock always seems to go off at the wrong time and why you always seem more rested on weekends when you wake up without the alarm? It is probably because the alarm clock that goes off during the week has no knowledge of your inner cycle, nor does it care whether it disturbs you from the deep or the light part of your cycle. If the alarm awakens you suddenly from the deep part of your sleep, you have a hard time getting awake. Whereas, if the alarm awakens you during the light part of your cycle, when your body is ready, you awaken feeling relatively rested. That is why that extra thirty minutes of sleep after the alarm goes off can seem so wonderful. That time allows your body to cycle from the deep sleep up to the lighter portion before you get out of bed.

TWO KINDS OF SLEEP

There are two kinds of sleep: REM or Rapid Eye Movement sleep and NREM or Non-Rapid Eye Movement sleep. REM sleep occurs when the sleeper is in an active, light sleep and usually dreaming, while during NREM sleep the sleeper is in an inactive, deep slumber. Look at Figure 15 again. We can say that the valley of each cycle is NREM sleep, while the peak of each cycle is REM sleep. All night long we move from NREM, to REM, to NREM, to REM, and so on. This is the same as saying that about one half of each cycle is composed of NREM sleep, while the other half is REM sleep.

Notice that in REM sleep you are almost awake—but not quite. In REM sleep, body signs and movements are close to those of an awake person, but the mind is not in a conscious state. Interestingly enough, it seems that most of the dreams that we remember occur during REM sleep.

TWO KINDS OF SLEEP

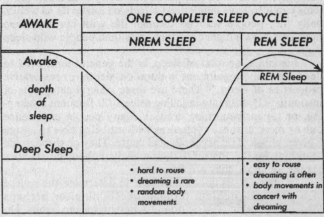

AWAKE	ONE COMPLETE SLEEP CYCLE	
	NREM SLEEP	REM SLEEP
Awake ↓ depth of sleep ↓ Deep Sleep		REM Sleep
	• hard to rouse • dreaming is rare • random body movements	• easy to rouse • dreaming is often • body movements in concert with dreaming

Karen Ann Atkinson

Figure 16: *Each sleep cycle consists of two kinds of sleep, NREM and REM.*

Even though the body seems restless at the time, REM sleep is a necessary part of the rest cycle. Experiments have shown that people who are artificially deprived of REM sleep for a period of time tend to make up for their lost REM after their deprivation is over by having longer periods of REM sleep and shorter periods of NREM sleep.

DISTURBED SLEEP—INSOMNIA

If we are to restore our normal reservoir of energy, we need the right kind and the right amount of sleep. A disturbance that keeps us awake too long, wakes us up too early, makes us sleep too much, alters our normal cycle, or affects our sleep stages will affect our energy balance.

When we are deprived of sleep for prolonged periods of time, we start to experience increased fatigue, irritability, and

187

difficulty in concentration. If we do not get rest, the symptoms progress to deterioration of motor function, decreased motivation, and even hallucinations. Long-term sleep problems can also have deleterious effects on longevity as well as daily life; people who go through life with chronic sleep problems have a higher mortality rate than people who sleep well.

Insomnia, or want of sleep, is the general term used to describe "any impairment in duration, depth, or restorative properties of sleep."[2] There are three general categories of insomnia: (1) difficulty in falling asleep, (2) frequent awakening, or (3) early-morning arousal. Many people experience one or more of these symptoms without being able to assign a given physical or psychological cause. They go through life searching for the answer to their malady without satisfactory results. In short, they are miserable.

In many cases doctors are able to determine the source of a person's problem through questioning, or perhaps through scientific observation of a person's sleep habits. Dr. William C. Dement, one of the pioneers in the field of studying the mechanism of sleep, told the story of one man who had been suffering the effects of insomnia for over thirty years.[3] The patient had been visiting doctors off and on for years. During that time, he had tried numerous drugs to induce sleep and had been psychoanalyzed. But nothing worked. He still could not sleep.

When Dr. Dement and his team at the Stanford University Sleep Disorders Clinic at Stanford, California, analyzed the man's sleep patterns, they found that he could not breathe while he was sleeping. As soon as he fell asleep, he would stop breathing and wake up to gulp for air. He was literally waking up every time he needed to breathe, which was hundreds of times a night.

This man's problem turned out to be a physical condition called sleep apnea. In sleep apnea, the central nervous system control over breathing abruptly ceases to function as the person goes from a waking to a sleeping state. However, the point of telling Dr. Dement's story is that it took the efforts of the sleep clinic to identify the source of the man's problem. The man had searched in vain for years for the answer to his insomnia. Often, the cause of insomnia can be found through the proper analysis of a patient's sleep patterns, but ordinary techniques available in a regular doctor's office are not sufficient to do the job. Specialized instruments and highly trained observers are often needed to make the correct diagnosis.

A number of sleep clinics have been established around the country. One of the most famous is the one at Stanford University mentioned above. These clinics are equipped to make measurements of patients' sleep habits and help identify the precise pattern of sleep dysfunction.

A typical visit starts with measuring the patients' responses during a complete night's sleep. Professionals at the sleep clinic then analyze the results to determine the characteristics of the sleep. Many times the results have shown that patients usually do not know really how much sleep they get or do not get, what the quality of the sleep is, or exactly what is disturbing the rest period. They only know that they are sleepy and tired.

Psychological Problems and Insomnia

Most of us know from experience that anxiety can disturb sleep. If we are busy thinking about a problem that we cannot immediately solve or shelve, we are not likely to doze off or to settle into a deep slumber. Women seem particularly prone to having their sleeping hours invaded by their daytime worries and responsibilities. Take Linda, a thirty-seven-year-old schoolteacher who is divorced and the mother of one child.

> "Another [incident of fatigue] was several years ago at school when I had a terribly difficult class to handle, teach, et cetera. I was always tired—worrying about what to do with them. I got up tired, pushed through the day tired, and then couldn't sleep at night. Mostly I worried. It was one of the worst years I've ever had."

Linda's case is not different from those of many women in nurturing jobs; they seem to carry home the burdens of their wards—even to the extent that it disturbs their sleep.

Linda's sleep improved when her psychological burden was reduced; her class and, therefore, her sleep were different the following school year:

> "This year, I had the best class ever. I spent most days enjoying teaching and never knew I was tired until I sat down at ten or so—and I really rested!"

Linda recognized right away that her fatigue and her sleep problem were related to her worry about the group of children that she was teaching. To her credit, she did not search for a simple solution, such as pills, for her sleepless nights.

Now that so many women are working outside the home, they also tend to bring home the problems of the office, the store, or the factory. Some women are not able to separate the relationships they have on the job from their private emotions and concerns. Studies are beginning to show that women's sensitivity to relationships and people makes them especially prone to personalizing the problems of others and, consequently, suffering from additional stress. A fifty-six-year-old mother of three said to me:

> "Even though the children are grown, I still worry. I'll wake up at four o'clock in the morning and not be able to get back to sleep; worrying about my son's promotion or my daughter's injury. My husband will roll over and say, 'You're awake again, what are you worrying about now? Go back to sleep.' And he's back to sleep in a snap. There I am wide awake and worrying about my grown children and I just can't seem to turn it off, although I wish I could."

When the time for sleep arrives, women often get into bed with their minds still ruminating about the day's activities only to find that their mate has lapsed into deep sleep. Men's lack of deep personal involvement with others seems to make it easier for them to block out the problems of the day and sink into their dreams. Sometimes women pay the price for their sensitivities through disturbed sleep.

We know that insomnia can be associated with psychological disorders. In fact, most serious psychological illness is accompanied by sleep disorders. Dr. Dement commented:

> At the very least, sleep is a sensitive barometer of psychic turbulence; it is virtually axiomatic that a disturbance of the mind will manifest itself in the sleeping state as well as in the waking state.[4]

Depressed people frequently have restless sleep and wake up too early in the morning. Early-morning wakening is an important indicator of depression; one of the first questions a doctor will ask a patient suspected of being depressed is "Are you waking up early in the morning?" Many such patients may go to bed exhausted but wake up early feeling generally anxious and not be able to get back to sleep.

Various other psychological difficulties can disturb sleep. It is extremely important in all such cases that the underlying psychological issues or illnesses get treated, rather than the sleep difficulty alone. For instance, if depressed patients are treated with sleeping pills alone, their difficulties may be intensified. However, when antidepressant medication and therapy are used to treat the depression, the early-morning wakening problem is usually resolved as the patient's mood improves.

Drugs and Insomnia

There has been a tremendous amount of progress in drug therapy for the treatment of various psychological ailments in recent years. Psychopharmacologists have learned a great deal about the biochemistry underlying the workings of the mind. New and more sophisticated medications have helped millions of people struggling with psychological problems. The judicious application of drug therapy can yield dramatic results in many cases.

However, side effects of drugs should be monitored carefully; they often cause more sleeping problems than they solve.

Mr. B. was studying for a civil service exam, the outcome of which would affect his entire future. He was terribly worried about the test and found it difficult to get to sleep at night. Feeling that the sleep loss was affecting his ability to study, he consulted his physician for the express purpose of getting "something to make me sleep." His doctor prescribed a moderate dose of barbiturate at bedtime, and Mr. B. found that this medication was very effective . . . for the first several nights. After about a week, he began having trouble sleeping again and decided to take two sleeping pills each night. Twice more the cycle was repeated, until on the night before the exam he was taking four times as many pills as his doctor had prescribed. The next night, with the pressure off, Mr. B. took no medication. He had terrific difficulty falling asleep, and when he did, his sleep was terribly disrupted for the rest of the night—he awoke often and had two disturbing nightmares. Mr. B. now decided that he had a serious case of insomnia, and returned to his sleeping-pill habit. By the time he consulted our clinic several years later, he was taking approximately 1,000 mg sodium amytal every night, and his sleep was more disturbed than ever. Yet he had been perfectly normal before the transient stressful episode! Patients may go on for years and years—from one sleeping pill to another—never realizing that their troubles are *caused* by the pills.[5]

As this dramatic story illustrates, drugs can disrupt the intricate balance of the sleep cycles, making it more difficult for a person to sleep. Studies on people who are regular users of hypnotic agents, such as barbiturates (e.g., Seconol), have shown disturbance of the normal sleep cycle, with sleep frequently interrupted by awakening, especially in the second half of the night.[6] In addition, barbiturates can cause daytime drowsiness, confusion, and loss of memory. Chronic use of barbiturates can cause the body to build up a tolerance so that larger doses are needed to achieve the desired effect.

As a result, barbiturates are only effective as sleeping pills for about two weeks.

Initially, sleep aids can help put a person to sleep, but she often enters the next day drowsy and below her maximum capacity. In fact, experiments have found that people who take sleep aids report that they enter the next day feeling washed out and are less productive than if they had simply slept poorly without taking any medication.

Benzodiazepines (e.g., Valium) can also affect the sleep cycle, in particular the REM portion of the cycle. Also, such drugs can be mildly addictive and produce the side effects of fatigue, drowsiness, and sedation. Once, when a friend of mine was under tremendous job stress, she had a severe case of insomnia. She tried the warm-milk routine, she went for long walks, she read dull books—nothing helped. Finally, after about two weeks of what felt like almost no sleep, she went to her doctor, who prescribed a low dose of Valium. On my friend's return visit, after a week of the Valium treatment, the doctor asked, "Are you sleeping better?" My friend answered, "No, I just feel pleasantly snowed all the time and I don't care if I am tired anymore."

My friend, of course, was referring to the tranquilizing effect of the Valium. It did not solve her sleep problem at all, but it did ease her anxiety about not getting sleep and her problem at work. Her fatigue was resolved only when the job pressure let up and she could sleep again.

The key to solving sleep problems is to get at the basic cause. Most of the time drugs will not solve an underlying problem. If a stressful situation, a disease, or a psychological problem is disturbing sleep, drugs may only mask the real problem. Using drugs in these situations is a classic case of treating the symptoms and not the underlying condition.

Another problem associated with sleeping pills is rebound insomnia. When patients are removed from drugs used to induce sleep, they may experience insomnia as a result of elimination of the drug. If patients withdraw from large regular doses of barbiturates or other depressant drugs, they may experience severe sleep-pattern disturbances with extreme daytime symptoms of nervousness, restlessness, or general body aches.

Mr. B.'s case was typical of withdrawal from barbiturates—and it only took the man two weeks to get "hooked." You should be very careful about your use of such drugs. If you are presently using them, get a doctor's help in tapering them off. Withdraw from drugs of this type very gradually and under the supervision of your doctor.

If you are on drug therapy, for insomnia or for a psychological problem, be cautious. Work closely with your doctor to monitor your response to the medication, including subtle side effects. Watch your sleep pattern carefully and record it in a sleep log. If you have a bed partner, ask that person to make observations too. Take the log to your doctor so that together you can examine any sleep difficulty that you may be having. Include in the log what medicine you took, when you took it, and in what dosage.

By all means, be faithful to your regimen, take your medicine regularly according to the schedule given to you by your doctor. When the doctor prescribes a change in dosage, make sure you understand the directions, ask for clarification, and then follow them precisely.

If your drugs are being prescribed to help you sleep, search for an alternative to drug therapy. Researchers have found that a regular regimen of exercise can be more effective than drugs in treating sleep disorders. Many of the women I talked to said that regular exercise helped them sleep better. One respondent put it very nicely:

"I refocused on an exercise program that allowed me to get sleep at night. When I have done some aerobic exercise, I sleep the minute I hit the pillow and I sleep soundly."

If drugs are being prescribed to correct your sleep problem, discuss the possibility of substituting a program of exercise and diet as an alternative.

Alcohol, of course, is just another drug as far as the body is concerned. Many people use a drink—the familiar nightcap—to help them get to sleep, thinking that the tranquilizing effect will ward off bad thoughts, calm their nerves, and send them off into a pleasant slumber. The depressant effects of alcohol actually do more to disturb sleep than to help it. Alcohol can have profound negative effects. Heavy consumption severely disrupts the stages of sleep, resulting in shortened REM-sleep periods and extensive awakening during the night. In addition, alcohol can upset the digestive tract, which may lead to sleep disruptions. The washed-out feeling that people experience the day after alcohol consumption is an indication that alcohol saps energy, disturbs sleep, and decreases effectiveness.

As with other drugs, people going through alcohol withdrawal also have sleep disturbances. They typically have difficulty getting to sleep and have other disruptions in the rest cycle. Even mild withdrawal (for example, after heavy weekend drinking or holiday partying) can cause such symptoms.

So, be careful with alcohol! It can create fatigue by disrupting sleep and by causing a subtle (or not so subtle) "hangover" effect the next day. If you want to be in top shape for an important day, you had best avoid alcohol altogether the night before. Beware of using alcohol to get to sleep; it may just keep you awake.

Eating and Insomnia

Margaret, a thirty-year-old woman, started having severe and chronic sleep disruptions. She would wake up in the middle of the night with stomach pain and indigestion. Antacid pills gave her relief in a relatively short period of time, but the interruption in her nighttime rest was causing her to be lethargic and tired on her job. She went to work feeling cranky and looking haggard; even her manager began to comment on her demeanor.

Margaret was an engineer, but it took the analytical capability of her doctor to solve the problem. The doctor's analysis turned up the fact that for years Margaret had been accustomed to a late-night snack before bedtime, a habit she developed as a young teenager. Margaret's snack consisted of peanut butter on toast with a glass of milk. Margaret's doctor prescribed no drug, simply the elimination of any food after dinner (especially peanut butter or milk—both upsetting to the stomach!). Margaret is sleeping just fine now.

Not all people eat peanut butter and drink milk at bedtime, but many do experience nighttime digestive problems. These can be in the form of just feeling too full, indigestion, reflux of acid from the stomach into the esophagus (wet burps), excessive gas, or severe heartburn. If you are having digestive problems that are affecting your sleep, examine your eating habits. As in the case of Margaret, you may be eating the wrong kinds of food too close to bedtime, or your diet simply may not agree with your digestive system. As we saw in Chapter 5, protein stimulates brain activity, while carbohydrates help put it to sleep.

Too much fat in the diet is likely to give you digestive problems. I have become aware of this since my husband and I changed to an extremely low-fat diet two years ago. Now, when I do eat something with fat in it at supper, I get indigestion and stomachaches a few hours later, which typically wake me up.

Also, watch for subtle effects of food. There has been a lot of discussion recently about the number of foods that contain caffeine, and I am happy to see that soft-drink companies are starting to market caffeine-free versions of their popular products. Hot chocolate may sound like a tastier way to get the soporific effects of hot milk before bedtime, but remember that chocolate contains caffeine. It also contains calories that are converted more quickly to fat at night than in the morning.

Go back and review the principles in Chapter 5, "Eat for Energy." Those principles will also help you get better sleep. If your digestive problems persist, check with your doctor. Your indigestion may be an indication of a physiological problem. In any case, be careful about what you eat and when you eat it if you want to sleep.

Illness and Insomnia

Various types of illness can disturb sleep. Pain, ranging from the aching of tired muscles to the severe pain of injury or disease, is a major cause of restless sleep. When the body is in pain, it must expend energy to fight back, but the resources available to fight the pain are diminished by the fact that the pain is disturbing sleep—a vicious cycle. The body is fighting pain from an energy pool that has not been restocked with the proper amount and quality of rest.

Special means must be used to deal with severe pain. Doctors have a wide variety of medicines to use today. However, painkillers—especially strong ones—have numerous side effects. Thankfully, progress is being made in research on pain and new therapies are becoming available. Centers have been established around the country for the sole purpose of dealing with pain. These pain centers are devoted to helping patients learn about their pain and how to cope with it, and have available a wide variety of subspecialty doctors who are adept at various treatments. If you have chronic pain that is not well-controlled, consider visiting a pain clinic to learn about your pain and to try some of the newer treatments.

For less severe pain, sometimes you can do simple things to reduce your discomfort. Aspirin or other over-the-counter pain relievers can help alleviate aching muscles or a headache. Exercise or a firmer bed could add more support to an aching back. Exercise, combined with a good diet, can really go a long way in helping you sleep better in the face of chronic pain. If you do not know the real source of your pain, consult your doctor.

There are a variety of other syndromes that are known particularly to disturb sleep. Some of these involve involuntary twitching of muscles, such as "periodic movements of sleep" and another associated condition called "restless-leg syndrome." People with restless-leg syndrome experience uncontrollable urges to move the legs. They feel an extremely unpleasant sensation on the inside of their calves. This can be extremely disturbing to the sleeper or the sleeper's bed partner.

Other sleep problems can be equally disturbing. Sleepwalkers may talk, sit up in bed, dress themselves, and walk around. The medical literature suggests that treatment consists of just waiting for the afflicted to outgrow the syndrome, since most sleepwalkers are children. I have known of cases of both child and adult sleepwalkers, and strangely enough, they seemed to sleep quite well.

Betty, a woman in her thirties, was often found by her family performing strange activities, such as crawling to the bathroom on all fours, standing on tiptoe to peer out of the window into the dark, or picking up imaginary items from the floor. If awakened, Betty would try to offer a seemingly logical explanation of why she was involved in the strange activity, such as, "I am just picking up these leaves" (from the floor!), or "I am just going to the bathroom" (on all fours!).

Luckily, Betty never crawled out windows or went outside in the cold, as some sleepwalkers have been known to do. Although her story may seem humorous, sleepwalking in adults can be an indication of a serious underlying psychological illness. If you are plagued by sleepwalking, persistent nightmares, or other such incidents, you should seek help to define the source of the problem.

TOO MUCH SLEEP—HYPERSOMNIA

Another major class of sleeping disorders is hypersomnia, or an extreme desire to sleep. Hypersomniacs may sleep well at night, yet still be very fatigued and sleepy during the day. Hypersomnia can be but one of the symptoms of a variety of physical diseases, such as liver failure, low thyroid activity (hypothyroidism), diabetes, chronic lung disease, and diseases associated with the brain, including multiple sclerosis and viral encephalitis.

Other diseases, such as the narcolepsy-cataplexy syndrome, have hypersomnia as their primary symptom. Narcolepsy is characterized by an uncontrollable daytime urge to sleep. An afflicted person may suddenly fall asleep while working, driving, or engaging in another activity. The period of sleep may last up to twenty or thirty minutes.

The cause of the disease is not known precisely, but is suspected as being a disorder of REM sleep. Ironically, narcolepsy patients have trouble with nighttime sleep. Persons who are unfamiliar with the disease may think that the narcoleptic is overly tired or suffering from severe fatigue.

I remember seeing the husband of an acquaintance fall soundly asleep in the middle of a small formal dinner party.

The wife went on talking as if nothing were the matter. Other people at the table began to show their discomfort in subtle ways, but no one mentioned the husband's dozing. He eventually woke up and joined in the conversation as if nothing had ever happened. Most people at the party assumed that the man was either just tired or impolite; but Tom was a narcoleptic. Narcolepsy is a difficult disease and may not be as rare as once thought. I have seen estimates that up to 100,000 people in the United States are afflicted.

Whether hypersomnia is the result of a disease like narcolepsy or a symptom of another illness, it can be an extremely debilitating condition and should be treated by a doctor. Hypersomnia is usually corrected by treatment of the underlying disease. In the case of narcolepsy, drugs (such as Ritalin and Benzedrine) are available to help keep the person from dozing off. If you are experiencing excessive sleepiness, you should have a thorough examination by your doctor so that the cause of your difficulty may be determined.

DISRUPTIONS OF THE SLEEP-WAKE CYCLE

Disorders of the natural daily rhythm of life, the sleep-wake cycle, compose another major type of sleep dysfunction. These problems are associated with the inability to sleep at the time that our bodies are naturally accustomed to resting—at night—and they normally take the form of external factors, such as shift work or travel through time zones.

We are rapidly becoming a round-the-clock society. Supermarkets are staying open all night, television stations broadcast to the late-night audience, the transportation industry runs all night, factories with expensive machinery run twenty-four hours, and, of course, hospitals tend to the ill twenty-four hours a day. About 25 percent of men and 16 percent of women who have jobs are on shift work, and it appears that the demand for "off-shift" jobs is increasing.

Shift work has a major effect on people's sleep and on their health. Working at odd hours stresses the body and the mind, and strains personal relationships. I am pleased to see that the public is beginning to show interest in this problem. One of the popular health magazines recently ran an article that acknowledged the severe impact that shift work can have on people's lives.

> Such time shuffling has its price. Breakfast at midnight won't fool your body; its inner clocks are not so easily reset. Fatigue plagues shift workers. So do digestive ailments, accidents, family problems and increased alcohol and drug use. And it is not just a personal problem. Many shift workers—doctors, nurses, pilots, air-traffic controllers, nuclear-plant and military personnel—are responsible for public health and safety.[7]

Work schedules have a big impact on sleep. Experiments have shown that people who work shift work have significantly more sleep problems and, as a result, sleep less than people with daytime working hours. The data have shown that persons working during the day sleep between seven and nine hours each night, whereas persons working during the night sleep only four to six hours each day.[8] *That means, on the average, a shift worker gets three hours less sleep than a person who works a normal daytime schedule.*

Up to 90 percent of shift workers report sleep disturbances, and it should come as no surprise that a major effect is fatigue. That fatigue takes its toll in work performance too. For example, night work has been shown to slow the response of telephone operators, cause meter readers to make more mistakes, make train engineers less alert to signals, and increase the single-vehicle accident rate of truck drivers.[9]

Nurses and doctors, performing critical patient care, work long hours and rotating shifts. I am well familiar with the bone-weary fatigue that comes after twenty-four hours of work in the hospital. The mind becomes foggy, every muscle in the body seems to ache, words are spoken sparingly so as to preserve energy—and through it all, one must make accurate, timely decisions that may spell life or death for an emergency-room patient. Studies have shown that doctors' judgment goes down rapidly after twelve to eighteen hours of continuous work. Thankfully, teaching hospitals have taken these studies into account when revising training programs for young doctors.

Somehow, many people to whom I talk have the image of a shift worker as a male factory worker who carries a lunch pail and tries to sleep while the wife yells at the kids to be quiet. This image is no longer accurate. While it is true that a larger proportion of men work on nonregular shifts, women seem to be catching up rapidly as the round-the-clock service industry grows. There is a growing demand for people to work at odd hours in jobs that have been traditionally held by women, such as waitresses and checkout clerks.

The most important impact of these unusual work schedules is that they disturb a person's normal sleep pattern. You would think that people who are on a steady nighttime shift would eventually get used to the schedule and readjust their sleep patterns. Well, they do sleep a little better than people on irregular shifts, but their pattern never seems to adjust to give them as much sleep as a person on a regular daylight schedule.

When I was working as the medical reporter for *The CBS Morning News*, I again experienced the disturbance of a demanding schedule. Although my on-air appearances were usually not until around 8 A.M., I got out of bed at 4 A.M. to make sure that I arrived at the studio early enough to go through the intricate preparation required of a network newscast. In addition, I had to look my best, so my morning routine always included hair setting, makeup, and clothes selection.

Of course, one should look alert to appear on television, so I also had to make sure that I was wide awake by the time the cameras rolled. My husband was working on a regular 8:30 A.M. starting schedule. Luckily, our schedules were similar enough that we could compensate with minor adjustments. We had a good warm breakfast together, after which I rushed off to the studio.

In spite of our efforts, I never really adjusted to the schedule; I was always tired. My sleep schedule was constantly changing, depending on how late I was editing a piece and whether or not I was on the air the next day. In retrospect

I should have tried to maintain the same earlier-morning schedule, but I reverted back to my old wakeup time at every chance. So I felt as if I was suffering perpetual jet lag. I spent every opportunity napping, and my nighttime sleep was almost always restless.

People naturally want to sleep during the night and work during the day. Our built-in daily rhythms provide us with optimum conditions, including the highest body temperature, cortisol levels, and energy levels, during the day. Hundreds of other factors cycle in a twenty-four-hour period, all converging to make us daytime creatures. To do otherwise is to really go against our natural bent.

We are just beginning to learn the intricacies of some of the hundreds of our daily (and seasonal) rhythms. It will take researchers many years to unlock all the secrets. However, the information that has already been gathered about daily rhythms can be put to immediate good use. For instance, a short afternoon nap can be a good restorer of energy. Scientists have found that an afternoon nap is more effective in making up lost sleep than a morning nap. If you have stayed up later than usual, or something has disturbed your normal sleep schedule (such as an infant), try getting up at approximately the normal time in the morning, then take a nap in the afternoon. You will probably have to experiment to find out the best time for your nap. The notes that you took about your natural rhythms in Chapter 2 can help you decide the best time.

When I was working at CBS, I was fortunate enough to have a couch in my office. After getting up so early in the morning and working intensely in the early-morning hours, I would go to the sofa and take a restful nap in the early afternoon. Afterward, I was ready to face the grueling task of getting ready for the next TV story. I know that everyone is not lucky enough to have a convenient sofa, but if you are creative, you can find a quiet place and some stolen time to put up your feet and close your eyes for a short nap.

Unfortunately, there seems to be no good overall solution to the sleep problems of shift workers, although recent research has revealed some important knowledge that can help substantially. For instance, workers who change shifts every three weeks rather than every week have been found to suffer less fatigue and to be more productive.[10] This is because it takes the body approximately three weeks to resynchronize all of its cycles. If shift changes occur more frequently than once every three weeks, the body's rhythms are constantly out of kilter.

Some people nap a lot and catch up by sleeping more on weekends. Be careful of sleeping too long on weekends; it can actually disturb your sleep pattern more than staying on roughly the same schedule as you are on during the week.

Besides shift work, other kinds of disturbances can severely disrupt the sleep cycle. Jet lag is being experienced by more and more women as they enter the world of international work. Jet lag is caused by traveling long distances, either east or west, in a short period of time.

The resulting discrepancy between the traveler's internal clock and the time in which she finds herself after her trip can have a profound effect on her ability to get enough rest. Her sense of time becomes disturbed, and her body does not know when to tell her to eat, sleep, or be active. She may try to sleep in concert with the time in the new place; but her circadian clock tells her to be awake. She feels fatigued and disoriented, and may have a slight headache. Her senses seem to be slow and she has little appetite.

In recent years, experts have learned a lot about how to cope with jet lag. Dr. Charles F. Ehret, one of the foremost experts on the subject, has gained worldwide recognition for developing a program to minimize the negative effects of crossing time zones. The program consists of changing a person's meal and sleep schedules before a trip in anticipation of the changing clock. (Dr. Ehret has also developed a similar program that involves a special weekend sleep and diet schedule that has been effective in helping shift workers adjust to new schedules.)

The jet-lag program is described by Dr. Ehret and Lynne Waller Scanlon in their book *Overcoming Jet Lag* (New York: Berkley Books, 1983). It helps you plan your trip, adjust your diet and sleep schedule before the trip, and adjust your schedule once you arrive.

Jet lag is an example of a sleep problem that is relatively easy to define; a person certainly knows if she or he has traveled across several time zones in a short period of time. Working a night shift or a rotating shift is another obvious case of disturbed sleep. However, other sleep problems, perhaps related to a subtle physical or psychological condition, can be far more difficult to identify.

Although there are many sleep problems that are difficult to diagnose and cure, many can be helped if you start to understand your habits and take some relatively simple actions. By understanding your sleep patterns, you will be in a better position to either solve the problem yourself or get professional help. Without the benefit of sleep, you cannot conquer your fatigue. Remember Mary, who has Mediterranean anemia, from Chapter 3? She summed it up very nicely:

> "Finally, sleep is the best way to eliminate fatigue. This is a luxury to me, but I make sure I keep a finger on my pulse and when the tiredness begins to creep in, I do not put anything on my calendar after the workday is over and make sure I get to bed early, or arrange to sleep late the next day, with breakfast in bed. Use of earplugs keeps out the noise. An understanding and compassionate lover or husband completes the picture."

WHAT TO DO

1. Become more sensitive to your sleep habits.

Keep a sleep log for a week (if you are on a rotating shift, keep the sleep log for at least one complete cycle of shift rotation). Record what time you went to bed, when you went to sleep, when you woke up, how you slept, what you dreamed, whether you woke up rested, and what drugs (including alcohol) you took. Also consider keeping track of when and what you ate before you went to bed. Ask your bed partner to pay attention to your sleep and add to your observations.

2. Watch your medicines.

I asked you to analyze the medicines that you take in Chapter 8. Take a minute to review those questions in relationship to your sleep habits. Record on your sleep log the medication that you took (whether or not it was to help you sleep), the time you took it, and the dosage. If you are taking drugs to help you sleep, consider whether the drugs are helping or exacerbating your condition (it may be hard to distinguish the difference). *Remember: Some sleeping aids can cause the very sleep problems they are meant to cure.* Do not taper off the dosage of such a drug without consulting your doctor. Rapid withdrawal may cause a variety of side effects, from withdrawal insomnia to convulsions.

3. Examine your diet and exercise habits.

Be careful about eating or exercising too close to bedtime. Both activities will stimulate you and make it difficult to drift off to sleep. Allow at least two hours to elapse between eating or exercising and bedtime. Watch out for caffeinated beverages after supper. You might try a high-carbohydrate meal at supper, to help induce relaxation and sleepiness. Review chapters 5 and 6 in the light of your sleep problems. By following the principles outlined in those chapters, you can alleviate fatigue and improve your rest.

4. Set a regular schedule for sleeping that takes your natural daily rhythms into account.

Set regular times for going to bed and getting up. Try to stick to your schedule even on weekends and holidays so you do not create a kind of jet lag from changing sleep times. Enlist your family or housemate(s) to help with your sleep. Ask them to be quiet during sleep time. Assert yourself to eliminate sleep disturbances. Wake a snoring partner up and turn him over. Set rules so that a loud TV or stereo is forbidden during sleep time.

5. Take naps for revival.

A thirty- to sixty-minute nap, at the right time, can really give you a boost. Afternoon seems to be the most effective time to revive most people's energy, but test that theory for yourself. Find out the time that is best for you. Set aside a small portion of the day to have a short nap. Do not feel guilty for wanting to catch up on sleep by napping.

6. Avoid shift work if you can.

If shift work is absolutely necessary, try to get a regular schedule that leaves you on the same shift. Adjust the rest of your schedule to compensate as much as possible. Try to stick to the same schedule on weekends. If you must rotate shifts, try to get your employer to let you rotate every three weeks; that schedule has been shown to be less tiring than rotating every week.

7. Consult your doctor or go to a sleep clinic.

If you are having persistent sleep problems and have been unable to solve them with any of the techniques you have tried, consult your doctor. Take your sleep log and discuss what you know about your sleep patterns. Consider going to a sleep clinic to have them study your problem through systematic measurements of bodily functions. Some sleep clinics are looking for volunteers to participate in their studies at no cost to the patient.

Part Three

EASE YOUR STRAINS

MONEY AND FATIGUE

Why is it that no amount of sleep seems to help?
Why is it just never enough?
Stops having to gain back is all that they ever do
Why can't they straighten up the mess that's

10
RESOLVE YOUR
CONFLICTS

When I was a child, I adored the score to the musical *My Fair Lady*. I had very little idea what the story was really about, but that didn't matter. It seemed to have such a magical effect upon my mother as she whirled around the living room, brandishing her duster and singing the tunes. The play had to be special if my mother liked it, so I believed in *My Fair Lady*.

Twenty-some-odd years passed, and I found myself living in New York City when *My Fair Lady* was revived on Broadway. I was so excited. I could not believe a childhood fantasy was coming true—to see *My Fair Lady* on Broadway, starring Rex Harrison! As Professor Higgins, he sings:

> Women are irrational, that's all there is to that,
> Their heads are full of cotton, hay, and rags,
> They're nothing but exasperating, irritating,
> fascinating, calculating, agitating, maddening, and
> infuriating hags
>
> Why can't a woman be more like a man?
> Men are so decent, such regular chaps,
> Ready to help you through any mishaps
> Ready to buck you up whenever you are glum,
> Why can't a woman be a chum?

Why is thinking something women never do,
Why is logic never even tried?
Straightening up their hair is all that they ever do
Why don't they straighten up the mess that's
inside?[1]

I have to admit I found some of the words of the tunes
hurtful. Unfortunately, the ideas Professor Higgins had about
women are still shared by many men today. Women are
objects that need to be fixed. I did not find the play romantic.
But do not get me wrong; I enjoyed seeing *My Fair Lady,* but
I left feeling irritated by the plot—man saves woman.

Unfortunately, it represents another version on the same
old theme—that women find ultimate fulfillment through the
love of a man, a knight in shining armor on a white horse who
will come and rescue each of us from the gutters of life. The
true route to happiness, we were told, was to catch a good
man, marry him, bear his children, and then live happily ever
after in wedded bliss.

Most women did exactly that; they found a man, married
him, bore his children—but they did not live happily ever
after. My mother was one of them. She was unhappy in her
marriage. Maybe that is why she sang the tunes of *My Fair
Lady* and *Camelot* as she was dusting; she was hoping that
Professor Higgins or, more likely, Lancelot would come to
rescue her.

Alas, as a girl growing up I learned that Professor Higgins and Lancelot never come. I outright rejected the role I
saw my mother in and promised myself that never, never
would the same happen to me.

What exactly is this role with which my mother struggled, I have had to struggle, and millions of other women
struggle? It is a deeply held notion of what we believe to be
feminine and good. The role is not something with which we
were born, that we intrinsically knew; it is something we
learned from our parents and the world around us when we
were very young and impressionable. The role became the
bedrock of our identity, and so it is all the more tenacious and
difficult to shake.

But the world has changed since you and I learned what it was to be "feminine"; how to behave, what to hope for, where to look for satisfaction. And with those changes new roles have evolved for women. Women's views of themselves and their places in the (men's) world has and is still changing. I think the changes represent real progress, but I am also very much aware of some of the prices women have paid. Many women are struggling with a deep identity crisis; the new roles are clashing with the old. And even though the new concepts may be healthier for our self-esteem, the old ones die very, very hard. This internal struggle of old against new is leaving many women exausted.

In this chapter, we will explore the old role. It is a role that creates a tremendous imbalance in the life of a woman—too much nurturing of others and not enough nurturing of the self. Consequently the traditional role is full of energy drainers but short on energy boosters. We will also explore some of the conflicts that have arisen in these changing times.

THE FEMALE EGO

Not so many years ago, psychiatrists, psychologists, and other behavioral experts believed that most of the traits we typically equate with femininity and masculinity were innate; that is, the traits were determined by biological sex and were present at birth. Because of these supposed innate traits and the pressures of society, stereotypic roles developed for each of the sexes.

Unfortunately, being born female was not as highly valued as being born male. Instantaneously, at the moment of birth, females were devalued because of their sex. Stop and ponder that a moment. The first question that most parents ask at the moment of birth is, "Is it a boy or is it a girl?" And from that time forward, everybody makes a lot of assumptions about the child based on the answer, especially about your child's capabilities.

Boys are taught at a very early age to develop their sense of self through their own achievements. They are rewarded for independence and assertiveness. They know that their success as men in the adult world will depend on their personal accomplishments, gained through work and mastery. They are encouraged to develop a strong ego.

Girls, on the other hand, traditionally have been negatively reinforced for this kind of behavior. Girls were given the message that the success of women in the adult world can only be had indirectly through relationships established with men. Girls very quickly learned that their self-worth depended on pleasing others, not on what they personally accomplished. The female ego was left vulnerable and undeveloped.

What is the ego? When we hear the word, we tend to think of the male ego, which represents pride, confidence, and self-seeking behavior. Or we may equate it with a big ego—something that is negative. Now when we hear the word, we should think of our own. How is it faring? Egos are something women have dealt with a lot, supported and fostered in others, but have little of themselves. Women need to develop stronger egos—a weak one spells chronic fatigue.

The ego is that part of the human psyche that allows us to interact with the environment and to meet all of our needs. It is our mental equipment that takes care of us. The healthy ego keeps tabs on our needs in life: food, safety, work, relaxation, laughter, intellectual stimulation, rest, love, sex, excitement. It is constantly setting priorities and making decisions about which need to satisfy at what time, deciding how to get the need met, and solving problems while doing so. The ego balances our life; it allows us to say "no" when demands become too great and seeks to rejuvenate itself without guilt. Many women's egos do not work well in balancing life and setting personal priorities. As one expert on the female ego said:

> If you are chronically sluggish, you may need to give your ego some challenges to sharpen decision-making skills. If your ego is not working well in this area, you need to ask a basic question: Am I overloaded with responsibility (burned out) or underloaded (unchallenged)? Many women who function poorly are either burned out yet pushing

themselves to do more, or underchallenged yet seeking rest from the exhaustion of boredom.[2]

A healthy ego would not allow these situations—which lead to chronic fatigue—to happen.

Unfortunately, most women are operating with a less-than-healthy ego. In other words, their internal psychological system is not doing a good job of meeting the needs of their person. They are not in touch with their needs nor do they have the skills to get them satisfied. Some women are so out of touch that they do not take care of themselves at the most basic level; they do not even rest.

Therapist Susan Price, author of *The Female Ego,* succinctly identified the crux of the issue. She wrote:

> My work and personal experience have led me to believe that the main thought pattern that gets women's ego in trouble is the desire to please other people. . . . Because a woman is often more concerned with pleasing others than with pleasing herself, she can find herself in a trap in which she hardly uses her ego to meet her needs. . . . Love or approval from others is more important than self-esteem to a people-pleaser. Approval from others is her self-esteem. Being a people-pleaser means that a woman lacks an ego that functions on behalf of the self. She surrenders her potential for happiness to others and is motivated not by her needs but by her fear of losing love.[3]

It is a very difficult, if not impossible, task to please everyone, and yet so many women still try. In some ways the situation has grown worse with the ideal of womanhood having been expanded to "Supermom." Women are attempting to do far too much for others and not enough for themselves. Consequently women are forever exhausted. One of the best ways to boost your energy level is by boosting your female ego.

DISCRIMINATION AND LOW SELF-ESTEEM

Women have developed a sense of themselves within a culture that, historically, has not only not supported their personal development but has perpetuated forces that severely impeded women's development. Discrimination is a reality, by now an old story. However, it is something with which women must continue to struggle—and where there is struggle, there is a great energy drain. Too few women realize that their chronic fatigue, in part, is a direct result of discrimination.

Our patriarchal culture conditions women to spend their efforts on supporting others and to gain their sense of self through relationships. Tragically, there are grave psychological consequences when women's identities are developed exclusively through attachments with others:

> Since men hold the power and authority, women are rewarded for developing a set of psychological characteristics that accommodate to and please men. Such traits—submissiveness, compliance, passivity, helplessness, weakness—have been encouraged in women and incorporated into some prevalent psychological theories in which they are defined as innate or inevitable characteristics of women. However, they are more accurately conceptualized as learned behaviors by which all subordinate group members attempt to ensure their survival.[4]

Not just women, but other subordinate groups, such as blacks, have been encouraged to take on certain psychological traits—passivity, submissiveness, dependency. I am reminded of a few lines written by Alice Walker, the winner of the Pulitzer Prize for fiction for her book *The Color Purple*, which touched me so deeply. She tells of traveling back to her childhood home, only to find it rotted and filled with hay. Nearby, however, Walker finds that the homestead of the white Southern writer Flannery O'Connor is in good repair and is being looked after by a caretaker. She wrote of her reaction:

> My bitterness comes from a deeper source than my knowledge of the difference, historically, race has made in the lives of white and black artists. The fact that in Mississippi no one even remembers where Richard Wright lived, while Faulkner's house is maintained by a black caretaker, is painful but not unbearable. What comes close to being unbearable is that I know how damaging to my own psyche such injustice is. In an unjust society the soul of the sensitive person is in danger of deformity from just such weights as this. For a long time I will feel Faulkner's house, O'Connor's house, crushing me. To fight back will require a certain amount of energy, energy better used doing something else.[5]

She was talking about her blackness and the injustice; she could have also been talking about her femaleness and the injustice. Women are consuming energy, fighting all the injustices they endure—a lifetime of them. Of course, some women endure more than others. Some women recognize the injustices, while others do not. But it drains them all just the same, because they have to use defenses to protect their sense of self-esteem. Low self-esteem is very common among women, even successful women that you would never dream had a problem with their self-image.

Nannette is an example of this. She is a forty-five-year-old married woman who runs a very prestigious art gallery in a major Eastern city. She started the gallery several years ago with almost no money. It has since grown into one of the most popular places in the city for cultural and political events to take place. Nannette associates with some of the most powerful people in the city, and is known for her beauty, taste, and social skills. But she does not feel self-confident on the inside.

> "I know what people think of me. My girlfriends sometimes tell me how much they envy

me. You see, supposedly, I have it all. I have a good marriage, lovely children, my own gallery, prestigious friends—but you ask about my self-esteem? I guess I don't have much of that. You know why I started that gallery? I didn't believe anyone would give me a job, and I am afraid if the gallery were to fold today, no one would hire me. I just feel that I am a nobody and I don't have much to offer."

One's image of oneself is developed during childhood. Messages come from our parents and others in the world around us about what kind of person we are. Many women have internalized negative images of themselves from the culture at large, which devalues women as a group. They may have seen their own mothers devalued in the position of a homemaker, a brother may have received favored treatment, or a father may have rejected them because he had hoped for a boy or they did not fit his image of a "good girl." These messages are powerful at such a young age and can leave a lasting scar. The negative images women have of themselves may no longer apply to them, yet because the image is so entrenched, it lingers. These negative images are extremely potent energy drainers and are destructive to women's mental health.

Experts in numerous disciplines are now reporting that the limited traditional role prescribed for women clearly has had dire consequences on women's mental health. It is true that women have more psychological problems and mental illnesses than men, but this is not because of some inborn fact of femaleness. It is the result of living under inequality. That is the conclusion reached by the Subpanel on the Mental Health of Women of the President's Commission on Mental Health:

The subpanel documented the ways in which inequality creates dilemmas and conflicts for women in the contexts of marriage, family relationships, reproduction, child rearing, divorce, aging, education and work. These same conditions of subordination also set the stage for extraordinary events that may heighten vulnerability to mental illness; the frequency with which incest, rape, and marital violence occur suggest that such events might well be considered normative developmental crises for women.[6]

It might surprise you that the highest rates of distress are found in married women. Marriage seems to exert a protective effect on men; married men who work have the best mental health. Conversely, marriage often has a deleterious effect on women; married women who do not work have the worst mental health. What is going on here? The difference seems to lie either in gender or work status. Studies have shown that employment has a positive effect on mental health by "improving economic status, increasing self-esteem and social contacts, and alleviating boredom."[7] The right kind of employment also alleviates the chronic fatigue that comes from boredom.

Women were taught, however, that employment was not a necessity for them. The family role of nurturer was supposed to satisfy all of their urges, desires, needs, and wishes. Complete happiness was to be had by giving to others. It turns out that this limited single role of homemaking is one of "frustration and low status and is incompatible with the needs, aspirations, and capacities of many women."[8] It is also exhausting.

I think that many of the binds in which women find themselves—struggling to feel good about themselves and develop their own identities while living in a society that continues to devalue them—are responsible for most women's psychological conflict and low self-esteem. These issues can be very painful and, in many women, they are driven beneath the surface; the real feelings are suppressed but they do not go away. Unaware, women struggle with them anyway, and that takes energy. It is the exhaustion from constantly dealing with the struggle, accompanied by a vague sense of unhappiness that bubbles up to the surface. Fatigue may be the only indication that discrimination and the old role are taking their tolls.

THE NURTURING ROLE

People pleasing—caring for others—is the essence of the nurturing role. Women are the keepers of relationships. This tendency to care for others, the nurturing imperative, is both women's strength and their weakness. One of the women told me that she was made vividly aware of her nurturing tendencies when she took a personality test. She said she did not initially believe in its predictability, and only took the test on a whim.

> "You know, it described me so well, it was eerie. It's really amazing, it really was. In the description it said, 'You tend to identify with people that are close to you, with their problems, to the point of losing your own identity . . .'—which I think is very true. I do tend to do that with my kids and my husband, and if they have a problem—oh, boy, I worry about it constantly. And it is so true, and it's not just with my family. Even friends, if they tell me their problems, I can take it on if I don't stop myself. I think in a way it is kinda weird, but it is helpful knowing that about myself, seeing it all written out, because I can try to control it a little bit."

This woman thought that what she was describing to me—her connectedness to others—was just an aspect of her own personality. But research is beginning to show that this nurturing imperative affects the way most women see themselves in relation to the world, which is very different from the way men see themselves. Because of women's concern about others, women tend to be more connected in their relationships. The line between themselves and others is often blurred. Men, on the other hand, tend to stand apart from the world as separate beings. They confront the world as a place to be mastered, conquered, and controlled.

Relationships and caring for others permeate the lives of women. I would think most women see this as women's greatness, something that men need a lot more of in their lives. But we must not lose sight of the fact that organizing life around relationships and trying to establish them and keep them can be detrimental to women. A therapist who works with women explained the consequences:

> As people pleasers, women do things for other people that they could do for themselves. When a woman overdoes on the giving to others, she gets tired and out of touch with herself. Her negative strokes are fatigue, anger, jealousy, and a sense of being cheated. She easily does more than 50 percent of the work in maintaining relationships, is taken for granted, loses her identity and purpose, and can find herself floundering. Then she is blamed for not being more together as a person.[9]

Many women often feel out of control and powerless in relationships with others, because they constantly attend to others' needs and not their own. To take control—and get one's own needs satisfied—is frequently seen by women as being self-centered, and thus they refuse to do so. But women who do not exert control over their lives find that they are totally exhausted, usually both emotionally and physically. The demands never stop. The family takes, takes, takes and often does not give back, or even appreciate the fact that they take so much! The chief nurturer rarely gets nurtured herself. No one else is taught the responsibility of caring for the needs of the prime caretaker. So many women end up overworked, emotionally drained, and unfulfilled.

Ella knows the feeling of endless demands on her time and endless giving. She is a forty-two-year-old married woman who works in the home, outside of the home, and takes care of her two stepchildren.

> "For a period of about two months last spring I was tired all the time. I went to bed late and was always early rising and rushing through the day. It seemed there was never sufficient time to learn all aspects of a new position the first year, the house

never seemed to be picked up, community activities and fund-raisers were always needing help, for just one more night. I felt I had little time for me when my husband always wanted personal attention but never wanted to help out with daily chores. Between his children and other relatives in both families, someone always wanted attention or money for some particular crisis. I'm glad that period of demand has slacked off."

Notice that Ella said that the period of demand had only "slacked off," she did not say the period of demand "is over." Women's caretaking is always in demand, if not by the children, then by our spouses or aging parents. I think it is wonderful that women do care and are connected to others, but I am concerned about the constant giving that leads to chronic fatigue. I asked Ella if during that period she had learned any new ways to cope that would prevent it from happening again.

"I have coped by really looking at the activities and issues in my life that I find stressful and often nonproductive. I'm learning to delegate responsibilities, to avoid situations that I know will be stressful by saying 'no' on the front end. I've learned not to have all the answers, to allow others to think through their ideas and arrive at solutions. I accept the fact that my house may never be dust-free and uncluttered. Most of all I've learned to worry about things in the order of their importance and to deal with them in time-related sequences. Someplace I read (1) 'Don't sweat the small stuff' and (2) 'Everything is small stuff!' It really helps when people are going nuts all around you."

It is so understandable why women become tired, irritable, angry, and even resentful. The traditional role calls for a lot of giving and sacrifice. To make matters worse, many women feel guilty when they experience ambivalent or negative feelings about their roles. They think, "What's wrong with me? Why can't I be happy with the proper role of a woman?" Sometimes it is difficult to get in touch with these kinds of feelings at all. That is because, according to the role model, the ideal woman does not experience any of these feelings.

The ideal woman is supposed to be selfless, eternally giving, and still never complain, which all makes it fairly difficult to get in touch with feelings about the role, such as dissatisfaction, unfulfillment, resentment, and anger. Consequently these feelings get suppressed and the only thing that many women may feel is fatigue. Consider this description of the "ideal woman":

> The "ideal" woman is supportive, self-sacrific-
> ing, always giving. She is the woman you see in the
> TV commercials, happily dispensing lemonade to
> all the kids on the block, getting up in the middle of
> the night to fetch the cold tablets for her husband
> who has the sniffles, rushing to the washing ma-
> chine to scrub the ring out of her husband's shirt
> collar. She is the Joan of Arc of self-sacrifice, immo-
> lating herself with everybody else's needs. She is
> also the woman who is a good candidate for the
> psychiatrist's couch or the Valium bottle, who com-
> plains of low energy levels, feelings of hope-
> lessness, and nameless anxiety and dread. The
> woman who always puts others first, who can't see
> that she deserves some of the "goodies" of life
> herself, may be particularly susceptible to depres-
> sion.[10]

Fatigue is particularly common in women who try to live up to this "ideal" role model, whether they work exclusively in the home or have employment outside the home. Much of the fatigue comes from overwork, both physical and emotional. However, I think the fatigue is also commonly a sign of boredom, frustration, low self-esteem, or inner turmoil.

You see, in society fatigue is allowable, at least to a certain extent. Some women will not even admit that they are chronically tired for fear that people will think they are failing

221

to carry out their responsibilities and fulfill their roles. Nevertheless, fatigue is a more acceptable feeling than, let us say, anger. Anger is particularly hard for some women to feel and express. As one psychiatrist explains, "In general, our culture and our psychological theories have viewed women's anger as inappropriate except when it is used in the service of others, as in a 'lioness defending her cubs.' Thus, most women experience considerable psychic conflict about anger."[11]

Because women's upbringing and subsequent role make it difficult for them to openly express anger, the feeling may get shoved aside or covered up, only to fester beneath the surface. Women often do this with many of the negative emotions that indicate how they really feel in situations. All of these telltale emotions are chronic energy drainers and get translated into fatigue. Fatigue is a more acceptable feeling. So it may be the only thing a woman is feeling, but in essence, it is an indication of all these other emotions bubbling beneath the surface.

Try to get in touch with some of these feelings. Feelings such as anger, frustration, boredom, and dissatisfaction are not "bad" feelings. They are feelings that are warning signals—they tell us something about our lives just as a pain on the right side may warn that an appendix is about to burst. These feelings say that something is not healthy and needs correction. You should listen to these feelings. It is not selfish to do so; it is practicing good health.

Examine the nurturing role you are in, write down what you like and what you do not like about it, and then make a change for the better. You do not need anyone's permission to do this. Women of all ages and from all walks of life are beginning to create their own personal identities. No one lifestyle is right for all women; it is a matter of discovering what is right for you.

If that sounds too selfish, if it makes you squirm to think of doing something for yourself, think of this: If you are not satisfied with your life, you really cannot hide it anyway. Your dissatisfaction with yourself or your life will display itself somewhere, for instance, as chronic fatigue. The fatigue might be simply telling you that you are tired of your life the way it is. And if that is true, the very people you are trying so desperately to give to and take care of will suffer in the long run. If you do things for them simply out of obligation and not because you want to, you will, with time, end up feeling you have no control over your own life and you will resent it.

It is far better to develop yourself and satisfy your needs, then your good feelings about yourself will radiate to others. This is what I call the positive domino effect. On the other hand, if you feel negative about yourself, you may have a negative domino effect going on right now with others in your life. You must take care of yourself before you can really take care of others in a healthy way.

CONFLICT—THE HIDDEN ENERGY DRAINER

Not only is the nurturing role itself tiring, conflict about playing out the traditional role is exhausting. And even though the women's movement—as we know it—is over twenty years old, role conflict is alive and well. I heard a woman say recently, "I'm sick and tired of hearing about role conflict, let's just get on with it." I sympathize with her feeling, but she has failed to realize that women cannot truly get on with "it" unless the conflicts are resolved. Millions of women still have not resolved their personal conflicts. I see women who are constantly at odds with themselves, running helter-skelter, trying to meet the demands of both the "old" and the "new" roles.

So many of women's aspirations, hopes, and ideals have changed, but many women fail to realize that their unconscious mind has not kept up; it is often a generation or two behind. Most people retain unconscious images of women that were created by views formulated in their childhoods. The new images women have painted of themselves often clash directly with the old etches in their minds. The battle might be the seven years' war, but to many women it often feels like the hundred years' war—the hidden conflict leaves them utterly exhausted.

The mental struggle to resolve a conflict consumes a

tremendous amount of energy. You can think of conflict as the conscious or unconscious struggle between two opposing desires or courses of action. You would expect anyone who fought in physical battles all day and night to be exhausted. Well, the same goes for anyone involved in psychological battles. Conflict—role conflict, sexual conflict, family conflict, work conflict—is such a battle. Most women do not realize that they may be experiencing conflict; it can rage beneath the surface without them being aware of it. They may only recognize the exhaustion that goes with it.

These struggles can be brought to the surface. They do not have to remain buried where they may sap your energy forever. In order to stem the energy drain, you will have to understand how the messages of the old role are in conflict with those of the new role. Then you can negotiate a "truce" between the two.

We are all part of a great social transition—and experiment—that is not easy on women. Women have moved into the work force in droves, but they have not resolved the inner desire to be nurturers and homemakers. The independent worker is at odds with the old self-image, molded by her upbringing, of a homemaker and mother. The conscience of her old role speaks in a voice that whispers "guilty" as the working mother kisses baby good-bye, cries "fraud" in the face of success, demands excessively high standards of cleanliness in the home, and screams "selfish" when she takes time for herself. The old conscience speaks with a voice that demands satisfaction of an old ideal.

Most women have not given up the old ideal, even though they think they have. They are trying to be true to the old image of the good, kind, selfless nurturing wife and mother, but at the same time take on the new responsibilities that are a full day's work for a man. Such women have three full-time jobs: their families, their careers, and their unresolved conflict.

Women are having difficulty dividing their time between career and family because, while women's aspirations have changed, the role of women in the family has not. Work, for men, kills two birds with one stone. They can derive personal satisfaction from their work, and fulfill their male role in the family. But work out in the work force does not satisfy the old notion we have of the female's role in the family. So as long as the old standard for both men and women calls for the old nurturing role to be played by women in the family, women will be carrying a tremendous load of responsibility, worry, and work, and be in a state of perpetual exhaustion.

The career-versus-family conflict is really a battle between the new voice and the old voice. Do not underestimate the power of that old voice. It gets you to scrub the kitchen floor at ten o'clock at night and it has you baking cookies and bread, even though you can buy them. Many of the women who appear to have resolved the career-versus-family problem are actually running themselves ragged satisfying both voices.

You must carefully examine your concept of what you believe is the role of the female today—in the family and in the work force. First, start thinking about your mother or your primary role model when you were young. What standards did the model set for you? Interestingly, a woman who had a mother who worked outside the home and had household responsibilities during her childhood does not suffer as much from these types of conflicts. Her model provided her with the notion that women work outside and also take care of families. On the other hand, if your mother was a housewife, chances are you are set up for a conflict.

Next, figure out what the old voice is saying to you; get in touch with it and listen to it for a while. If you want, have some fun, give it wings for a few days and try to act out the old role in its entirety. If it calls for you to be feminine, passive, dependent, and to bake cookies and bread for the family, do it and have fun. Then find out what the new voice is saying. What do you want to do to further develop yourself? Fantasize about new careers, promotions, recognition, money, and power. Where would you like to go in life and what would it take to get there?

The next step is to achieve a new identity, to resolve the struggle between the two consciences. This will take time. Talk about your conflicts with your mother, sisters, aunts, friends, and especially your spouse. Figure out what each role is asking of you. Determine where the two clash and where they overlap. Discover what you cherish and would like to keep from each role and what parts you would like to discard. Decide what is truly special and good about each role, point out what is counterproductive and energy-draining, and then change to integrate the two.

For some women, it is relatively easy; for others, it is extremely difficult. But no one can "have it all" in the sense of totally fulfilling the demands of the old role and the new role. Yet I firmly believe women can—and should—"have it all" in the sense of having a warm personal life and a rewarding job, if they work out their priorities. To do so, however, requires resolving the conflict: not just running around like a chicken—an exhausted one—with its head cut off, trying to live out the two roles.

THE HEALTHY RESOLUTION: BALANCING MASTERY AND PLEASURE

I have heard many young college women, new at struggling with role conflict, say that they plan on solving the dilemma by giving 100 percent of themselves to either a career or a family. In frustration, they feel they have to choose one or the other. However, this is not the answer, because an unbalanced life—which is what they are describing—is an unhealthy one. We have seen how the old role, which directed women to concentrate on the feeling side of life—relationships—has many unhealthy consequences. Chronic fatigue is only one of them.

An unbalanced life—consisting of all family *or* all work—or a life of conflict between the two is full of energy drainers and is missing some energy boosters. All of us need a balance of love and work to be energetic, productive, happy, and healthy. This concept has been lent great support by an excellent study recently completed by social scientists Grace Baruch and Rosalind Barnett.

They set out to discover what contributed to a sense of well-being in women. After studying over three hundred women—housewives, career women, divorced women, some with children, some without—they discovered that what makes a woman feel valued and in control is not necessarily the same thing as that which gives her enjoyment. So the belief that the traditional role fulfills all of women's needs was not borne out.

In their superb book *Lifeprints,* written in collaboration with writer Caryl Rivers, they report:

> Our study documents the fundamental importance of both love and work—what Sigmund Freud saw as the twin pillars of a healthy life—to a woman's mental and emotional well-being. When either is ignored, a person's development becomes lopsided. The man who shuts off the emotional side of his life and throws himself entirely into activity becomes the workaholic. But we hear less about the other side of that coin—the woman who only pays attention to the feeling side of her life, and who becomes what might be called a "lovaholic." The workaholic can wind up overworked, exhausted, and emotionally sterile. The lovaholic risks feelings of worthlessness, dependency, and depression.[12]

Based on their findings, Baruch and Barnett have proposed a model of well-being that has two major components, mastery and pleasure. They delineated the elements that are associated with each. Mastery—or a sense of feeling important and worthwhile—consists of good self-esteem, a sense of control over one's life, and low levels of fatigue, depression, and anxiety. These mastery elements usually come from doing and achieving. Pleasure—or finding life enjoyable—consists of satisfaction, a feeling of happiness, and optimism regarding the future. These pleasure elements typically come from the development of intimate relationships. The authors stressed that the sense of mastery and pleasure come from distinctly different areas in life:

> The ingredients in life that provide a sense of mastery for today's women typically center around involvement in the work of one's society. Most often—but not always—this means paid work. A

sense of pleasure usually comes from intimate relationships—feeling lovingly connected with others. This doesn't necessarily require marriage and children![13]

Baruch and Barnett's findings are very important to any woman, but especially one struggling with chronic fatigue. It is so important for women to understand that they need a balance of both mastery and pleasure to maintain a sense of well-being. Women have traditionally lived within the world of pleasure, or relationships, but they have not developed the mastery elements. (By contrast, men have traditionally excelled within the world of mastery, failing to develop the pleasure side.)

The Baruch-Barnett conceptualization really helps to explain much dissatisfaction, boredom, low self-esteem, and chronic fatigue in the lives of women. It appears that women have been taught to expect too much from their relationships and family. Uncountable women have found themselves with good marriages, secure homes, and lovely children, but also a feeling of malaise. This feeling is often confusing for the women, who might think, "Here I have everything I could ever want, but I'm so exhausted all the time. What's wrong with me?" Family life may satisfy the sense of pleasure, but it cannot serve to satisfy the need for mastery. Mastery can only come from one's own doing, not from vicariously experiencing the achievements of one's spouse or children. This is exactly what Baruch and Barnett found: Homemakers are doing just fine in the area of pleasure, but mastery tends to be a problem for them. The women who rated the highest in both mastery and pleasure are married working women with children.

The traditional role of women is firmly rooted in nurturing, taking care of others' needs. Caring about others is one of women's great strengths; but it can, unfortunately, become a weakness. The ideal role calls for so much giving and self-sacrifice on the part of wives and mothers, that if women live up to it, their mastery needs are forsaken and chronic fatigue and dissatisfaction often become a way of life. I want to see women go on giving, but not to the extent that they give away their own self-esteem and lives.

Women must continue to struggle with the role conflict until we discover how to balance pleasure and mastery in each of our lives. Pleasure and mastery are both energy boosters—a life without one or the other is missing a primary component of well-being and is unbalanced. Remember that fatigue is a lack of well-being and a signal of that imbalance. Do you need more pleasure or more mastery in your life?

The internal conflict between our old role as nurturers and the new one as competent workers is probably the major cause of fatigue in American women today. This conflict is particularly fatiguing because the psychological struggle creates a situation where you are physically and emotionally overworked from trying to do it all. Thus, the conflict itself causes fatigue, and the overwork obviously leads to more fatigue. It is a double whammy. Do not let it be! Resolve your conflict by learning how to balance a healthy dose of both pleasure and mastery in your life.

WHAT TO DO

1. Get in touch with your feelings.

Often fatigue is the only indicator of a host of other feelings beneath the surface. Are you dissatisfied? Are you angry? Are you resentful? These kinds of feelings are symptoms, just like physical aches and pains; they mean that something in your life is off. Search for the cause. And be patient! Sometimes it takes a while to figure out what you are really upset about, or dissatisfied about, or resentful about. Just letting the feelings come to the surface, however, is a great start. You will begin to feel better and more energetic. It will release all the energy you have been using to keep the feelings bottled up inside. Remember that unexpressed feelings can poison your life. Feeling is one of women's great strengths; use it. Feeling is good for your health.

2. Boost your ego.

Developing your ego is one of the best actions you can

take to improve all aspects of your life, let alone alleviating chronic fatigue. A strong ego is bursting with energy. With a healthy ego, you will take charge of your life and learn to fulfill your own needs. You will then be able to give more and to achieve more in life.

One of the first steps in developing your ego is learning to say yes to yourself and no to others. When you nurture, make sure you are on the list too—and not always last! Take time-outs from the "give, give, give." The woman who sets no limits with others is going to become a doormat. The people in your life certainly have the ability to take more than you can possibly give. Trying to meet all of their demands and needs is a sure way to exhaustion and despair. By taking care of your own needs and developing yourself, you will actually be giving the people you love more than you ever imagined. You will be more confident, more energetic, and have higher self-esteem which will reflect on them.

An excellent "how-to" book on boosting your ego is Susan Price's *The Female Ego* (New York: Rawson Associates, 1984). Read it!

3. *Develop your own identity.*

So often, women drift in relationships, letting others have control so as to avoid a feeling of being selfish. I have had so many women tell me that until they took control, their lives were a mess. Now, however, after taking full control and responsibility, these women are happy, fulfilled, and growing in all areas of their lives. There is no one role or blueprint for life to make all women happy. There is no one "right" way to live.

Now that doors are swinging open, each woman will have to work a little harder to discover what is best for her as an individual. If a woman really wants to be a homemaker, then that is the place for her; but to be in that role because of a cultural decree is dangerous to one's mental health. Women now have choices available, which at times can lead to confusion and insecurity; however, they also provide the opportunity for personal growth and satisfaction. Use the new freedoms available to women to develop your own identity.

4. Identify and resolve your conflicts.

Almost every woman is struggling with one conflict, if not several. Most of these conflicts have been created by the changing role of women in society. Try to identify your conflicts—there are conflicts over the role itself, work inhibitions, sexual conflicts, interpersonal conflicts, just to name a few. Write them down in as much detail as you can. Identify the "old voice" and "new voice" for each conflict, then see if you can list what each voice demands of you. Once you have a pretty good idea of the tug-of-war going on inside you, decide how you would like to integrate the two voices.

Be patient! Resolving conflicts takes time. Share your conflicts with a confidant. You can learn a lot about yourself by talking to a friend about the kinds of issues discussed in this chapter. Studies are demonstrating that confiding in others is good for your physical and mental health. Pick someone whom you can trust and who can relate to the issues with which you are concerned.

Consider joining some sort of women's group to talk about issues that concern you and your conflicts. Millions of women have used women's self-help groups for problems involving eating, smoking, alcohol, drugs, rape, incest, divorce, wife beating. One of the most important things women learn in these groups is that their feelings are not "crazy"— they have been experienced by other women. To have such validation of your feelings is a tremendous relief.

These groups also provide a lot of emotional support for women going through difficult times or trying to work out feelings over a traumatic incident. Look for such a group by checking with local churches, schools, the YWCA, and the community mental-health program.

If you are having trouble identifying your conflicts or difficulty resolving them, try consulting with a professional. Too often conflicts avoid our best attempts to bring them to our consciousness where we can wrestle with them more easily. Unconscious conflicts left unresolved continue to drain energy. A therapist can be of tremendous help in this situation.

A variety of types of professionals such as psychiatrists, psychologists, and social workers, are available to help.

Therapy is a wonderful opportunity for growth, and should be taken advantage of if at all possible. No one type of professional is preferable over another. The choice depends on an individual's specific problem, the mental-health resources available, and a person's financial situation. The best advice I can give you is that you should try to visit the most highly trained person you can for the initial visit (i.e., a psychiatrist). That person can assess your situation and, if necessary, refer you to another therapist whose specialty is dealing with your type of problem and whose fees are affordable.

5. *Balance your life*.

Examine your balance of pleasure and mastery. Which are you lacking? Are you trying to get all your needs filled through a relationship? If you are anxious to be in a relationship, ask yourself what you really want from it. Make a list of what you hope your relationship, in the future or now, will bring you—love, intimacy, caring, money, status, security. If you are listing objectives that you would be or are now getting indirectly through a man, such as status, money, self-esteem, be careful. Expecting total fulfillment from a relationship can be damaging to both your self-esteem and the relationship.

Examine your own life and see what you can do to start directly satisfying your needs of control, self-esteem, money, security, and competence. Much of women's fatigue is due to frustration born of underutilization of their capacities. Their mastery needs have gone unfulfilled. Do something for mastery—the most effective source is paid work, but other work can suffice. Working for a cause or charity organization can also give you a sense of mastery. Go back to school or try to improve your present job skills. Whatever you do, be sure it is something that develops your skills and self-esteem. If trying to move outside the home into the work world creates problems in the family, remember that we are talking about your mental health, which ultimately affects the rest of the family. Do not be so willing to sacrifice your self-esteem in order to build someone else's up.

6. Read the book Lifeprints.

Lifeprints is a wonderfully practical book that discusses what gives women a sense of well-being. By examining how life turned out for women who made various life decisions, it dispels a lot of myths and gives you facts about various lifestyles. Anyone who is searching for their identity in life can be helped by reading this book.

The book is by Grace Baruch, Rosalind Barnett, and Caryl Rivers, *Lifeprints: New Patterns of Love and Work for Today's Women* (New York: New American Library, 1983), paperback $8.95.

11

LIGHTEN YOUR WORK LOAD

Women have always worked. Yet judging by some of the stories in the media in recent years, you would think that it is a brand-new activity in which women are engaging. I guess "the big deal" is that women are now working outside the home, as well as in the home, in record numbers. I think the gains women are making in the work force are great news. However, I cannot help but feel that there is an underlying assumption that women's labor in the home does not qualify as work. And that is wrong.

Millions of women are now working in the home and outside the home—and the exhaustion that comes from it is like an old, faithful friend. The fatigue is there day after day after day. And many women see no end in sight to the work and the exhaustion. Stella is one woman who no longer suffers from chronic fatigue—but she remembers the day when she did.

> "In my first months as a working mother I was constantly tired. I felt that my body was trying to tell me that I was incapable of effectively managing a career and a family. It took a lot of convincing on my husband's part to get me to believe that I was

being very impatient with my body's ability to recover from a caesarean delivery.

"Hindsight makes me think I was trying to prove I could be Supermom, and since this was six and a half years ago, that wasn't a topic you heard much about. I was ready for a mental adjustment which wasn't a problem—in dealing with the guilt feelings of leaving an infant—and hadn't thought of the physical adjustment in recovering from pregnancy and surgery as well as keeping a baby's night schedule."

So many women can relate to Stella's trials and tribulations as an employed mother with a child at home. Probably no single area has a more widespread and profound effect on women's fatigue as does work and the conflicts about it. If our grandmothers said, "Women's work is never done," what would they say about all the work women are trying to do today—"Mission impossible"? There just does not seem to be enough time: time to get all the work that needs doing done, time to develop good relationships, quality time with the children, time to run the household, and personal time.

Stella did something very atypical to control her fatigue—she protected her personal time.

"I learned during my pregnancy and continue today—although the baby is nearly seven—to take time to unwind when I first get home, no matter how late it makes dinner.

"Taking some adult time, quiet time, alone or with your spouse, has a wonderful payback. It cuts down on the quantity of family time, but it definitely ups the quality of that time.

"It helps to separate the two worlds. Work problems can be erased before conquering family ones. It enables me to get a second wind and start the family time with a clear slate and enjoy it rather than looking forward to bedtime.

"I also found that forcing myself to be involved in a physical-fitness program—it is not my natural bent—helps increase my energy level. Since a lot of my fatigue is mentally caused, the physical exhaustion makes me very tired and therefore I sleep better."

Personal time is the block of time that typically disappears first. Studies have shown that working mothers give up any spare time that they would devote to themselves and reduce their hours of sleep in order to get all their work done.[1] (Men, on the other hand, rarely give up their personal time. No matter how busy they are, they seem to make time for themselves.) However, when women give up sleep and relaxation time it only makes it more difficult to complete all of one's work, because fatigue is brought on more quickly. The fatigue decreases one's work capacity, leading to a vicious cycle. It is no surprise that working women report that they are chronically tired.[2]

Work is not new to women; women have always worked hard. Now, however, they are working more than ever and at jobs that bring added stresses. In America, women have entered the work force in record numbers. Between 1947 and 1980, the number of women in the labor force increased by 173 percent—four times the rate of increase of male workers![3] The Bureau of the Census has projected that over 70 percent of women between the ages of twenty-five and fifty-four will be working outside the home by the year 1990.[4]

And here lies the source of most of a working woman's fatigue. As women have moved into the labor force, they have not swapped their traditional female responsibilities as homemaker for worker; rather, most women have taken on new work burdens as they struggle to do the old ones.

There are a myriad of reasons why women are so overloaded in both roles, the traditional bread*maker* role and the new bread*winner* role. Women are often overburdened in the home because either their spouses or society, or they themselves consider homemaking a female obligation. Furthermore, working women usually experience more stress in the labor force than men because of role conflicts and discrimination.

In this chapter, we will explore some of the burdens

working women have in common (both in the home and on the job), the primary difficulty that arises because of women's new working status—being overworked—and, most important, what can be done to lighten your work load.

FROM HOUSEWORK TO THE LABOR FORCE

Women as a group have moved outside the home and into the labor force for a variety of reasons. To a certain extent, lower-class women, single women, and widows have always had to work for wages. But more and more middle- and upper-class women have been moving into the work force in recent decades because of economic inflation. In order to maintain the same standard of living, many families have been forced to become two-paycheck households.

The most recent trend, which has been making head-lines, has been women working for mastery—a sense of self-esteem and personal achievement. Of course, it is assumed that men will be fathers and workers, yet women who want to be mothers and workers are often thought of as "selfish" or "greedy," or they "want it all." Even as I write, "working mothers" is the vogue topic. Three magazines that I receive had covers this week showing a working mother with a child by her side, the headline asking the biggest question of the decade (if not the century), "Can she do it all?"

Why do women want to work outside the home so much now? We are beginning to understand that human beings, whether female or male, need to do productive work in order to feel fulfilled—to have that sense of mastery. Sigmund Freud thought work attached a person to the real world, "Work . . . gives him a secure place in a portion of reality in the human community."[5] No doubt, when Freud wrote "him" he was speaking only about men and their need to work. Freud admitted he did not understand the psychology of women and asked the famous question, "What do women want?"

Women want the same thing as men, to be fulfilled as human beings and valued within the human community.

Work provides a sense of personal identity, status, achievement, and an outlet for one's creativity and talents.

Rose, a forty-six-year-old twice-divorced woman, tried finding fulfillment through homemaking but never could. Homemaking just did not satisfy her creative urges and her intellect. She spoke of her homemaking days with a delightful sense of humor, although the despair Rose felt still came through. Chronic fatigue was always high up on her list of physical complaints in those days.

> "For a majority of my life, I have suffered physical problems from stress and emotional-related causes. I have always had a difficult time designing my life in the classical roles of women—both in thoughts and in actions. I have attempted wife (passive), homemaker, schoolteacher (elementary), community volunteer, et cetera. All of these created hysteria."

For twenty years, Rose was in and out of treatment with a number of doctors for symptoms of fatigue, dizziness, muscle cramps, and anxiety attacks. Depending on which doctor or psychologist Rose consulted, she got a wide variety of diagnoses ranging anywhere from being told she was a homosexual who needed shock treatments to a hopeless neurotic who needed a lifetime of psychotherapy. She underwent various treatments.

> "I was snowed for seven years with Librium (100 milligrams) gasp! I probably don't have a liver left. I also had several surgeries done to remove various things, which never helped me. Then of course, over the years I was seeing male psychologists who told me my problem was penis envy and I should learn to accept my place as a woman. Finally, I got to a female psychologist who worked with my feelings and my symptoms. Biofeedback and relaxation techniques helped me control my anxiety attacks and I came to understand that I was in conflict over my role as a woman—that I was, on

the one hand, trying to play out the passive good woman, but on the other hand, I wanted to go out and do something in the world."

Rose was able to solve her conflict and did go do something in the world—she went back to school. She now loves her work as a state administrator and no longer has any physical symptoms. She enthusiastically participates in tennis, golf, running, and skiing. Rose says that she has learned that physical activity is "an antidote for anger, depression, and fatigue." Rose is much happier now. She is not alone. Millions of other women have discovered the satisfaction of having a paid job—but they have discovered that the job has brought on chronic fatigue as a way of life, not alleviated it.

MORE WORK AND NO REST

As women enter the work force, they have less and less time and energy to put into "making the home." Yet someone has to perform the household tasks, and in America that someone is still the woman. One historian aptly described the present situation as follows:

> The transition to the two-income family (or to the female-headed household) did not occur without taking a toll—a toll measured in the hours that employed housewives had to work in order to perform adequately first as employees and then as housewives. A thirty-five-hour week (housework) added to a forty-hour-week (paid employment) adds up to a working week that even sweatshops cannot match. With all her appliances and amenities, the status of being a "working mother" in the United States today is, as three eminent experts have suggested, virtually a guarantee of being overworked and perpetually exhausted.[6]

Millions of women can directly relate to this situation. They constantly suffer a huge energy drain from overwork. However, most women fail to do anything to increase their energy supplies. As time becomes more precious, women meet all of their responsibilities before they attend to their individual needs. Time that would have been used for their own rejuvenation is spent getting more work done—but this in turn actually decreases the amount of energy available. Sleep is diminished, exercise gets canceled, eating occurs on the run, and personal time no longer exists. It's work, work, work, and emotional needs often go unfulfilled.

All of these factors create fatigue, but I think the last one is the straw that breaks women's backs. Certainly the sheer physical load that many women are carrying is reason enough to be tired. However, when women work within an environment of not being recognized or appreciated for their work, being taken for granted, or not being nurtured themselves, it makes the work almost unbearable.

Luanne, the mother of a five-year-old girl, is one of these women who feels unappreciated and taken for granted. She said that ever since she started working outside the home, she is now tired all the time. Her husband does not help around the house at all.

> "He comes home and spends the time on the telephone and talking and reading. He doesn't even go to the store to buy a loaf of bread. He doesn't think about how tired I am . . . tired, lonely, exhausted, no attention . . . all I do is work, work, work. I am tired of doing the laundry, cooking, helping our child with piano, schoolwork, making my husband's lunch. I go shopping, I do it all. I spend the weekend cleaning house and I never do anything for myself. I don't go to the spa to relax. I am tired of it all."

Luanne does not have any mechanisms to counteract her tiredness and had given up two very important activities that offset fatigue: her exercise at the spa and her own personal time. Women should not give up their personal time. And if you have, you should take it back. You should "pay yourself first," because you cannot do anything else effectively if you do not first take care of your own needs. If you find that taking time out for yourself is difficult, or makes you feel a little guilty, that is okay. Millions of other women feel the same way.

Sonia is a twenty-three-year-old married woman without children, and she is so busy all the time, I cannot imagine how she would cope if she had children. She works six days a week during the day, and on many nights of the week, she sings with her husband in nightclubs. The couple is trying to make it big in the music industry and uses any other spare time writing and recording their own tunes.

> "With my job and singing at night, sometimes I can't even tell when fatigue has arrived, but others can see my steps drag. So does my speech. I never have enough sleep. That's when you need another person to let you know, that is the time to pull the plug and say STOP.
>
> "I think every woman should find something to get away with at least once a week: look at their old school albums, paint, read . . . something that just puts the emotions and thought patterns on hold— not having to think or do anything for a while. There's nothing wrong with doing nothing once in a while. I find that if I do that, I can handle anything that comes along. My mind and body has had a time to cleanse themselves and rejuvenate. I feel less tired, under less stress and more relaxed."

I think Sonia offers some good advice, but I am struck by how many women feel guilty for taking some personal time and want (or need) other people's permission (such as their husband's) to do so. You get a sense that Sonia will push herself until someone else tells her she should or may stop. And she calls for personal time only once a week! I would like to see women take personal time at least once a day. Ten percent of the day should be yours—even it if gets spent taking a l-o-n-g hot bath. When your husband or children call in, "What are you doing in there?" tell them you are washing. Actually, many of the women I talked to said they spend their personal time reading. When I asked one woman how she alleviated her fatigue, she said:

> "In fatigue due to pregnancy, overwork, et cetera, I have learned to set aside a structured time for rest. One doesn't have to lie down—a good example is when I was driving a car pool, I used to rush madly to the store and the market while the kids were taking music lessons for forty-five minutes. After I learned my lesson, I stayed in the car and read a book."

Another woman, a working married mother of two children, said she also reads to alleviate her stretches of tiredness.

> "I lose myself in reading a good book, usually a romantic novel. I find that it helps me forget about all the stresses at work or an extensive disagreement with my husband, which are the situations when I really feel my fatigue. I guess a good romance novel, in a way, rejuvenates me."

Millions of women across America receive a boost from this genre of book. Why is the romantic novel so popular with women? I stumbled upon a study that helped me understand why romances are so appealing to women. The author explained how a bookstore clerk, Mrs. Evans—a local adviser to the romance-novel readers who were studied—understands the books' appeal.

> She talked at great length about the benefits these books provide the traditional wife and mother. The typical woman, she said, has many, many caretaking duties that are part of those intertwined roles, but her labors are inadequately appreciated by her family. Because individual family members do not sufficiently recognize her efforts nor compensate her for them by "taking care" of her, Evans believes such a woman must find a legitimate way of

releasing her from her duties temporarily and of replenishing the energy that is constantly being drained in performing them. Romance reading, she explained, is the perfect solution.[7]

Luanne, Sonia, and millions of other women do not think there is a solution to the constant energy drain. Overwhelmed by her fatigue, Luanne told me, "Women need to either work at home or work out. If women work outside the home, husbands should do half of the work, share the work." Even though that is what she believes, Luanne does not have the choice to stay home and she does not have a husband who shares the work.

SHARING THE WORK

Married women with jobs or careers are trying to work out a life-style that gives both wife and husband a feeling of worth and accomplishment as well as providing the comfort, security, and love of home and family. We are plowing new ground—and it is hard. There is almost no historical precedent on which to model our new life-style, and the societal and institutional supports are lagging far behind.

There is no question that the dual-career couple faces extreme and unique pressures in both work and family life today. It has been said that the word *career* means "a demanding, rigorous, preordained life pattern, to whose goals everything else is ruthlessly subordinated. . . ."[8] (Who needs to go outside the home to find this? A homemaker fits the definition, as far as I'm concerned.) Studies have demonstrated that typical male executives spend fifty to seventy hours per week on the job.[9] While everyone seems to take it for granted that men can have careers and be fathers, it has been assumed that women have to choose either a career or motherhood.

Of course, women have been actively challenging this notion for some years now; they are supposedly "trying to have it all," combining the rewards of professional life and the joys of family life. You might think that it is this group of women who are the most harried and exhausted, running from responsibility to responsibility. Actually, studies have shown that motherhood is a major source of stress to women, while a career—rewarding work—seems to be a key to well-being.

In *Lifeprints,* Baruch and Barnett report that women who have high-level jobs, husbands, and children have the greatest sense of well-being.

> Why is it that married mothers in high-pressure jobs seem to be so well-off? Certainly it's not that they don't have strains in their life, or that they never feel that they have too much to do. But the notion of balance applies here: the rewards far outweigh the problems. What might be called the "recharge your batteries" model of energy is probably operating rather than the "limited" model. The variety and richness of these women's jobs gives them a sense of vitality, rather than draining them.
>
> There is another likely explanation. Some theorists believe that adding roles to one's life is only a process of addition; you simply add on extra tasks to all the ones you already have. But a "revisionist" view of this process is emerging, and our study further confirms the new idea. What actually seems to happen is that when they take a paid job, women drop off many of the things they did before. They cook less elaborate meals, they say no to a request to chair a fund drive. They don't have to accompany a mother-in-law on a shopping trip. Often a paid job is a great excuse for a woman not to do the things she didn't want to do in the first place. And the more prestigious the job, the easier it is to shed the unwanted aspects of other roles.[10]

Women with high-paying jobs may find it "easier" to shed some of the aspects of the role, but it is still difficult. Society is still operating as if the only responsibility women have is homemaking. And this is the crucial point. Women were left the responsibility of homemaking when the industrial revolution took men away from home. But women today are still left solely with the responsibility for the home and children when a new revolution is taking them away from home! Homemaking has become synonymous with "feminine" over the last few decades, so many women feel responsible (and the men expect it too) for fulfilling the home obligations by themselves, without help, in addition to holding down a job outside the house.

Many women feel that before they are entitled to have a job or develop themselves, they have to fulfill all the demands of the homemaking role. Otherwise, they will feel guilty and bad about themselves. You can clearly hear the voices struggling inside of Jean, a twenty-nine-year-old housewife.

"This past year I felt extremely fatigued for a two-month period. I was juggling several responsibilities at once and gradually became very rundown. I was attending school at the time, determined to achieve a 4.0 GPA [grade point average]. I was also working on an internship through school and maintaining a home. I am guilty of taking on all the housework and not delegating any of it to my husband. I imagine it's my way to compensate for not bringing in an income even though I work just as hard throughout each day as he. To top it off, I am a neat freak and try to keep a clean and orderly environment. So along with school full-time and an internship, was the cooking, cleaning, shopping, laundry, dishes, banking, bills, and those many tiddlywink errands us housewife suckers get left with."

So many women express similar frustrations. Because their husbands bring home the money (or the bigger paycheck)—in essence fulfilling the male role in a marriage—the wives feel they have to do all the housework to fulfill the female role (even if they have a job that pays). Jean admitted that she was guilty of not delegating housework because of her own guilt; yet at the same time she was angry about all the work she was doing.

Happily, Jean was able to resolve some of her conflicts, get her husband involved in the struggle, learn to say no to the old voice that was setting unrealistically high standards.

> "My schedule eventually simplified, for the internship came to an end and I no longer did all those house chores it was assumed I'd always do. No clean underwear on a weekday morning can really shock a husband into verbalizing 'I just assumed you'd take care of it.' Although not as balanced as I'd like, we are swaying towards a team effort when it comes to house chores."

For most couples, the distribution of work is a major problem. Most surveys are indicating that, in spite of the rhetoric surrounding sharing of household responsibilities, the woman still carries the lioness's share of the work load of managing and running the home. She is the floor manager and the floor sweeper! The data indicate that in addition to her outside job, the typical working wife is spending somewhere between fifteen and fifty extra hours a week in household and child-care chores. One study reported that a mother with preschool children who has a forty-hour-a-week job outside the home, "works an average of 77 hours a week."[11]

Those additional thirty-seven hours a week are spent doing household chores: the laundry, cooking, cleaning, shopping, child care, house decorating, et cetera. (Working thirty-seven hours a week on household chores is at the low end of the scale. Other studies have shown that the housewife who does not work outside the home spends about one hundred hours a week working at twelve different chores.[12]) The same study reported that the amount of time husbands spend doing housework has increased less than thirty minutes a week in the last ten years!

It is not simply a matter of hours, either. Wives tend to do the most undesirable housework and child-care chores, such as cleaning and bathing, whereas the husbands spend more time playing with and entertaining the children. Even when women are engaging in leisure time, much of it is consumed by tasks that are useful to the family, such as sewing, knitting, or baking.

Not only do the women perform the most undesirable tasks, also they tend to retain "executive" responsibility for the family. They carry the burden for school relations, social schedules, shopping, health care, education, and emotional nurturing. And working women report that they are very concerned about the lack of time and emotional energy they have left for children.[13]

Does it really have to be this way? While women have expanded their responsibilities, most have not been able to give up or share their traditional chores with someone else. Why? I think it goes back to our notion of who is responsible for homemaking. Although we are in the midst of change, most men and women have been raised with strong male and female identities that tend to categorize chores as either male work or female work.

Many women do not realize why it is so hard to get a team effort going in the home if they have a partner. Sometimes it is because the men refuse to help. More often, however, it is because women are their own worst enemies. The men get a message from their spouses "to stay out of the kitchen." Again, women's role conflict raises its ugly head. On the one hand, women may want the help and resent all the work they have to do; but on the other hand, they often fiercely protect their domestic territory or simply do not demand help.

Home and family have been the traditional turf of women, where women got their identity and self-esteem. Many women have difficulty, whether they want to or not, letting go of this turf and witnessing their husbands performing quite adequately in the role. Relegating the traditional tasks of mothering to a father can be especially threatening. Motherhood is the most valued aspect of the female role. Splitting up domestic tasks is actually tinkering with one's identity as a woman and a mother, which explains why it can be so difficult.

The next time you have an argument with your spouse over domestic chores, ask yourself what you are really fighting about. It just might be that your self-esteem is involved in the struggle. Even though you may find aspects of the nurturing role mundane, you probably cling tightly to it because your sense of femininity comes from it. And the more your mother was consumed by the role, the more difficult it will be for you to give it up. One woman executive said to me, "I feel guilty when I see my husband cleaning the house. I just can't sit still, so I might as well do it myself."

Rather than face the conflicts and work out some of the major issues involving the division of household tasks and child care, money, and power, many women try to keep the peace—and assuage their guilt—by attempting to "do it all." Other women are forced to "do it all" because their spouses refuse to help or they have no spouse to help them.

I think "How can women do it all?" is the wrong question. I do not think women should have to do it all. Unfortunately, the old and the new roles are being merged into one, called "Women Do Most of the Work." We must not let this become the new role of women, shouldering most of the responsibility at home and working full-time in the work force. A truly new role must emerge that throws out some of the old role and shares the rest with the men. Our entire society would prosper if men were more involved in the home and shared more parenting with women.

The question should be "How will the responsibilities get divided?" I do not mean chores either, I mean responsibilities. Consider the phrase, "My husband helps around the house a lot." The verb is *help*, which implies that the primary responsibility for the task is the woman's; she does the worrying. Perhaps he may help with the shopping, but does he carry the worry around in his head? He may pick up the children from after-school practice, but does he keep track of the household calendar and see to it that everything gets done? The concept should be "share" instead of "help."

If you are exhausted from overworking, the first place you must look for a solution is inside yourself. You must examine your notions about homemaking and working outside the home. Realize that many of the rules that drive you are unconscious and linked to your concept of femininity and goodness. You must begin to let go of some things, such as some of the standards you have for cleanliness.

The advertisements for household cleaning products are playing upon your assumptions about what a good homemaker should do and setting the standards at the same time. Do not let them! Next time you see the ads on television, listen to them closely. What are they trying to tell you? That you are a bad homemaker if your kitchen floor does not shine like a mirror? Nonsense. You should see my kitchen floor. No one will eat off it, including our dog. I have really lowered my standards. But let me tell you, I know it is not easy. My husband has often heard me mumble to myself, "Holly, lower your standards." I use that line on myself when something is bothering me, which I would like to see done but just do not have the time to accomplish. As time has passed, letting go of my standards has become far easier. You must start to lower yours.

Look realistically at all of your tasks. Make a list of the chores you do (you may be shocked when you write them all down—I was) and divide them into four groups—cleaning (dusting, vacuuming, beds, laundry); food preparation (shopping, cooking, dishes); child care; and other (bills, decorating, car, garbage). Then make some decisions about each chore. First of all, does a particular task really have to be done? For instance, when I was a child my mother taught me to iron my father's handkerchiefs; she did the sheets and pillowcases. My husband's handkerchiefs and our sheets and pillowcases are as wrinkled as prunes. In this case, I refuse to waste time upholding the standards my mother taught me.

Second, if the chore needs doing, try to decrease the number of times you have to do the task. Either reduce your standards (like how clean the kitchen floor should be) or change some behavior. We use paper plates and cups when both my husband and I have intense schedules. What a joy to throw dirty dishes away rather than wash them!

Do you have a huge load of laundry to do every day because people in your house use a clean towel every time they dry, or pitch their clothes in the heap after they have worn them once? I cringe when I remember the loads of wash my mother did for my family. I grew up on a lake with two other sisters and a brother, and we all must have used three towels a day between swimming in the lake and taking showers, not to mention the changes of clothes we would go through. Certain clothes can be worn more than once, and towels should not be washed after only one use. Set some rules—and stick to them!

Third, decide what chores can be delegated to others. Maybe a youngster cannot do the bills, but he or she can clean a bathroom, dust, vacuum, and so on. Children will automatically lower your standards; let them help you set new ones! I have found that doing chores together in a playful way can also be family time spent together. I hate grocery shopping, but I have learned to enjoy it now because my husband and I almost always do it together. Try getting your spouse to help you clean the bedroom and change the sheets (a loving pillow fight is always a good way to break the monotony). Get creative.

Many women have told me that they have done away with all the drudgery that could possibly be erased from their schedules. I do not believe that. Women's schedules are still full of the tasks the old voice demands be done, tasks to which women cling. It is hard to let go of those tasks, but I know that many of them can be tossed out or shared with someone, including children. The notion that adults work and children play is not only fatiguing to mothers but damaging to the development of a child's sense of responsibility; the new voice should start saying that everything is "our" responsibility. Create a team spirit in your home.

Try to determine with your family what they expect out of you. If you feel overworked or unappreciated, you must begin to communicate this to those around you. If your husband does not share responsibilities, or does not "help" around the house, you two need a conversation (or several) about the issue.

Discuss these issues with the entire family. Do they consider taking care of the house and all the people in it "Mom's" responsibility? Do they simply "help Mom" when they (finally) do something around the house? Or does everyone believe that the home belongs to the family and caring for it is a family's responsibility? Attitudes are important to achieving the right kind of sharing. Once again, the family should talk and work together.

I do not believe that only women should be responsible for homemaking; everybody living in a home—including the children—has the responsibility to make that home a warm, nurturing place to live. I know mothers who are teaching their children at a young age how to cook simple meals and use the washing machine. It is good for Mom, and the children learn to be responsible and independent. (Giving children responsibility is not synonymous with deprivation and poor mothering!) Taking care of the house, no matter what the chore, should become a family matter.

That message must begin to come from you, because up until now everyone has assumed that homemaking is a woman's job. If you are working outside the home, you should not have to do everything or even most of the work just because you are female.

I know this means change; and change in itself takes work. But working for a change that will bring you some rest and relaxation is rewarding, not exhausting. Talk about your needs, assumptions, and priorities; then work out a mutually agreeable solution whereby you truly share the work with the other people in your life. Be patient. It will take some time to change attitudes, but most likely you can get others to share your work. I did it with my husband—when I met him he could hardly make me a cup of instant coffee. Now he is—among other things—the (marvelous) cook in the family. Everything gets shared in our household, including the worry. Who said you can't teach an old dog new tricks?

DOING IT ALL—ALONE

Millions of working women—sadly—have to do *all* of the housework because there is no spouse with whom to share the chores. At the beginning of this chapter I mentioned three recent magazines with lead stories devoted to working women. All three used married professional career women as examples. Not one of the articles addressed the plight of a divorced woman, a single mother running a household and working, or the problems of the underpaid woman with "just a job."

Most women do not have the luxury of deciding whether or not they will work outside the home. I get sick and tired of the implication that women have this cushy decision to make and are rather selfish if they try "to have it all." Women are working because, for the most part, they have to.

Millions of women are carrying the entire burden because they are alone. The number of households headed by women almost tripled from 1960 to 1980. In 1980, 17.5 percent of American households were headed by women.[14] There are a number of trends behind that increase. Women are marrying later in their lives than they did thirty years ago, unmarried women are setting up their own households, older single women are less inclined to live with their adult children, and women are divorcing.

Divorce has done as much as anything to change the American familial landscape. According to a study done in 1980 by the National Center for Health Statistics, a couple married in 1952 had about three chances in ten that their marriage would end in divorce, while a couple married in 1977 was estimated to have about a fifty-fifty chance.[15]

Many divorced women find that they are thrust into the labor force with little or no training or work experience. They are faced with the hard economic necessity of working to maintain their home and their children. This must be done in the face of perhaps the biggest stressor of all, the feeling of betrayal and personal devastation. The new work stressors are combined with the stressors of lost status, loneliness, and feelings of fear and panic. Exhaustion is often a symptom of these overwhelming stressors.

Liz, fifty-four years old, went through such a separation fifteen years ago (you met her in Chapter 2). She now works full-time outside the home, but there was a time she was a full-time homemaker. I should say Liz was an overtime homemaker; she had eight children. She lived with chronic fatigue for five years after her husband deserted her.

"My marriage was kaput. What I thought was solid and secure turned to vapor. I felt betrayed—hurt beyond recovery—confused—frightened. I was tired all the time simply because I was tired of my life the way it was. I still had small children to care for—no man of the house to share the care, as he had moved to a bachelor apartment. I knew what the problem was. I figured out that I really was fine physically; my body wasn't tired. My soul, mind, emotions—whatever—were exhausted. My means of coping were to immerse myself in a discipline, in my case, stage work—acting. There was no other world from the time I entered the theater until I left it, and it was better than a good night's sleep. I was refreshed—better able to see objectively, to cope."

Liz is doing just fine today. She seems to accept life so gracefully. I asked her what she had learned during those five bad years and the fifteen that have gone by since. She said, "Patience—not so much with other people as with yourself. Sometimes we expect more from ourselves than we are capable of delivering at the time." Liz had discovered a great truth, that most of us are sabotaged by our own internal expectations and standards, rather than somebody else's.

Liz's story—unfortunately—is not rare. Over two thirds (69.3 percent) of the households headed by women in 1980 included children under the age of seventeen. In fact, the Census Bureau estimated that 45 percent of children born in 1978 would be living in one-parent homes before they were eighteen years old. Millions of women are and will be carrying heavy responsibilities for jobs, children, and maintaining their homes.

Single women with children have enormous responsibilities. They must work to support the family and they must carry on the traditional job of homemaking with its myriad chores of child care, budgeting, cooking, cleaning, laundering, shopping, et cetera. Many women find that the responsibility—the mental worry of managing all the activities—is actually more tiresome than performing each chore.

Facilities to help women organize all these tasks and carry them out are woefully inadequate in most areas of the United States. The family structure in the country has changed drastically, but our institutional and sociological support organizations have not yet responded. Working parents find that day care for small children is extremely difficult to find.[16] Not enough employers have created on-site day-care centers, let alone instituted part-time and flextime work schedules or longer vacations.

Today, separation, divorce, or death of a spouse usually means a plunge into poverty for many women and their custodial children. Of all the female-headed households below the poverty level, almost 46 percent are run by a divorced woman. One sociologist reports that "a woman's standard of living generally falls by 73 percent in the year following a divorce, while a man's typically rises by 42 percent."[17]

For the most part, women do not receive alimony anymore under the new equitable-distribution divorce laws. Only 14 percent of divorced women are being awarded alimony, and only 7 percent receive what they are entitled to. Furthermore, of those women who are awarded child support, less than half of them receive the full amount due them, and one quarter get nothing at all.[18]

Mothers are forced into the nouveau poor because they cannot get a good job with decent pay, contrary to what the media may make you think. Displaced homemakers lack the occupational training or the years of experience to compete with men for better jobs. Even in equivalent jobs, women earn less than men because of the wage gap, now 63 cents to every dollar. The median income for families headed by women in 1980 was only $9,927 compared to $21,150 for families where the husband was in the labor force or $25,552 where both husband and wife were working.[19] The old saying is "The rich get richer, and the poor get poorer." I think the new saying should be, "The men get richer, and the women get poorer."

If the median income for families headed by women is so low, it is obvious that women have less-than-desirable jobs. Economist Sylvia Ann Hewlett reports:

"Eighty percent of American working women are employed in traditional 'women's jobs.' They spend their days waiting on tables, typing letters, emptying bedpans, and cleaning offices. These women are not only badly paid (on average they earn just over $10,000 a year), they are also expected to bear and raise children in their spare time."[20]

Furthermore, more than half of all working women hold jobs that sociologist Arlie Russell Hochschild calls emotional-labor jobs. These jobs have three characteristics in common.

"First, they require face-to-face or voice-to-voice contact with the public. Second, they require the worker to produce an emotional state in another person—gratitude or fear, for example. Third, they allow the employer, through training and supervision, to exercise a degree of control over the emotional activities of employees."[21]

The emotional aspect of the job is rarely recognized as a stressor, and rarely appreciated or honored. But the emotional energy women may be expending on such jobs can result in considerable fatigue.

All too often, women are huddled in low-paying "female" occupations that offer little opportunity for advancement, provide inadequate benefits, and use their emotions to provide a service to strangers. In these jobs, women earned only 60 percent of the salaries of their male counterparts. Furthermore, the more an occupation is dominated by females, the less it pays. The lower wages earned by single working mothers have a profound effect on the amount of work they have to do and subsequently on how much fatigue they experience.

I know several women who work as nurse's aides seven days a week, sometimes two eight-hour shifts back to back, in order to bring home enough money to pay the rent, buy the food, and clothe their children. If they do not work a second job in order to spend more time raising the children, they must settle for a standard of living that is substantially below the poverty level.

I have listened to the stories and seen the tears of mothers who are worried about the neighborhoods in which their children are growing up or the schools they attend. These mothers are willing to compromise themselves, such as their own nutrition, leisure activities, or health care, but it disturbs them terribly to have to compromise their children's well-being.

A black single working mother shared with me her struggles—and her concern for her five-year-old son. Germaine works for a Fortune 500 company located in a very posh skyscraper in downtown New York City. Even though she works for a good company, her pay is not very good. The only housing she can afford is in a very bad section of New York that is forty-five minutes away by subway. Germaine worries about James growing up there.

> "I'm working for the day I can get us another place to live. Sometimes it just keeps me awake at night—then I open a book and read—why there's water coming through the ceiling and the landlord does not care. There is garbage in the halls.
>
> "And I'm afraid of James copying what he sees the other boys do—just like pulling *it* out and going to the bathroom anywhere, in the elevators, in the halls. We got in the elevator the other day, and he went to do that and I said to him, 'Oh no you don't!' It is no place for any boy to grow up—it is no place for a person to live, but I have to because I can't afford anything else. I am *so* tired of trying to do it all alone, but I'm the type that will never, never give up. You can't give up. I'm determined that one of these days I will make some more money, and I will get James and me out of that dump."

Poor wages and wage discrimination are also indicative of other pressures women are under, pressures on the job. Germaine told me what discrimination was like for her, being both black and female. She said it absolutely drains her emotionally. Women clearly must work harder than men to reach equivalent goals of recognition and pay. So often, when

I am confronted by a situation involving or I hear a story about a working woman, I think, "We have to be gold to pass for copper."

Women must often face sexual discrimination and sexual harassment on the job. It is discouraging to know your performance is good, but to look around you to find that others are making more money and getting promotions and recognition and for less effort.

Furthermore, when a woman does get a promotion, especially in a job that is traditionally male, she is under great pressure to prove herself. Such women are scrutinized by peers, management, and customers to see if they can "cut the mustard." The list of stressors resulting from discrimination could run on and on, they all drain women of energy in a myriad of ways. And the fatigue that results from the stress is the type that will not go away with a night's sleep, because we cannot make the problem of wage discrimination and its underlying cause—sex discrimination—go away overnight. Both discrimination and the fatigue that comes from it are chronic problems.

Unfortunately, some of the changes that are necessary to alleviate the fatigue and other stress-related illness from overwork and underpay cannot be brought about by individual effort. As a group, women must struggle for appropriate recognition and wages on the job; we must encourage young women to get the education and training that prepares them for jobs that are in high demand and pay well (such as science and engineering); women must seek programs in the community that help provide domestic support; they must press for the proper working conditions to allow them to perform in the best possible way; and they must join with other women to seek their rights and fair treatment. There are many problems to be overcome if the wage gap is to be narrowed, and it will require long-term effort on the part of business, government, institutions, and women and men.

I firmly believe that single working mothers, beyond making individual changes, need outside help, from the support of friends to a local day-care center. So many women are trying to make it on their own—as individuals. There are other options! One way you can get help is to band together with other women in similar circumstances; share burdens, talk, get ideas, share babysitting, share shopping, share chores, share living facilities.

Look for a "Y" exercise program that provides child care. Call your church or temple to see what kind of programs it has. Look for agencies that provide counseling services or that help with the children. Communities can help. Get involved with community efforts to bring about needed changes. They need to provide more facilities that take single mothers into account.

Unfortunately, communities can also hinder. For example, some housing laws make it difficult for single-parent families to form joint living arrangements. These laws need to be changed. Work to get them off the books! We need community agencies that provide counseling services, financial advice, legal advice, housing advice, and assist in establishing contact between single parents. Communities need to recognize that the structure of the American family is no longer a mother, a father, 1.87 children, and a dog (if it ever was). We need to rethink who makes up our communities and provide services to the real constituents.

One of the services that is sorely lacking in the United States is day care for children of working parents. In 1977, when one of the last big studies was done, statistics showed that a little less than half (45 percent) of the mothers with children under age six worked. That translates into more than 8 million children under the age of six who have employed mothers. Who cared for these children while mother was out working? About 43 percent of them were watched by father or another relative, and about 9 percent of the children were taken by their mothers to work. That means about half of the children (over 4 million) were watched by nonrelatives who were paid for their child-care services.[22]

Yet in 1982 there was room for less than 500,000 children in publicly supported day-care centers.[23] "A recent survey found that most working parents must piece together two or three different private child-care arrangements per day for each pre-school child."[24] It is disgraceful that this country does not have better day-care facilities.

Of course, many people still say that "a woman's place is

in the home" with the child. This view belies the facts that most women in the work force must work for economic reasons and, furthermore, for most women work leads to a sense of well-being. Work is not an avocation or a diversion for most women today; women are dedicated to their vocations. They are no less dedicated to their families and children. Women are concerned about what effect their working will have on their child(ren); it is probably the primary stressor of working mothers and the main reason society is concerned about the growing trend of employed women.

Are women's psychological (and economic) needs now in conflict with children's psychological needs? Are our children being irreparably damaged because their mothers are out working? Contrary to expectations, the studies are showing that children of working mothers suffer no ill consequences and most likely reap positive benefits. A recent study indicated that there were "no negative effects on children's social, emotional, and cognitive development attributable to maternal absence due to employment."[25]

This country desperately needs more child-care facilities. When doing the research for this book, I was struck how often experts in all fields cited the lack of child-care facilities as an impediment to women's efforts: efforts to receive good health care, to attend drug and alcohol rehabilitation programs, to receive counseling, to attend school, and to go to work to support their children.

If we are ever going to improve the lives of millions of working women—whether single or paired—and their children, make progress on the wage gap, and allow women to fully participate in their occupations and careers, something must be done to provide competent and readily available day care.

It is hard for a mother to concentrate her attention and talents on a job when she is constantly worried that her child(ren) is not receiving the proper care. As one writer said, "Forced into a variety of job compromises in their childbearing years that permanently depress their earning capability, the only feasible option for many women becomes a third-rate job with short hours close to home."[26]

Employment, and all of its attendant problems, is a

major issue for women today. Because most women have not been able to effectively shed or share their traditional role of homemaker, many women are substantially overworked (and, I might add, underpaid). And even though we still have many, many social barriers to overcome, there are some remedies that fall within the individual's grasp; something can be done to alleviate the situation. You must have faith, that no matter how grim your circumstances are and no matter how dead-end your life may appear from the inside peering out, there are always options and choices you can make to improve your life.

WHAT TO DO

1. Build leisure time into your life.

This may sound impossible to a tired working woman, but if you take back some of your personal time, you will find that it will increase your energy level. Pay yourself first—take care of your own needs so you can effectively love and work. If you are dissatisfied with your life or worn out, it rubs off on others anyway; children are especially good at picking up on these kinds of feelings. Take some personal time—find something that you enjoy that relaxes you and rejuvenates you. No leisure time will eventually catch up with you in the form of exhaustion, sickness, and unhappiness, which will cost you far more time than I am asking you to take for yourself.

2. Lower your standards.

Most women have standards for the home that are far too high for their own good. Get in touch with the fact that the rules that drive you in your own housework are, for the most part, unconscious and part of your identity as a female. You must start to separate your standards from your sense of womanhood and goodness. When it comes to housework, women are their own worst enemies. You may think you have already lowered your standards; but look harder. Make it a challenge to see how low you can get your standards. You might be joyfully surprised at how low you can really get them and still live happily!

LIGHTEN YOUR WORK LOAD

If you need further incentive, read Ruth Schwartz Cowan's book, *More Work for Mother* (New York: Basic Books, Inc., 1983), paperback, $7.95.

3. Lighten your work load.

Identify all the chores you usually do in a week by making a list. Then set your priorities. Decide which chores can be thrown out totally (ironing sheets, making beds, et cetera), which ones can be delegated to others in the family, and which ones you choose to handle. Try to cut down on the number of times you repeat a task in a week—make the sheets or clean floor last a few days more. How do you do that? Simply ignore them.

4. Communicate more with your family.

Begin by talking with your spouse. Let him know how you are feeling. This is not always easy, but I have found it is most helpful to make what I call "I" statements instead of "You" statements. Start with something like, "I feel _____," or "I need _____." "You" statements usually put people on the defensive, such as "You don't help me enough." The second you hear yourself say, "You—," try to stop yourself. If you really cannot get a word out, or in edgewise, consider writing your thoughts down in a letter and giving it to your spouse. Sometimes I find writing is the easiest and most effective way of saying something very difficult.

Change your idea about housework being women's work. Foster an attitude among your family members, especially young children, that everyone in the home has a responsibility for homemaking—making the house or apartment into a nice home—not just Mom. Giving them everything you can, including all that you can spare of yourself, is not good for their own development. Work is good for children. It teaches them obligation and responsibility. Set reasonable rules and guidelines in the house—and stick to them.

5. Do not feel guilty about child care.

Rest assured; the studies are showing that day care is not detrimental to your children. Some studies are even reporting that there are positive effects to having children socialize with other children and adults. Keep informed about the day-care situation in your area and support all efforts to improve the number and quality of facilities. Get involved and, if you possibly can, help start a center at a school, in your church or temple, in your place of employment—talk to your employer. Women and children need day-care facilities!

6. *Purchase any homemaking chore you can afford.*

Many women, even if they can afford it, will not purchase household help. If you could, would you? And if you can, do you? To have someone come in the home—even once every two weeks—to assist in cleaning and washing is a tremendous help. Consider it; the money is well-spent. If you cannot afford hired help, consider other ways to alleviate burdens. Buy whatever you can afford: day care, diapers, paper plates, laundry service for shirts, cleaners. When we do not get the laundry done, my husband goes to the dime store and buys underwear and socks.

7. *Support efforts to improve the lives of women.*

There comes a point when individual effort is not enough to change the circumstances of life. Many of the problems that women, especially single working mothers with young children, face are firmly entrenched in our culture. Women have made great strides in the last several decades, but we have far to go. By working together, we can all make it better for each individual woman. Social gains eventually do touch all of us. Lend your support to efforts aimed at improving the lives of women and their children; write a letter to a representative or senator for a good cause, join a club; get involved on the community, state, or national level; fight for day care whenever you can.

12

SURVIVE YOUR LOSSES

> Our joys as winged dreams do fly;
> Why then should sorrow last?
> Since grief but aggravates thy loss,
> Grieve not for what is past.
>
> —Anonymous,
> *The Friar of Orders Gray,* st. 13

But grieve we do when we suffer a loss. It is a human reaction over which we have no control. If we try to stifle grief, as the anonymous author of the verse above suggests, we only prolong the mourning process. Whenever we lose something dear to us—whether it is a person, our health, our youth, or our hopes and dreams—we must mourn. Sometimes, however, we may be in a state of mourning without exactly knowing what we have lost. In this situation, a woman may feel pain, an emptiness, a loss of interest in the world, fatigue—and she may be confused about what is wrong in her life.

I think women, more than men, go through life repeatedly suffering losses. They not only endure their own personal losses, but because women place great value on relationships and care so much about others, they also react to the losses incurred by their loved ones.

At some point in their marriages, many women have grieved the death of dreams and hopes that were never fulfilled. Women mourn as their children leave home, one by one, until the nest is empty. Divorce has forced countless women into long periods of grief, leaving them to mourn not only the loss of an intimate relationship, but also the loss of financial security, status, and identity.

As the aging process begins to take its toll, women pay a bigger price than men when they lose their youth, looks, and sexuality. And of course, death imposes untold grief on women as they live their final years alone, without spouse or parents.

Sigmund Freud, the founder of psychoanalysis, was the first to clearly link the mourning process with these types of losses. He wrote brilliantly about it in his 1917 essay "Mourning and Melancholia." Although the language is a bit archaic, the definition can hardly be improved upon:

> Mourning is regularly the reaction to the loss of a loved person, or to the loss of some abstraction which has taken place of one, such as fatherland, liberty, an ideal, and so on. . . . It is also well worth notice that, although grief involves grave departures from the normal attitude to life, it never occurs to us to regard it as a morbid condition and hand the mourner over to medical treatment. We rest assured that after a lapse of time it will be overcome, and we look upon any interference with it as inadvisable to even harmful.[1]

Freud recognized that the mourning process is the normal reaction in response to a real loss in the world. If left to run its natural course, the grief will slowly and gradually fade. The length and depth of the mourning period depends upon the severity of the loss. Another psychoanalyst explained, "The major work of mourning often occupies one year or more and is completed during the second year as the mourner relives the first anniversaries of meaningful occasions previously shared with the deceased as birthdays or holidays."[2]

Some people, however, never seem to stop mourning, especially in cases where there was a strong feeling of dependency upon the person who was lost. Their unresolved grief goes on for years. The feelings of sadness and fatigue are especially strong at anniversaries, holidays, or birthdays. Such people find it difficult to speak about the lost person without crying or may experience other crying spells, especially when alone. Women who are in the perpetual state of grieving seem to have little interest in life and are chronically fatigued.

Why is the human reaction to loss so predictable? Why is fatigue ever-present during the grieving period? Freud explained that we must mourn a loss in order to go on with life. During this time, all of our energies are devoted to separating ourselves from whatever we have lost, be it a person or a dream. This is a terrible struggle, for on the one hand, we do not want to let go of, say, our dead loved one; yet, on the other hand, we know we must let go to resume living. We must slowly and gradually cut all the mental ties that attached us to the person (or whatever was lost). That results in a tremendous expenditure of energy. Freud wrote:

> The task is now carried through bit by bit, under great expense of time and cathectic [emotional or mental] energy, while all the time the existence of the lost object is continued in the mind. Each single one of the memories and hopes which bound the libido [love energy] to the object is brought up and hyper-cathected, and the detachment of the libido from it accomplished.[3]

During the "work of mourning," as Freud called it, a person has little energy left over to devote to anything in the outside world. As the mourner relives each memory to cut each tie, she will feel pain, dejection, loneliness, a loss of interest in the outside world, and fatigue. These symptoms are a sign that the work of mourning is going on. So, whenever you have suffered a loss, it is perfectly normal for you to feel fatigued. Once the work is completed, energy and interest in life will return.

We live in a world that makes it increasingly difficult for people to work through their losses. In days gone by, birth, sickness, and death were truly part of life. The newborn child took her or his first breath in the family home, and Grandma and Grandpa took their last breath there too. The family gathered together during those times and shared their happiness and grief. Now these great events usually occur in a more mechanical and depersonalized setting, in rooms behind doors marked AUTHORIZED PERSONNEL ONLY, that keep the family away. Everyone suffers in silence, trying to deny the loss.

I vividly remember so many patients that I have taken care of in their final hours, behind the imposing doors of an intensive-care unit. With visiting hours almost nonexistent, the relatives were always waiting in some small room far removed from the sickbed. I was repeatedly struck by how cold and cruel dying can be in the middle of humming machines and white-sheeted stainless-steel beds. The sicker the patient became, the more the family was kept away and the more obsessed the medical staff became with tubes and drugs and numbers and machines. Death often became a welcomed relief to the suffering and loneliness the actual dying process had brought to the ill. I always murmured that it should not be that way.

The more technically advanced our society becomes in science and medicine, the more we seem to deny sickness and death—and loss and grief. If this is true, and I really believe it is, then many of the feelings involved in these life experiences get denied too. That is not good. These feelings need to be expressed or they will fester beneath the surface to cause physical and psychological illness.

Some of the feelings that often attend the mourning process are confusing, frightening, and guilt-provoking. It is no wonder that it is difficult for people to talk about them. So many women, who are suffering a loss of some kind, fail to share their inner turmoil, thinking that they should not "burden" others with their problems. I have seen so many suffer in unnecessary silence. How much better they would have felt had they discussed their feelings with others—family, friends, a member of the clergy, a social worker, a doctor!

LOSS OF PEOPLE

Losing a loved one in life—a parent, spouse, or child—is the greatest loss we can suffer. Many never get over the loss of people in their lives, and this often takes its toll in chronic fatigue. People, and their doctors, fail to realize the fatigue is actually a sign of prolonged and intense grief. Women, understandably, have a difficult time cutting the ties with people because they have been the nurturers of relationships.

The Empty Nest

Frances is a forty-eight-year-old divorced mother of three who now works as a social worker. She was particularly fond of her youngest daughter, who lived at home while attending college. As Elsa's college years were coming to a close, Frances began encouraging her to go on to graduate school and offered to help with some of the finances. Elsa did apply and was fortunate to get into a good school, but one that was a long way from home. Elsa was afraid of letting such a distance come between her and her mother, although Frances reassured her the distance meant nothing and reinforced Elsa's ambition.

When Elsa left for school, Frances was the one who had a hard time. She became withdrawn and dejected, lost interest in her job, and was tired all the time.

> "I felt so sad and lonely. It was as if the end of the world had come and there was nothing left for me. I had no one and it seemed as if there was no reason to do anything, especially around the house. I left the bed unmade, the dishes were not done, and when I got home from work at night, sometimes I didn't even make dinner. I just slumped into my chair. I was tired all the time, I felt like I just couldn't get going. Sometimes I called in sick to work because I felt so tired and lethargic."

267

Frances's grief deepened as she tried to stifle her feelings instead of coming to grips with them. After about two months, she became significantly depressed and finally went to one of the psychologists who worked with her.

She told the psychologist how she was feeling but did not bring up Elsa on her own. When the psychologist mentioned her daughter and the fact she had gone off to school, she tapped into the anger Frances had been suppressing.

> "I didn't realize it until Kathy forced me to see it. I was so angry with Elsa for leaving me, I thought, 'That ungrateful child.' I have given my whole life and now I'm giving her some of my money too and she ups and leaves me. I came to realize I was infuriated—which was very difficult for me to admit. I can't tell you how bad that feels, because I felt so guilty about saying those things, feeling like that about her. I thought, 'What kind of mother am I to feel this way about my daughter?' I'm really so proud of her and I wanted her to go. It was all so confusing."

Once Frances started to voice her feelings to her co-worker, they started to make sense to her. Her depression also started to fade once she started talking about her feelings with someone. It took a few more months for her to work through the grief of her loss; then she was able to start making a new life of her own.

Frances, like millions of other middle-aged women, was suffering from what has been called the "empty-nest syndrome." The syndrome occurs at a time in a woman's life when she must adjust to reaching the end of her child-rearing role. After years and years of child rearing being her main occupation, the loss of that role and the child can be extremely stressful and is usually mourned. The woman must find a new way of life, explore new roles for herself, and find other means to obtain emotional gratification. Some women have more difficulty than others, but it is normal for all women to have a period of feeling fatigued, low, sad, and empty when children leave the nest.

Women have a particularly difficult time making this adjustment when their only or last child leaves home, when the relationship with the child has been very close, or when there is no spouse available to provide emotional support. It is important to remember that no matter how prepared one is for the occasion, a child leaving home is a loss that is mourned.

Divorce

A loss-laden occasion for which we never plan is divorce. When we marry, we carry the hopes and dreams of romantic love into the union. Even if there are problems at the beginning, we hope that "things will work out okay." None of us ever expects to fail at our marriage.

The first time Marion considered that her marriage might be failing was even before her first child was born.

> "I married way too young; I was only eighteen. Within the first few months of my marriage, I knew I had made a mistake. I found that he had another side to him at home with me than he had for other people. He was terse, brusque, short, taciturn, and noncommunicative. He resented if I wanted him to share anything with me. He wanted to go in the basement and be by himself.
>
> "I would have gone along with anything he wanted to do, but I felt that he wanted to be left alone. I thought something was wrong with me, because he didn't want me around. It made me feel terrible about myself. I should have left then, before it was too late, but I was too scared."

Then the family started to grow, first one child, then another, and another. Marion tried to make the best of it; she tried to make a good home for the family; she tried to work on the relationship, but it slowly got only worse. Years passed and the children grew.

Finally, Marion started contemplating divorce. Sometimes when the thought came into her mind it was comforting; it gave her a sense of hope. At other times, the thought terrified her and made her panic. She started setting deadlines for herself, "I'll leave when the children are out of school," "I'll leave when my mother is over her illness." Marion struggled with balancing the pros and cons of staying and leaving. She had never worked for wages before in the outside world and was terrified that she could not support herself.

Then one night she and her husband got into a particularly bitter fight. She realized, as she listened to him, that she was hearing the same old attitudes of twenty years ago. Nothing had changed, and she was convinced that nothing was going to change. Her hope died as a result of that fight, and she walked out the next day with her youngest child, carrying a little bit of money and a suitcase. She had no idea where she was going, she had no job, and she had no hopes or dreams.

When she got settled two weeks later, she wrote the following to her husband:

> I am sorry, so sorry about the hurt, frustration, and anguish that we are all going through, but a decision had to be made regarding our own slow death of spirit and life. I am not coming home. I do not want to come home on just promises and years of heartaches. Not only we but all our kids were suffering from our poor relationship . . . I think I love you sometimes; I hate you other times; I'm lonesome; I don't ever want to see you again; I go through the whole gamut of emotions. I love our house, especially in the summer; I love the patio, the garden, and my plants on the porch. There is so much I miss. Ann misses you, her animals, the house, her room, her friends—so much too. Yet to not have the dissension, the quarreling, the angry tones is all such a relief.

Everything that Marion missed was turned into losses to be mourned, because she and her daughter never went back. She was not only mourning the loss of a relationship, she was feeling the loss of her home, her hobbies, even the household pets.

However, Marion's losses did not stop there. Like millions of other divorced women, she also faced losing her financial security and her status and identity. Marion lost the security of her husband's income, her "job" as a homemaker, many of her belongings, her neighborhood, the proximity of her friends, and her identity as a housewife. Now she was a separated, lonely woman waiting for a divorce and hunting for her first job.

If a divorce is not mutual, women also must struggle with personal feelings of rejection and a loss of self-esteem. This is especially true when another woman complicates matters. Marjorie, a forty-three-year-old mother of three grown children, said that her world fell apart within a few hours. She discovered her husband was seeing another woman. When she confronted him with it, he asked for a divorce. After a few months of terrible bickering and fighting, he moved out and filed for divorce. Marjorie sank into a state of profound grief, fluctuating with intense periods of rage. Given all her losses, many similar to those that Marion suffered, Marjorie discovered that her loss of self-esteem was a major problem during her transition period.

> "I put my whole life into being a good wife and mother, and now I feel like a total failure. I'm obviously not a good wife—and at forty-three, what chance have I got at starting over again? I never did go to college, and somehow I always think he held that against me. . . . Sometimes I am afraid that the children blame me for him leaving."

There are so many losses and fears to cope with in divorce. Most people fail to realize just how many losses occur in the divorce process. It is not simply a matter of losing a live-in partner. There are profound losses involved in the breakup of even those marriages in which both partners desperately want to get out of the relationship. Often these women, and men too, are surprised when they feel grief after their divorce. When a marriage falls apart, women must mourn many losses besides the loss of the relationship, such as the dreams and hopes of having a good marriage.

Some losses are greater than others; however, all of them are grieved accordingly. And the grieving takes time. This is why the crisis of divorce and the transition period can go on for what seems like a long time. It is a time filled with turmoil and confusion. The feelings of loneliness, fear, anger, pain, hopelessness, guilt, and fatigue are strong.

As Freud said, the grieving process is normal and, left alone, will run its own course. You might think that there is nothing to be done to alleviate some of the distress. This is not true. Talking can help make you feel better and can facilitate the grieving process. Talking about your situation and feelings to someone you trust is the best action you can take.

Death

Perhaps the ultimate crisis in life that involves loss is the death of a loved one. As we mourn a death, we have great needs. We need people to listen to our pain, we need companionship to ward off loneliness, we need people to understand our self-absorption and our need for emotional support. Most of all, perhaps, we need to understand that grieving is a normal process, that it is to be expected, and hence we should be more tolerant of and gentle with ourselves during this period.

Irene faced the unforeseen death of a loved one. Her pain was intensified because she did not know what to expect after her tragic loss. If she had known that mourning is natural and desirable, her grieving would have been less painful. In remembering when she suffered from chronic fatigue, Irene shared this with me.

> "You ask about stress and fatigue. One of the reasons I go to my bed is that it has become a sort of sanctuary. I can doze and perhaps not be aware of all the problems that are confronting me, and time passes that way. Like the time my mother passed away in the car with my husband and me.

"It all happens so quickly (in half an hour) that you do not really know what is actually happening and by the time you do, traveling on the road, you can't reach anyone. We had two funeral services for her, one in [the city] and one in her hometown, and I remember sitting through both of them thinking if I can live through this, I can live through anything.

"I went along normally after that for two weeks and suddenly one night my heart started to go like a trip-hammer, and I was sure I was about to have a heart attack also. My heart continued like that for I'll bet two weeks and I went to my family physician, who merely informed me that I had gone into shock and it might last a month.

"He never did have much of a bedside manner. He never adequately explained my sense of depression for me and I floundered around for maybe a month, going to different doctors and discussing it with people but never reaching any solution.

"I even went to a psychiatrist because I felt I was so different from my normal self that perhaps I was losing my mind. I had a five-year-old son and I didn't even have the energy to get him up in the morning to go to school. I just wanted to lay in bed and not ever get up. . . . Also during this time I could hardly eat anything. The only time I could eat was when I first awakened and all the grief was sort of out of my mind. . . . I eventually found a doctor who was very sympathetic and was able to explain to me that there was nothing wrong with me and it was a perfectly natural reaction."

Irene thought she was losing her mind when in fact she was going through a normal process after losing her mother. Once she was told that, she accepted her feelings and was able to do the work of mourning over two years.

Studies are now showing that confiding in others, rather than shouldering your grief alone, is good for your health. We are now learning that people who bear their burdens in silence pay a price by developing more physical illnesses. It seems as if the relief we experience when we "get a load off the chest" is more than just a feeling; sharing our burdens seems to have a positive effect on our bodies as well.

One study, which investigated the effects of confiding in others, looked at how well widowers and widows were coping a year after the death of their spouses. Those individuals who kept their sorrow to themselves tended to have more ailments than those who shared their pain with others. The study showed that those who talked out their grief were just as healthy as people who had not suffered the loss of a loved one.[4]

We seem to have a pretty good physical explanation for this result. People who do not confide their troubles in others are under more stress than those who talk things out. Stifling grief takes a great deal of mental energy and produces stress. Stress causes numerous changes in the body. Over the long run, this leads to health problems, including chronic fatigue.

LOSS OF PERSONAL ATTRIBUTES

So far, we have been talking primarily about the loss of people; children moving away from home, the end of an intimate relationship through divorce, and death of a loved one. There are other types of losses as well, such as the loss of personal attributes. Some of the losses experienced in divorce are included in this category, such as status, identity, self-esteem, and the sense of security. Other personal attributes that are commonly grieved when lost are youth, beauty, health, and sexuality. While covering a story for CBS News, I was made vividly aware of how devastating such a loss can be to a woman.

Faye was a very attractive blond woman who worked as a waitress in a hotel. She was single, fun-loving, and extremely content with her life. Then tragedy struck.

Faye was working the night that the hotel went up in a blaze. She escaped with her life, but she suffered permanent damage. Although she never saw flames, she was bathed in acrid smoke from the burning plastics. Faye was left with scars on her face, chest, and hands, and severely burned mucous membranes in her throat and eyes.

I had been briefed on her story before I met her, so I knew that she had suffered some disfigurement in the fire. But she looked nothing like the description that was given to me. Before me sat a very attractive, well-dressed middle-aged woman with blond hair, blue eyes, and a big warm smile. She had a delightful personality and a wonderful sense of humor. I had to strain to see any of the scars and yet, in telephone conversations, she had made it sound as if she had suffered gross disfigurement.

I was perplexed at first. She was clearly feeling much more disfigured than her outside appearance indicated. Her sense of loss was out of proportion to her visible scars. I was searching for the physical losses, obviously because they would be the easiest to see, but also because she concentrated on her physical losses in our earlier conversations.

As I sat speaking with Faye in person, I began to understand what she was grieving. She talked about herself as having become an old and unattractive woman who was unlovable. It was clear she linked these changes to the fire. Faye was mourning the loss of several of her personal attributes that, although mostly intangible, she closely associated with her good looks.

She equated the scars on her face to not only the loss of her good looks, but also the loss of her youth and her sexual desirability. In one tragic stroke, Faye felt she had lost her youth, beauty, sexuality, health. All of these losses had destroyed her sense of well-being and gave her much to mourn. She was still grieving three years after the fire, and had not yet completed the work of mourning. She was doing a good job at it though, because she was talking about it openly.

Many women suffer the kinds of losses Faye was grieving when they go through the menopause. In this youth-and-beauty-oriented society, women become concerned over the effects of aging. And because women have traditionally been valued and rewarded for good looks more than men have, this is a period in life that can be filled with losses.

First, the menopause marks the loss of the ability to bear children. When so much of women's lives has focused upon childbearing and child rearing, this loss can be especially painful. If a woman's sexuality is closely linked with her childbearing function, a woman may also feel the loss of her sexual attractiveness at this time.

Second, the menopause may bring about body changes that accentuate the aging process and clearly make a statement about the passing of years. If ours were a culture that venerated old age, women would not suffer a loss with the passing of youth. Unfortunately, there is no reward for aging in American culture and so the passage of youth is something we mourn. Our culture's concept of beauty is narrowly and tenaciously linked to youth. Hence, not surprisingly, women usually perceive the loss of youth and beauty as one in the same.

Menopause is a time of life that is filled with personal losses, whether it be one's health, youth, or sexuality. Some of the losses, such as our health and sexuality, can be lessened through life-style changes. Smoking, drinking alcohol, poor nutrition, and no exercise seem to take a greater toll on postmenopausal women than on premenopausal women. When losses occur, such as the loss of one's health through sickness, try to be gentle on yourself. Be aware of the grieving process and take an active role in doing the work of mourning your loss by confiding in others close to you.

LOSS OF HOPES AND DREAMS

Not only must we mourn for things we have had and lost, we must also grieve for things for which we have hoped but will never be. We all have hopes, dreams, and fantasies about how we would like our lives to be. Some of our expectations come from the early days of childhood, while others have been formulated during our adult years. We nourish them and keep them alive as long as possible. However, there often comes a time in life when we realize that an important dream or hope cannot possibly come true, and then the hope or dream dies. It is a loss that we must mourn, the loss of an ideal.

Another story I did for CBS News poignantly demonstrated how painful the loss of a dream may be. I reported on the hope offered by new medical technology to couples who had previously been unable to conceive a child. However, no matter how advanced our technology has become, there are always those who cannot be helped. Sometimes couples go through years of medical procedures while trying to conceive, only to find out that they are still sterile. They cannot have children.

As part of the story, I was allowed to sit in with a group of couples who met on a regular basis to discuss their sterility. They were helping one another mourn the loss of a child that would never be. So many people tend to take having children for granted in this age of birth control. Most people have the dream or expectation of bearing children, and almost take the ability to do so for granted. The couples that I saw taught me the depth of loss that they felt when the dream is shattered by reality. What they had to say made me cry. And their pain made me think a long time.

Many women today are choosing not to have children, even though they had hoped or expected to have them. Contrary to the traditional notion that equates motherhood with femininity, many women have discovered their identity through their work or other pursuits and are very satisfied with their lives.

Some women have decided that they do not want to sacrifice their careers or close relationships with their husbands to have a child. Others may be in a bad relationship and know a child would not thrive in such circumstances. Other women may never develop that intimate relationship for which they had hoped.

Whatever the reason may be, the choice to remain childless is accompanied by a feeling of loss for many women. It is the loss of the hope or expectation of experiencing pregnancy and motherhood. Many women go through a period of decision making, and then grieving.

Marlene, a very successful lawyer, is just beginning to enter that period of her life. She is divorced but has always hoped to find a man with whom she was compatible. Now she faces a serious illness that is forcing her to think about children and marriage.

"I'm getting up there in age, I'm thirty-six. But the funny thing, when I started looking at 'Do I want children?,' and I chose not to up to this point even when I was married, I always thought in my mind that I wanted kids between the ages of thirty-seven and forty-two. So I actually set a period of time for myself in which to have children, which has not yet arrived. But if I get to that point in life without having them, I think I will feel a great loss. I think I will be really upset.

"A couple weeks ago I found out that my ovary has something on it. And it has grown remarkably fast. I have been told I probably have a tumor there, because it has grown 4.75 centimeters in two months. So I face the possibility of not having the choice to have kids. I do not like the idea of them taking one [ovary] out of me, and I could even lose all my reproductive organs. What does that do to me as a person?

"I never realized that some of the things I have been doing really have been hidden and linked to some old values. I still live, and have chosen to live, in a rented apartment complex. Many people have advised me to buy a house for investment purposes and I retort 'No, that means permanence. I am in a temporary situation.' But I have been in that 'temporary' setting for eight years.

"Maybe I did have some hidden old values even though I am the single, career woman. I now realize I was equating being single with temporary, and being married with permanence. I have been sitting in an apartment, hoping a man would come along and change my housing situation. There must be an old value in me that says hitching up with a man is necessary in order to be in a permanent situation. I was putting off something I might want to do because I did not have a man, and you see I was never in contact with what I might want to do, which is permanence. I never faced that. I was convinced I wasn't in a holding pattern. I was convinced I was making a full choice based on a new value of temporary versus an old-fashioned value of permanence, and only when it came down to losing the possibility of having children did I realize that my temporary living arrangement is connected to other things that really do mean permanence—a husband and a family."

Even though Marlene is satisfied with her life as a single career woman, it is clear that the old values of love, marriage, and motherhood are bubbling beneath the surface. She had little idea how much these "old-fashioned values" were affecting her decisions. Only when an illness threatened her with the loss of her reproductive organs and hence the loss of the choice to have children, did she begin to realize how much she has longed for a good marriage and children. Marlene is just beginning the mourning process for those lost dreams in preparation for the drastic surgery that may take place.

Throughout our lifetimes, we experience many losses. Some are easily recognized, such as the loss of a loved one. Others are not so apparent. Sometimes we may find ourselves feeling pain, emptiness, dejection, and fatigue without being aware that we are mourning the loss of something. Personal attributes and ideals are not often thought of as things we lose, but actually when you stop and think about it, these are some of the losses we grieve most deeply.

I have covered several of the major losses women must face: the empty nest, divorce, death, aging, and unfulfilled dreams. There are many more. A woman, after being a homemaker for many years, may decide to begin an education or train for a job. She may mourn the loss of years and a chance gone by. Another woman may grieve the loss of a job.

Yet whatever the loss, the grieving process is basically the same. The work of mourning must be done and, unfortunately, there are unpleasant aspects to it. It is natural to experience distressing emotions and to be drained of energy. However, rest assured that this normal reaction will pass if it is allowed to run its course. You can survive your losses.

WHAT TO DO

1. Learn to recognize your losses.

Your feelings of loss may not always be on the surface, in your conscious mind. However, when a grieving person has the question "Have you suffered a loss?" put to her, she can usually identify one. Ask yourself: Am I suffering a loss? Have I lost a person: a child, husband, lover, friend, or parent? Am I grieving over the loss of my looks, youth, sexuality, or health? Have I lost a position, my status, my security, or my way in the world? Have any of my dreams or hopes or ideals recently died?

2. Accept mourning as a natural reaction.

When we suffer a loss, we must grieve over it. It is human to do so. Accept the mourning process as a normal and healthy response, recognizing that it means you will feel bad for a while. You must work through your feelings, which means expressing all of them without apology. As each feeling gets expressed for what it is, you will then be able to let go of it. This work of mourning takes time, so be patient and gentle with yourself. Be aware that if you attempt to stifle your grief, you will prolong the process and burden yourself with emotional baggage.

A person in mourning may be in pain, lose interest in the world, lack energy, and complain of fatigue. These may be accompanied by a wide range of emotions including sadness, guilt, resentment, rage, anger, envy, and loneliness. Some of these emotions may predominate over others; not everybody suffers the same emotions or the same intensity of feelings. The mourning period may vary considerably in length. However, the worst of it should be over after one or two years.

3. Confide in others.

Share your grief, it is good for your health. Bearing your burdens alone will make the process more difficult, create more internal stress, and ultimately lead to illness. Be discriminate in your choice of a confidant. Pick someone with whom you are comfortable and you trust: your spouse, a friend, a religious counselor, a therapist. Try keeping a diary. Confiding on paper can be beneficial also. Writing can help get a load off your chest perhaps as well as talking. Try writing about your feelings for fifteen minutes at least four times a week.

4. *Read* On Death and Dying *by Dr. Elisabeth Kubler-Ross (New York: Macmillan Publishing Company, Inc., 1969).*

This is a remarkable book that I hope everybody reads in her lifetime. It is a must for anyone suffering with a dying loved one. The book is primarily about helping the terminally ill die a more peaceful and dignified death. The book explores the mourning process that both the patient and the family go through in the final struggle. Dr. Kubler-Ross offers insight on how to cope with the losses that death imparts. Although this book is specifically about death and dying, many of the concepts can be helpful to a person mourning any kind of loss.

5. *Seek medical help if grieving turns into severe depression.*

If instead of improving with time, grieving gets worse and includes symptoms of severe depression, you should be evaluated by a competent professional. Besides feeling down or blue, these symptoms would include physical disturbances (such as a change in sleep habits, a change in eating habits, headaches, extreme fatigue, menstrual problems, or impaired sexual functioning), feelings of helplessness, hopelessness and/or thoughts of suicide. Depression is a very painful illness, and one need not suffer the agony of feeling this way. A wide variety of treatments is now available and one should not hesitate to seek assistance. In the next chapter, we will be exploring depression in detail.

13

BEAT YOUR BLUES

When does ordinary sadness become depression? Often the
line between everyday sorrow and depression is blurred. We
all have periods of feeling low, blue, or sad, and accept them
as a normal part of the human condition. As we saw in the
last chapter, a period of grief is considered normal after a
permanent loss. Perhaps, though, on some occasions those
moods have left a person wondering whether or not she is
normal or abnormal. What is normal? When should one go
for help? Too often these questions remain unanswered, and
people suffer in silence.

A person should be able to distinguish between normal
mood changes and abnormal mood states; there can be serious consequences otherwise. It is estimated that only 20
percent to 25 percent of those suffering from depression
receive treatment.[1] This is a tragedy, for depression can
cause terrible suffering and disability, and it can lead to
death. It is responsible for at least 25,000 suicides a year, and
suicide now ranks as the tenth leading cause of death in the
country.[2,3] Most important, people do not have to suffer the
agony of depression anymore. Most depressions can be very
successfully treated today with help of new antidepressants.

Depression is a mood that people seem reluctant to talk
about or admit that they experience. (I think that is because
people have a difficult time facing despair and because depression has the stigma of being considered a "mental ill-

ness." I hope both reasons disappear in time.) If you judged on the basis of the amount of talk you hear about it, you might suspect that depression is relatively rare.

Unfortunately, depression is widespread. It is one of the most common conditions doctors see; it is certainly the most common problem psychiatrists treat. And most of the patients are women. Somewhere between 20 percent to 30 percent of all women will experience depressive episodes in their lifetimes.[4] Some experts have even called depression a disease of women. It is at least two times more frequent in women than it is in men.

The word *depression* can conjure up different meanings for different people. Some may use it to mean feeling blue, while others (especially doctors) use the word *depression* to refer to a severe condition that requires medical intervention. Obviously, there is a range of states between these two extremes and the term *depression* can be appropriately applied to all of them. At times, such a broad usage of the word may be confusing to us, but it does serve a purpose. Depression refers to, in all of these cases, a disturbance in mood. It is only the degree of severity that differs. Psychiatrist George Engel talks about the range of depressive reactions and their causes:

> The adjective *depressive,* as used here, refers to a wide range of reaction patterns, including the mood swings of everyday life, normal and pathological grief and loss reactions, and the major affective disorders (neurotic depressive reaction, psychotic depressive reaction, involutional melancholia, and manic-depressive illness).
>
> In a broad sense, the depressive reactions all occur in response to a real, threatened, or fantasied loss of sources of emotional gratification, be it a loved person, home, job, status, strength, physical attractiveness, or even ideals or goals. Such losses may include illness, death, marriage, graduation, military service, or any other real or threatened separation from a loved person; or they may involve

any life change, including chronic illness or disability, which requires one to give up or modify relationships or way of living. Especially important are the crises of middle and later life . . . women [may become concerned] about fading attractiveness, loss of childbearing capacity, and decline in the importance of their maternal functions. The fading of life goals reduces motivation and incurs a feeling of futility often experienced primarily as fatigue.[5]

Fatigue is inseparably linked to depression. In many cases, especially in women, fatigue is the primary way a depression is expressed. The more severe the depression, the more profound the fatigue. Thus fatigue, as part of the depressive reaction, can be triggered by the normal blues of daily living, the grief reaction (as we saw in the last chapter), or more serious depressions. In this chapter, we will look at the connection between fatigue and depressive reactions, I will have you answer a simple questionnaire to rate your mood, I will tell you when you should get concerned about depression, and, of course, give you some tips on what to do about it. First, let us put depression into the context of our everyday moods.

A SPECTRUM OF FEELINGS

Mood is defined as a state of mind or of feeling. The feelings experienced in life can range all the way from utter despair to euphoria. We can plot this on a line, with despair at the far left and euphoria at the far right (see Figure 17).

Normally our mood is somewhere in the middle, and based upon what life has in store for us, we dip down into the blues or pop up into happiness. Many times it is difficult for a person to describe her mood in precise terms; so it is not easy to determine exactly where a person fits on the scale.

Depression is simply another name for the range of sad feelings and can be seen as a continuum on the scale. A

THE MOOD SCALE

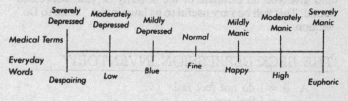

Karen Ann Atkinson

Figure 17: *Mood is represented by a spectrum of feelings, with severe depression representing one extreme.*

person can be mildly depressed, moderately depressed, or severely depressed. Or, using the everyday words, the feeling could be described as "blue," "down," or "despairing."

We can say that a mood is abnormal—a disorder—when a person experiences an extreme feeling, either high or low, for a prolonged period. Not only is the intensity of the mood important, the length of time a mood persists is very useful in judging whether or not it is of a serious nature. We have all experienced moments of despair and euphoria, although we do not remain in those moods for a long time. We may feel devastated by a failure to get a promotion or upon being told we have done one of our tasks poorly. Nevertheless, the feeling passes relatively quickly and we can still feel good about ourselves.

A SELF-RATING DEPRESSION SCALE

Now that we have developed a scale of moods ranging from the abnormal to the normal, let us see how you are faring. The following is a self-rating scale that measures depression. It is called the Beck Depression Inventory and will take you only about ten minutes to complete. Simply circle the number that represents your choice on each letter item. After you have finished all items, add up the encircled values. The total score will indicate whether or not you are depressed and give you an estimate of the severity of your depressed mood. This will be very useful to us later in the "What to Do" section.

THE BECK DEPRESSION INVENTORY[7]

A. 0 = I do not feel sad.
    1 = I feel sad.
    2 = I am sad all the time and I can't snap out of it.
    3 = I am so sad or unhappy that I can't stand it.

B. 0 = I am not particularly discouraged about the future.
    1 = I feel discouraged about the future.
    2 = I feel I have nothing to look forward to.
    3 = I feel that the future is hopeless and that things cannot improve.

C. 0 = I do not feel like a failure.
    1 = I feel I have failed more than the average person.
    2 = As I look back on my life all I can see is a lot of failures.
    3 = I feel I am a complete failure as a person.

D. 0 = I get as much satisfaction out of things as I used to.
    1 = I do not enjoy things the way I used to.
    2 = I do not get real satisfaction out of anything anymore.
    3 = I am dissatisfied or bored with everything.

E. 0 = I do not feel particularly guilty.
    1 = I feel guilty a good part of the time.
    2 = I feel quite guilty most of the time.
    3 = I feel guilty all of the time.

F. 0 = I do not feel that I am being punished.
    1 = I feel that I may be punished.
    2 = I am disgusted with myself.

3 = I hate myself.

G. 0 = I do not feel disappointed in myself.
   1 = I am disappointed in myself.
   2 = I am disgusted with myself.
   3 = I hate myself.

H. 0 = I do not feel I am any worse than anybody else.
   1 = I am critical of myself for my weaknesses or mistakes.
   2 = I blame myself all the time for my faults.
   3 = I blame myself for everything bad that happens.

I. 0 = I do not have any thoughts of killing myself.
   1 = I have thoughts of killing myself, but I would not carry them out.
   2 = I would like to kill myself.
   3 = I would kill myself if I had the chance.

J. 0 = I do not cry any more than usual.
   1 = I cry more now than I used to.
   2 = I cry all the time.
   3 = I used to be able to cry, but now I can't cry even though I want to.

K. 0 = I am not more irritated now than I ever am.
   1 = I get annoyed or irritated more easily than I used to.
   2 = I feel irritated all the time now.
   3 = I do not get irritated at all by the things that used to irritate me.

L. 0 = I have not lost interest in other people.
   1 = I am less interested in other people than I used to be.
   2 = I have lost most of my interest in other people.
   3 = I have lost all of my interest in other people.

M. 0 = I make decisions about as well as I ever could.

1 = I put off making decisions more than I used to.

2 = I have greater difficulty in making decisions than before.

3 = I can't make decisions at all anymore.

N. 0 = I do not feel that I look any worse than I used to.

1 = I am worried that I am looking old or unattractive.

2 = I feel that there are permanent changes in my appearance that make me look unattractive.

3 = I believe that I look ugly.

O. 0 = I can work about as well as I could before.

1 = It takes extra effort to get started at doing something.

2 = I have to push myself very hard to do anything.

3 = I can't do any work at all.

P. 0 = I can sleep as well as usual.

1 = I do not sleep as well as I used to.

2 = I wake up one to two hours earlier than usual and find it hard to get back to sleep.

3 = I wake up several hours earlier than I used to and cannot get back to sleep.

Q. 0 = I do not get any more tired than usual.

1 = I get tired more easily than I used to.

2 = I get tired from doing almost anything.

3 = I am too tired to do anything.

R. 0 = My appetite is no worse than usual.

1 = My appetite is not as good as it used to be.

2 = My appetite is much worse now.

3 = I have no appetite at all anymore.

S. 0 = I haven't lost much weight, if any, lately.

1 = I have lost more than five pounds.

2 = I have lost more than ten pounds.

3 = I have lost more than fifteen pounds.

I am purposely trying to lose weight by
eating less:
Yes_____
No_____

T. 0 = I am no more worried about my health than
usual.
1 = I am worried about physical problems such
as aches and pains, or upset stomach, or
constipation.
2 = I am very worried about physcial problems, and it's hard to think of much else.
3 = I am so worried about my physical problems, I cannot think about anything else.

U. 0 = I have not noticed any recent change in my
interest in sex.
1 = I am less interested in sex than I used to be.
2 = I am much less interested in sex now.
3 = I have lost interest in sex completely.

To determine your score, add the numbers you circled in
items A through U. The highest score possible is 63. I would
consider a score of around 10 means "not depressed";
around 20 means "mildly depressed"; around 25 means
"moderately depressed"; and over 30 means "severely depressed." Mildly depressed can be considered to be part of
everyday mood swings; it would fall within the normal range.
Moderately depressed makes me concerned, and I think
people who fall within this range should be evaluated by a
doctor so that the depression can be treated. Those who are
severely depressed definitely should be seen by a doctor.

These numbers and categories are not hard and fast.
This questionnaire is simply a means of providing a person
with a general idea of whether or not she is depressed and
how severe it might be. It does so by measuring the presence
and severity of twenty-one of the more common symptoms
seen in depression, listed below.

Mental symptoms: Sadness; pessimism; sense of
failure; dissatisfaction; feel-

289

ings of guilt; sense of punishment; self-dislike; self-accusation; self-harm; crying spells; irritability; social withdrawal; indecisiveness; change in self-image; difficulty working.

Physical symptoms: Sleep disturbance; fatigue; appetite change; weight loss; decreased interest in sex; and other problems, such as aches and pains, headaches, upset stomach, or constipation.

It is important to remember that there is a large variety of symptoms that a person can have while depressed, and, of course, not all people will react to depression in the same way. Some people may have many symptoms, while others may have only a few. However, the more severe the depression, the greater the tendency to experience several symptoms.

FATIGUE AND DEPRESSION

Fatigue is almost always present in depression. It may take a variety of forms, as psychiatrist George Engel explains:

Depressive reactions characteristically are dominated by various expressions of fatigue, including weakness, tiredness, drowsiness, lack of energy, loss of interest, apathy, discouragement, a sense of weight or heaviness, and a general feeling that it is no longer worthwhile to exert oneself.[8]

To many people, depression *is* fatigue. More than just feeling sad, these people experience their depression primarily as a loss of energy and a loss of interest in the world and cannot really differentiate between the feelings. Some doctors question whether all chronically fatigued people ought not to be diagnosed as being depressed.

In some people fatigue will be the predominant symptom of depression although other symptoms are usually present. Sometimes, however, chronic fatigue is the only symptom of an underlying depression. This kind of depression is called a "masked depression." That is because it is hard for both the person suffering from it and the doctor to see it. Often, upon detailed questioning by the doctor, a person with a masked depression will become aware of a recent disappointment or loss, and the presence of some of the more common symptoms—sleep changes, appetite changes, and feeling glum.

Fatigue may also herald a depression. Chronic fatigue may persist for weeks or months before the other symptoms of depression become obvious. Darlene's story really illustrates this.

"I think I was fatigued for years. I always felt like I never had enough energy. No amount of sleep could fix it. Then, when I was in my late twenties, I noticed over a period of a few months that I was getting more and more tired. I really had to push myself to do things, but I was going to bed earlier and taking naps whenever I could, like on the weekends. I just didn't have the energy to do anything I didn't have to. I saved my energy so I could get through my day.

"Then I got depressed, but I didn't know what it was at first. I had crying spells for no particular reason, I lost my appetite—and, subsequently, about ten pounds—I was nauseated some and had constipation, and I wanted to sleep all the time. And I felt terrible about myself, I thought I was totally useless in the world.

"It got so bad that the only thing I could do is get out of bed, go to work, fake my way through the day, and come home and collapse in bed. I don't even know how I managed that. Through it all, I think it was the fatigue that bothered me more than anything else, even more than the feeling blue and down on myself. The fatigue was the thing that held me down."

Many women know depression as Darlene has described it. They may be chronically fatigued for months and then slide into a full-blown depression. Studies have shown that fatigue is one of the most consistent and overwhelming symptoms depressed people report. And this statement appears to be truer for women than for men. Some studies have concluded fatigue is much more common in depressed women than in depressed men.[9]

Why is this so? No one really knows. We do not understand the biochemistry of fatigue, nor have researchers fully worked out the biochemistry of depression. I will hazard an educated guess, however, and say that we will probably discover the two phenomena are intrinsically linked. The missing link may explain why women are more susceptible to both fatigue and depression.

In one sense, we can view depression as a withdrawal response, a type of protective mechanism. In severe depression, a person totally withdraws from the world. It is almost like wrapping up oneself in a protective coat and hibernating. Perhaps depression is simply an extreme extension of everyday fatigue; they both act as mechanisms to make us stop and recover.

Maybe fatigue is "minimal depression," somewhere between normal mood and mild depression on the mood scale. When I get extremely fatigued, I experience many of the symptoms of depression: bad mood, irritability, low motivation, loss of appetite, stomachaches, headaches. Granted, they are not as severe as one would find in depression, but they are similar.

WOMEN AND DEPRESSION

Why women and depression? What causes so much depression in women? Researchers have tried to explain why depression itself is more common in women by citing the sex-hormone theory of causation. We learned in Chapter 2 that apparently any time a woman's hormones are fluctuating, she is more likely to experience fatigue: for instance, during her premenstrual days, after childbirth, and during menopause. The same appears to be true for depression. Minor feelings of depression are commonly reported during periods of premenstrual tension. Furthermore, up to 50 percent of all women suffer some degree of depression—the "baby blues"—within ten days after giving birth. About 10 percent of them experience severe depression.[10] In none of these situations, however, have researchers been able to find a responsible hormone.

Depression has also been said to occur more frequently around the time of menopause. Now experts are saying that the data suggest that menopausal depressions, if they do occur, are not caused by hormonal changes, but rather that psychological stresses related to the event may be responsible. However, other experts report that hormone-replacement therapy does alleviate the depressions (and fatigue) that seem to develop around the time of the menopause. So even though there is some evidence to suggest sex hormones may be linked to depression, research has yet to identify any specific mechanism, and the mystery is unsolved.

Researchers have also tried to explain female susceptibility to depression by looking at genetic and biological factors as well as hormonal factors, but none of these seem to account for the predominance of depression in women. Now researchers report that they "have turned to the area of life stress to explore the apparent vulnerability of women to depression. Certain life events can be correlated with depression and psychophysiological symptoms, both of which predominate in women."[11]

People who suffer with depression have probably undergone more stress in life. The stress does not necessarily have to be of any certain type, although certain events tend to trigger depression more readily than others. Myrna Weissman and Dr. Eugene Paykel, who conducted a study on depressed women, found that, "These [stresses] include separations and losses (both physical and interpersonal), arguments and difficulties with loved ones, blows to the self-esteem, and other events categorized as undesirable. Separation from close persons is the most common event reported."[12]

For every category that Weissman and Paykel list, studies are beginning to show that women experience more stress than men. I say "beginning," because initially, stress studies could not demonstrate any difference between women and men. Critics of those studies have pointed out that the early scales used to measure life stress were not asking the right questions that would tap into the areas that women found particularly stressful. For example, early stress scales measured personal stresses and did not ask about events happening in the lives of significant others, such as one's children, that might stress women. Life-event scales also did not measure events that are major stressors in women's lives: menopause, children leaving home, physical assault, sexual abuse, incest, rape, abortion, and sex discrimination. Furthermore, these scales were not sensitive to chronic conditions that affect women's lives, such as poverty, large families, divorce, or ill health. The stress scales were biased toward men's lives, and not particularly relevant to women's lives. Once the scales were rewritten, women's stress scores started to reflect the depressions they were feeling.

June remembers only too well the stresses she was under when she was depressed, and she told me one of the greatest difficulties during the whole period was coming to terms with her bad marriage.

"I felt like I physically (not mentally) couldn't cope for at least a year. I was so tired I'd have to say sometimes out loud, 'get moving,' 'no one else can do this but you.' All this at a time when I was getting enough sleep by the books, eight hours a night. Life circumstances at that time? I was continuing to hold together a marriage of twelve years that shouldn't have gone past the seventh year. I was also working on a Ph.D. and teaching full-time in a community college. I also did all the household chores. A vivid thought that always came to me at night was, 'I wish I were at least sixty-five years old. That way, this wouldn't have to go on so interminably.' Understand please, I wasn't suicidal, I just couldn't even see that life would be different and I was so tired."

294

I think the feeling that June had during her depression is one that women experience often. And that is the feeling that life will never change and that there are no options available. There are always options. When you are feeling depressed or otherwise, try to remember that there are always options to choose from in life. They may not be "free" but they are there. June found that out.

> "I found that once I decided to take control of my life, I was no longer exhausted. I began seeing a marriage counselor, came to terms with my feeling about divorce and went through with that. Then I made the commitment to finish the Ph.D. and get it off my list. Result—more time for me and more control over my time. I find I get very tired and down when I let my life and actions be under the control of others rather than taking charge. When I have my life under control, my energy returns."

I have to admit, I was a little surprised by the number of women who told me, as June did, that they conquered their feelings of depression and fatigue when they took control of their own lives. Taking control usually meant setting limits on the demands others were making of them and striking out to develop themselves and their career.

A thirty-six-year-old working woman gave me her key to beating the blues and tiredness: "Stay in control of as much of your life as possible. Be as self-directed in your life as possible, as opposed to other-directed."

So often in the past, it was assumed that when a woman was depressed, it was due to difficulties in one of her relationships, because it was perceived that that was the only source of a woman's satisfaction and happiness. Researchers Baruch and Barnett tested this assumption in their study on what contributed to the well-being of women. In their book *Lifeprints,* they contend that depression in women is not intrinsically linked to relationships. Quite the contrary.

> We found symptoms of depression and low self-esteem among women with few difficulties or depri-

vations in their relationships but with major problems in their work life. Conversely, many women—for example, divorced women with satisfying jobs—reported serious problems in relationships, yet were not depressed. When one's sense of selfhood and role in society is intact, one can usually tolerate a reasonable amount of unhappiness or dissatisfaction in relationships without developing symptoms of depression and anxiety . . . merely being employed, regardless of the kind of job, helped protect women from developing psychiatric symptoms. We would argue that this is because work can provide a sense of self-esteem, meaning and *control* often hard to come by in the thorny area of human relationships. [13]

What is the link between the lack of control and depression? This is an important question because it may give us some insight on why depression is so common in women and some hints on what to do about depression. Many researchers are now focusing on women's disadvantaged status as a possible contributor to their depression. Women have been raised and taught to be helpless and depend on others, especially men. Such learned helplessness, one expert writes, "suggests that the expectation of powerlessness and inability to control one's own destiny, whether real or perceived, prevents effective action on one's behalf." [14]

In other words, if a woman feels that she has no power over her life and can do nothing to change her situation or feelings, she may use withdrawal—fatigue or depression—to protect herself. Women often shut themselves down, for weeks or months at a time, because they feel they have no right to an emotion, to have a need fulfilled, or to make a change in life. To a certain extent, I think depression is a learned coping mechanism for women. If a person is confronted by a dilemma, she can fight or withdraw. If fighting is not perceived as an option, there is only one alternative left—withdrawal through fatigue and depression.

CONQUERING FATIGUE AND DEPRESSION

What can be done on a personal level to combat depression? There really is a lot that can be done. First, women have to ask themselves if their fatigue or malaise is depression. Often, fatigue is the major symptom of depression and it is not clear to an individual that other minor symptoms, such as restless sleep, decreased (or in some cases increased) eating, boredom, and feeling a little blue or down, are all connected.

Depression usually develops slowly and insidiously, and sometimes the depressed person is the last one to know it. Family members, friends, or coworkers may be the first to notice something is wrong. Try to get in touch with your feelings and listen to the comments of others. Depression can be very subtle and hence very difficult to recognize.

How did you do on Beck's Depression Inventory? Are you depressed? Sometimes it is hard for people to admit that they are depressed. I have had many women patients breathe a sigh of relief when I have given them the "permission" to feel their depression out in the open. They felt guilty about being depressed and did not want to burden others with how they were feeling. Repression of feelings takes energy and may even make the feelings worse. By the sheer fact of becoming aware and admitting to feeling blue or downright depressed, you will begin to take control of your life.

Try to think back to when the depression began and recount what was happening in your life. Often depression starts when feelings—the type a woman thinks are unacceptable—are repressed and go unexpressed. Depression is usually a reaction to some emotional event in life. Perhaps someone hurt your feelings and you did not express your hurt and anger. Once you figure out what that event is, then you will have the power to fight your depression. The feelings that caused it must be expressed. Depression results when expression of feelings has not occurred and energy is being consumed to keep the lid on them.

First, admit your feelings to yourself. Then try to share

your feelings with those close to you. It will not only relieve you of the burden of trying to cover them up, it will bring you needed support and also help your loved ones understand you. Talking will make it easier on everyone. If you can identify an event that involved a particular person, express your feelings—no matter how difficult—to that person in a constructive way.

I once solved a big problem by admitting mild depression to my husband. I always get a little blue before my menstrual period, and early in my marriage I found myself getting into stupid arguments with my husband. Of course, they always ended with me being hurt, feeling wretched, and crying. When I finally realized what was happening, I sat down with him and explained how I felt. Now we tread lightly during my premenstrual blues, and I give him warning if I'm feeling particularly sensitive—I *growl* at him. He growls back and cracks me up. Laughing is a great remedy for the blues, at least for a moment.

As we saw in the last chapter, confiding in someone you trust is good for your health. This appears to be particularly true in the case of depression. Studies have shown that women who do not have an intimate confidant or who do not have casual, less intimate friends have more severe symptoms.[15] Do not neglect your social support system when you are feeling down. That is when you may need your friends the most. Make an extra effort to keep in touch and pay them a compliment by sharing with them.

Talking about your feelings—if you cannot identify what is causing them—may assist you in pinpointing exactly what is bothering you. Try to determine what the thoughts are behind the feelings you are having. There is something going on behind those feelings, although sometimes it is difficult to discover what it is. Write your thoughts—especially the negative ones—down on a piece of paper. Those are the culprits. Then, once you have a firm idea of what is bothering you, what you are unhappy about in your life, take action. This is part of taking control.

Taking control is particularly difficult when you are feeling blue. I think the motivation is often there, but it is often extremely hard to initiate an activity that you may want to do or a chore you want to tackle. Pick one thing each day you really want to accomplish and put your energy into that. You will feel a sense of reward when you can do it, and that will help beat the vicious cycle of feeling bad.

Another activity that will help is exercise. Exercise is a very powerful weapon against all degrees of depression, from mild to severe. Exercise exerts its antidepressant effect precisely where it is needed—in the brain. It boosts the amount of norepinephrine, the neurotransmitter that is depleted in depression. The body derives a host of other benefits from exercise, too, if you recall from Chapter 6. It helps your energy level, decreases anxiety, raises your self-esteem—all of which can only be both psychologically and physically beneficial for someone who is depressed.

Remember that drugs can cause depression. Review the drugs you take and if you have any questions, check with your doctor to see if the medications you use could be responsible for your depression. Be particularly wary of alcohol, diazepam (Valium), and marijuana. Often women will use more diazepam or alcohol as a means of coping when they begin to get depressive symptoms, without being aware that the drugs only make the depression worse. If you are feeling depressed or routinely experience premenstrual blues, try to avoid these drugs altogether. You really will fare much better without them.

GETTING HELP

There are some blues and depressions we can handle by ourselves, along with our families and friends. Others are more serious and should be treated by a doctor. At first glance, this may appear to be an obvious statement; however, most people with depression who should be treated do not seek assistance. You should never hesitate to ask for help if you do not think you can handle your depression on your own. Sometimes, when you are in the middle of a depression, it is hard to see the forest for the trees. How do you know when to ask for help? When does feeling blue become a depression that needs to be treated?

If you recall, earlier I talked about two factors that can be used to judge the seriousness of a depression: the severity of the low mood and the length of time it has persisted. Generally speaking, if the depressed mood is intense and prolonged (over one month) and it interferes with the activities of daily living, then it should be treated.

I have provided you with Beck's Depression Inventory to assess the intensity of a depression. I think anyone who scored "moderate" or "severe" should see a doctor. If you scored "mild" and prefer to try to cope on your own, give yourself one month. If you have not improved in one month, you should see a doctor also.

Why see a doctor? First, the cause of the depression should be sought. A thorough physical examination should be conducted to determine if an underlying physical disease (several directly cause depression as part of the disease process) is the source of the depression. Furthermore, all current medications should be reviewed as possible causes or complicating factors of a depression. Once these two major sources, physical disease and drugs, are ruled out, it is then appropriate to consider antidepressant drug therapy.

Second, depression can be very successfully treated today by doctors. Unfortunately, only 20 percent of depressed people receive treatment. Most are suffering longer than is necessary! Depressions can be cut short by the use of medications. These treatments are sometimes augmented with psychotherapy, which helps a person gain insight and control over her life. Often depression is caused by unresolved losses and conflicts from the past and it will take the help of a trained therapist to work them out.

Treatment for depression is very good, and most people suffering with it can expect an excellent recovery. And yet depressed people often have an inappropriately bleak outlook on treatment and their future. If you are depressed and contemplating seeing a doctor (which I hope you are), try to approach the experience with an open mind and see it as an opportunity to get better and grow as a person.

Be willing to consider all treatment methods, including psychotherapy or hospitalization, if your doctor suggests it. I have seen a week's stay in the hospital change many women's lives. It obviously cannot fix everything, but the time out, protection, and support offered in a hospital setting can give a depressed woman needed rest and time to think about her life and what changes need to be made.

I still hear the voices of so many women who shared with me the feelings of despair and hopelessness they have had about their lives and about themselves. There is one word that continues to echo loudly in my memory: *control*. When they took control of their lives, then fatigue, anxiety, and depression all started to fade from their worlds. I asked, "But HOW did you take control?" Many of them laughed, and said that things just got so bad, they were forced to do something. Others could see a major crisis coming, so they made a change beforehand. But all of them suffered emotionally, and some physically, before coming to terms with making a change.

Maybe that is it. Maybe depression, and all the fatigue, is nature's way of giving us a message. It says, something is wrong in life. Women should listen to that message, as painful and as hard as depression can be sometimes, and then try to do something about it. Take control and do something, even if it means getting yourself help with the depression. I cannot quite tell you the secret of taking control; we each have to discover it on our own. I just hope this chapter will make you think about it and help you do it sooner than later. If you are depressed, do not let it turn into a crisis.

WHAT TO DO

1. Learn to recognize depression.

The classic picture of a depressed individual—looking sad, disheveled, not speaking, and slumped in a chair—is not the most common form. Depression can be very hard to recognize at times, often appearing primarily as fatigue, with perhaps a little bit of insomnia, an appetite change, and a loss of interest in the world. This is especially true for middle-aged women. Here is a simple checklist of the eight symptoms that form the core of depression:

- fatigue or loss of energy
- difficulty sleeping
- change in appetite
- loss of interest in formerly pleasurable activities, especially sexual activity
- feelings of worthlessness or guilt
- poor concentration
- thoughts of suicide or death

A person is considered to be depressed if five out of these eight symptoms are present for one month or longer. A person with four symptoms is probably depressed.

2. Admit depression to yourself and to those closest to you.

It is so much easier to cope with depression and chronic fatigue if you are not trying to hide your feelings from your family and friends. Although it may be difficult at first, try to tell others how you are feeling. It will make you feel a little better, relieve you of a great burden, and it will help them give you the support you need and understand your behavior. Depression can be stressful on others in your life, particularly when they do not understand what is going on.

3. Confide in others and maintain a good social support system.

Other people can be very comforting when you are feeling blue or depressed. They can help you put your feelings and thoughts into perspective at a time when you are probably being very hard on yourself. You might also find that others who know you well can offer suggestions on how you might effectively deal with a problem or make changes in your life. Recognize that depression is hard to talk about, so pick the person with whom you feel most at ease. You might even start by telling them how hard it is to talk. Make an attempt to talk every day with your special person about how you feel.

4. Exercise regularly.

In order to get the antidepressant effect or preventive medicine effect from exercise, you must do aerobic exercise.

This means taxing your heart and lungs at least three times a week (preferably five) for a minimum of thirty minutes. I know that it is particularly hard for anyone to exercise when feeling down, but it is very important that you try to do so.

I have found that the easiest exercise for women to do while depressed (because it takes the least amount of motivation and you are more likely to succeed) is brisk walking. Begin by thinking of it as a pleasant experience, a time for relaxation and reflection. Start the walk slowly, and try to pick up the pace as you go. Let yourself feel good about the fact that you succeeded in getting out. If you have trouble getting going, a family member or a friend can be enlisted to help prod you along and be a sympathetic listener on the walk. If you would be better off alone, do not hesitate to explain that to your family and take the time for yourself. You will get a mental and physical boost from your walk.

5. Stay away from drugs.

Drugs can cause depression and drugs can make a depression worse. Two of the drugs used most widely by women, alcohol and diazepam (Valium), are the biggest culprits. Initially, you might think you get relief from feeling sad, anxious, or irritable by using these drugs; however, in the long run they will only make things worse. Check with your doctor about all other drugs you use.

6. See a doctor.

Depression can have serious consequences. You not only have to suffer through the mental pain of it, it can lead to physical ailments, loss of job, loss of relationships, and loss of life. Sometimes people can cope quite effectively with mild depression; other times they cannot. You should seek help if you have had symptoms of depression longer than one month. Also, if you scored a "moderate" or "severe" on Beck's Depression Inventory, you should be seen by a doctor. Remember: Treatment is very successful.

7. Take control.

This may be the hardest step, but it is the most important step. You have more power than you think you do, all you have to do is take control. Examine your frustrations and your negative voices, and then make a change. It can be scary at first, but once you start making decisions for yourself, you will feel so much better and you will wonder why you waited so long. Do something to improve your self-esteem. Get a job, go back to school, improve the skills you already have—do something for you. Act on that dream of yours.

Part Four

GET YOUR PHYSICAL

DISCUSS YOUR
FATIGUE

Talking to doctors is often difficult—even for me. Whether we are aware of it or not, we all bring a set of assumptions and a code of behavior to the doctor-patient relationship. Doctors are expected to behave in certain ways, while patients are expected to behave in others.

I have come to understand the differences very well, because I have experienced both roles. Not all of the behaviors assigned to each role, however, are conducive to the patient's best health. Patients have been taught to be compliant and, for the most part, not to question medical authority. Women have become particularly sensitive to being labeled a "hypochondriac" or "hysterical," and as a result, they often avoid seeing doctors or refuse to press for a diagnosis. Women pay heavy prices for such behavior, and must learn to be more assertive.

When I had appendicitis, I had abdominal pain for one full week before my appendix ruptured, but I did not do anything about it. At first, I thought I had menstrual cramps, but then my period was soon over.

Next, I thought the problem was a ruptured ovarian cyst. I knew that if I went to an emergency room and was diagnosed as having a cyst, the doctor could not do much for me. I briefly considered the possibility that I might have appendicitis or an ectopic pregnancy (a pregnancy that occurs outside the womb, usually in the fallopian tube—a rupture in an ectopic is very often fatal), but quickly dispensed with the ideas because I figured I was not having "enough pain" (whatever that is). I should have gone to an emergency room, but I did not.

You see, I was fearful of showing up in an emergency room, only to have some (male) doctor look at me and say, "So you have belly pain, do you, dear?" And then after a few hours of waiting, have him return to the examining room where I was lying, freezing to death with no clothes on or blankets, and say to me, "Well, the tests seem to indicate that everything is okay." Bells go off, and what does a woman hear? She hears: DIAGNOSIS—HYSTERICAL FEMALE. But, it is worse for me because I hear, DIAGNOSIS—HYSTERICAL FEMALE DOCTOR, AND SHE SHOULD HAVE KNOWN BETTER! So instead of taking the risk of having this nightmare come true, I foolishly avoided medical care and my appendix ruptured.

I hope you never have to pay that sort of price for fear of having an interaction with medical professionals. This is the reason for this chapter. In it, I would like to prepare you for some of the experiences you might have when consulting a doctor about fatigue, so as to improve your chances of getting a reliable diagnosis. I will be discussing some of the attitudes you might run into, how to talk with your doctor in a more effective way, and what you can expect to happen during the evaluation of fatigue.

WOMEN AND THE COMPLAINT OF FATIGUE

Unfortunately, fatigue in women is one of those complaints that are often unfairly labeled. Many women have told me that they are afraid of being called "neurotic," "hypochondriacal," or "hysterical" by a doctor, simply because they complain of a symptom, such as backache or headache or fatigue. I think this is a legitimate concern, for doctors have the right to "name." A tremendous amount of power lies in the privilege of naming, because diagnoses made by doctors can have considerable social, economic, and political repercussions, especially for women.

Too often doctors go unchallenged in their assumptions and in their name-calling. Women are accustomed to being dependent on authority figures such as doctors. That is because the doctor-patient relationship is modeled on the parent-child relationship. The parent has most of the power in the relationship and is supposed to use it in the child's best interest; the child is not supposed to question the authority of the parent and is to do what she is told. We have got to start changing that power balance in the doctor-patient relationship so that women are not so much at mercy of the medical authorities.

The doctor-patient relationship is also modeled on the traditional male-female power imbalance. The practice of medicine happens within a cultural context; it is not without the same prejudices and biases that pervade the rest of our society. Medicine discriminates against women in a myriad of ways.

Physicians have different perceptions of men and women. Studies have shown that doctors believe women to be more emotional, have more psychological problems, and provide less reliable information.[1] Furthermore, "Stereotypic notions about women are reinforced in medical school training, textbooks, and medical advertising. Little attention is devoted to female sexuality, and women's psychological illnesses and need for mood-modifying drugs are emphasized."[2] Hence similar symptoms may lead to different diagnoses depending on the sex of the patient. Women's symptoms are more often attributed to psychological inadequacy, while men's symptoms are more often thought to be the result of an organic illness.[3]

One study attempted to assess directly the response of male doctors to vague complaints from men and women. The medical charts of fifty-two married couples, 104 men and women, were reviewed to see how extensively the doctor worked up the complaints of back pain, headache, dizziness, chest pain, and fatigue. The authors of the study reported, "the physicians' workups were significantly more extensive for men than they were for women. These data tend to support the argument that male physicians take medical illness more seriously in men than in women."[4]

Some researchers believe that the differential treatment patients receive appears to be a result of the interaction between physician expectation and patient behavior.[5] The way in which patients present symptoms may influence the diagnosis. It has been shown that women report more mental-health symptoms in the medical interview than men, and use more psychological language to describe their problems. If the doctor expects women to have more mental disease and hears such symptoms, a diagnosis of a psychological problem is more likely. There is something to be learned here. Women might carefully think about the way they communicate with doctors and be on the lookout for such obvious bias.

Uncounted women have told me that when they went to a doctor, complaining of fatigue, they always received sympathy and adequate treatment if a physical cause was found. But not one woman told me that she received sympathy or guidance when the diagnosis was psychological (unless the doctor was a mental-health professional). My sister said to me, "I think the physical doctors should also suggest psychological counselors to their patients and work more closely with mental-health professionals in joint conferences, seminars, or workshops. Perhaps they could even practice together in clinics." Bravo!

If a doctor finds that a symptom cannot be explained by any physical disease process, I think it is incumbent on that doctor to help the patient see that it is a psychological problem and what area of her life it entails, and to assist her in solving it, which could mean simply referring her to the right place to get the assistance she needs, if that is what it takes.

Chronic fatigue is a symptom; it should be evaluated by a physician as such. You may think that you are, for instance, young and healthy, and without "reason" to have a physical disease. This does not mean, however, that you could not have a disease process or physical ailment that is the major source of fatigue or adding to your fatigue. I strongly feel that all women with chronic fatigue should be medically evaluated to rule out disease.

During the evaluation, you will probably encounter some sexual bias. Chances are your doctor will approach your complaint of fatigue with the assumption that its cause is psychological. If you are aware of the biases and assumptions, you can make them work in your favor. If, after a complete physical, your doctor tells you that your fatigue is psychological, I hope you will be better able to handle it and work to resolve the issue.

THE WORKUP OF FATIGUE

The symptom of fatigue is one of those vague complaints that are actually quite challenging to doctors. First, it can be caused by almost anything in life. As we have seen throughout the pages of this book, chronic fatigue can be the result of what we put in our mouth, sedentary living, disturbed sleep, overwork, internal conflicts, the grief reaction, and, of course, illnesses. That is a lot for any doctor to consider in trying to determine the cause, especially if he or she does not know you. That is why it is so important for you to understand your own fatigue and communicate the details.

Second, fatigue is a subjective feeling. For all practical purposes, it cannot be touched with the fingers, seen by the eyes, heard through a stethoscope, or measured with expensive technological tools. The doctor can only listen to your description of your fatigue. This is why the interview is particularly important to the doctor who is evaluating fatigue. Expect many questions, similar to the exercises you did in Chapter 4. Remember, all of those exercises were attempting to get at a piece of information I would ask from you if I were able to see you in person.

The subjective nature of fatigue makes it very easy for a doctor's bias toward psychologically induced disease or sexual bias to creep into the evaluation process. Since fatigue cannot be seen or measured, the doctor can always wonder if it is "real." The doctor may wonder, but you should not forget; your fatigue is real.

Keep notes, start a diary. The more specific you can be with regard to explaining the nature of your fatigue, the better the response from your doctor will be; you will put that wondering mind to rest. It is important to demonstrate that you have taken time to think about your fatigue and that you are concerned with the amount of fatigue in your life.

Indicate that you are very willing to make some changes in life and you do not want pills as a Band-Aid solution to the problem. Also be willing to discuss the psychological aspects of your life—without apology. A doctor has not taken a good medical history unless you have discussed areas such as your love relationship, your sexuality, or your work pressures. All of these profoundly affect our health. So, in the initial workup of fatigue, talk is going to be the doctor's best tool. Expect a lot of it.

The Interview

The first step your doctor will take in approaching your problem of fatigue is to interview you about it. The goal is to delineate as much as possible the characteristics of your fatigue. That means the doctor must ask penetrating questions to get at the fine details of the complaint of fatigue, such as when it started, the length of time that you have had the symptom, the physical setting in which it occurs, any associated symptoms or factors that aggravate the fatigue.

The following questions are the ones that I would ask you about your fatigue. Be prepared. Spend some time thinking about them so that you are able to answer them for your doctor.

1. What does your fatigue feel like? How and where in your body do you experience fatigue?
2. How severe is your fatigue and how much does it interfere with your life?
3. When did your fatigue begin? How abruptly did it begin? How long has it lasted? Has it been constant, or does it come and go? How often does it occur?
4. Is there any setting in which you feel more tired? (Describe your surroundings when you feel most

fatigued. Where are you? Who is around you?
What are you doing?)

5. Is there anything that aggravates or alleviates
your fatigue? (Describe conditions that make it
better or make it worse.)

6. Are there any other symptoms that occur with
your fatigue? (Describe in as much detail as you
can any other physical or mental sensations that
usually accompany your fatigue, for example,
headache, backache, muscle weakness, irritability.)

Because fatigue is such a vague symptom, the doctor
will spend time determining what other symptoms you have
to see if they all point to one disease. For instance, the doctor
might ask, "Have you had any abdominal discomfort? Have
you had any constipation? Have you had any black stools?"
You might wonder what this all has to do with fatigue. What
the doctor is attempting to do, is rule out iron-deficiency
anemia as the cause of fatigue. The anemia could be the
result of a bleeding ulcer, which one would suspect if the
symptoms of pain, constipation, and black stools were present.

Most doctors ask an abbreviated form of the Review of
Symptoms, which you took in Exercise 14 in Chapter 4,
during the interview. It is a checklist to help ensure that
nothing gets forgotten during the discussion. The long list of
symptoms helps the doctor determine if disease is present
and what part of the body or organ system is involved.
Remember that investigating the symptom of fatigue may be
like looking for the needle in a haystack. Your answers to the
ROS will lead to areas in which additional discussion and
tests may be necessary.

The Physical Examination

After completing the interview, your doctor will do a physical
examination and then decide what laboratory tests to order.
The physical exam should be a complete one, including a
breast exam, a pelvic exam, and a full test of your nervous
system. Your doctor will be looking for clues to ailments that

313

might cause fatigue; fatigue per se is not associated with any specific findings. There is nothing that can be found on a physical that will substantiate that you have fatigue; remember, it cannot be heard through a stethoscope or seen with the eye. The doctor can only find evidence of disease processes.

Frequently, no abnormal findings will be noted during the physical. This still does not mean that an ailment is not present. For example, you could be dragging around because of an iron-deficiency anemia without any signs evident on your physical. Only a laboratory test can definitively determine if you have anemia.

Laboratory Tests

The final step in a workup of fatigue is determining what laboratory tests to order. Do not place too much hope that such tests will provide you and your doctor with the complete answer. The few studies that have been done on fatigue show that laboratory tests yield relatively few results. The history and physical examination usually reveal more. Nevertheless, this does not mean lab tests can be totally forsaken.

Because of the vast array of tests and procedures available today, they must be selected thoughtfully with the individual patient in mind. Your doctor will use the information gathered from the interview and physical exam to decide which tests to order. But there are some basic tests that should be included in a workup for fatigue. You are likely to have many of the following done:

Blood Tests

1. *Complete blood count (CBC)*. The CBC will determine the number of red blood cells, white blood cells, and platelets in your blood, the hemoglobin content, and the overall health of your blood. This test is especially important for picking up blood disorders, such as anemia. It will also show signs of an infection in the body.

2. *Biochemical screen*. This "test" of the blood is really a battery of tests conducted with automated equipment. One of the most common screens used in medicine (the SMA-6, or M-6; various labs have different abbreviations) combines

six blood values: sodium, potassium, chloride, carbon dioxide combining power, blood-urea nitrogen, and glucose. These six constituents of blood are among the most important and often are the first numbers a doctor is interested in seeing. Another combination that is often ordered is the SMA-12 (or M-12); this includes determinations of calcium, phosphate, proteins, uric acid, liver enzymes, cholesterol level, triglyceride level, albumin, and bilirubin. Abnormal values for any of these blood chemistries should be evaluated further.

3. Monospot. This is a test to diagnose infectious mononucleosis, one of the most common physical causes of fatigue. Doctors often forego ordering this test. However, I think it is extremely important. In one study on patients with fatigue, the monospot proved to be the most frequently positive laboratory test of all the tests ordered.[6] Twenty percent of the patients had a positive result and were not suspected of having mononucleosis by history or physical exam.

4. Sedimentation rate. This test, called the sed rate, measures how quickly the red blood cells in blood settle in solution. When this value is above normal, it indicates that a disease process is probably taking place in the body and needs further evaluation. Pregnancy can also affect the sed rate.

5. Thyroid-function tests. Several tests are available to assess, either directly or indirectly, the thyroid gland. One of the most reliable means of confirming a diagnosis of hyperthyroidism or hypothryroidism is by measuring the concentration of T4 and T3, the hormones made by the thyroid gland, in the blood. These tests are referred to simply as "a T4 or a T3."

Other Tests

1. Urinalysis. In this test, the urine is examined for the presence of cells (i.e., white cells indicating infection), bacteria, blood and spillage of glucose, ketones, proteins, potassium, and sodium, among others. A urinalysis is a simple and relatively inexpensive test that will quickly check for urinary-tract infections and kidney problems, as well as some metabolic problems such as diabetes.

   2. Urine culture. Urine cultures are done to either sub-stantiate the suspicion that a urinary-tract infection is present or determine the kind of organism causing the infection. This entails getting a specimen of urine from a "clean catch" void (uncontaminated from the body's opening) and incubating it in special growth media in a lab.

   3. Glucose tolerance tests. This test, called the GTT, determines your body's ability to handle a carbohydrate load, sugar. Both high blood sugar (diabetes) or low blood sugar (hypoglycemia) can cause fatigue. You can be checked for both conditions with the same test. After eating a standard amount of glucose, your blood-sugar level is drawn two hours later. If the value is below normal, you are probably hypoglycemic; if above normal, you are probably diabetic. (I say "probably" because stress can produce an abnormal response to the test.)

   4. Electrocardiogram. The EKG measures the electrical activity of your heart and is a fairly good indication of its general condition. It is an excellent screen for picking up heart problems.

   5. Chest film. This is an x-ray of your chest that reveals to your doctor the state of your lungs and heart. Occasionally it will also give clues to other problems in the area, such as in the neck, shoulders, upper portion of the stomach, and part of the liver.

   6. Pregnancy test. This test should be done on all women who are able to conceive, no matter how remote the possibility of pregnancy. Fatigue is one of the earliest symptoms of pregnancy, which oftentimes is not suspected by the woman for a variety of reasons. Failures occur with all forms of contraception, and pregnancy has occurred during the menopause. So, if you are sexually active, a pregnancy test is warranted.

GETTING AN ANSWER

This is the most important part of your communication with your doctor and, unfortunately, it is probably the area that needs the most improvement. All too often, patients leave the doctor's office with only a vague sense of what is wrong with them or no answer at all. And when I say answer, I do not mean simply a name for your condition, such as diabetes mellitus or a psychological problem. The answer I am talking about is an understandable explanation of what is causing the fatigue and, most important, an explanation of how it is going to be treated and a description of your responsibility. I can hear you mumbling, "Fat chance."

Such skepticism is probably warranted. In a study conducted in Denver, Colorado, the records of 176 patients with fatigue were evaluated to determine the cause of fatigue in each case and whether or not the doctor communicated the final diagnosis to the patient.

In many cases, the patient met with or talked with the physician only once, even though the subsequent results of the lab tests gave the doctor the probable cause. It concluded that, "Despite the fact that 92 percent of the cases reviewed had one or more diagnoses associated with the fatigue, 51 percent of the cases had no documented follow-up visit or telephone call to the patient to clarify the problem of the patient."[7]

Based upon what people have told me about their experiences with doctors, this study is probably representative. I recently overheard a young woman say in a restaurant, "I hate doctors. They never explain anything to their patients." I think most of us are probably like her; smart and experienced but in the dark when it comes to our own well-being. If you do not get a satisfactory answer from your doctor, you must ask for it. Ultimately, your health is your responsibility. Do not stop until you have your questions answered.

You must set out with the idea that you are entering into a partnership with the doctor to solve your problem of fatigue and that you are determined to get an answer, not just a name. Ask questions until you are blue in the face. Women, particularly, are so accustomed to being quiet and docile when faced by a physician. How many times have you left a doctor's office wishing you had asked the question, or just as you hit the street all the questions you forgot started rushing into your mind?

Many people think doctors are purposely vague in their

explanations. I do not think it is purposeful, but I agree that they are often vague. Often doctors think they are being crystal clear in their explanations when in fact they are talking gobbledygook. I have interviewed countless doctors on television and I always forewarned them that they had to speak in terms everyone will understand. Few of them ever did. Many times, even when doctors think they are speaking in a manner that laypeople can understand, they are not communicating effectively. They seem to forget everyday language.

You have to tell them you do not understand. You have to ask for more clarification. I hear doctors talking a mile a minute, using medical jargon in such a way that it makes the patient feel as if she should know what those words mean. People may assume that because the doctor is talking that way, everyone else understands the words except them. Wrong. Most people do not understand the lingo and why should they? Do not feel bad for not understanding. Do not be afraid to say, "I don't understand." Getting a satisfactory answer to your problem of fatigue should be your goal; do not stop short of it.

WHAT TO DO

1. Select a good doctor.

Try to find a doctor with whom you can talk and feel comfortable. Shop around. It is best to try to find either a family-practice doctor, a general practitioner, or an internist to do the initial evaluation for fatigue. You might need to be referred to a specialist if you have a special problem, but you would do best to start with a generalist.

Some doctors are better than others. Better educated, progressive, congenial physicians are less likely to simply treat the symptom of fatigue without searching for the real cause. You do not need to put up with doctors who are not willing to explore the real cause of your fatigue if no physical ailment shows up in your tests. Nor do you have to deal with doctors who will not answer questions, are obviously sexually biased, or are patronizing in any way. If you are offended by a statement such as, "Now, dear, you just let me worry about that" in answer to one of your questions, let the doctor know. Ask him or her not to refer to you as "dear." Doctors need feedback about their behavior. They do not always know when they are doing something offensive. Some will be grateful for the information and try to change. Others will not.

If a doctor is not responsive to such a request, do not put up with it. How do you "not put up with it"? Do not go back (or if a situation becomes intolerable, leave). You are essentially hiring a doctor as a consultant to your health. Do not hand over all control and power to the doctor. Keep some for yourself. Remember, you always have the right to fire a doctor. Do not be afraid to do so. Do it in person, call, write a letter, or simply, just do not go back.

2. Be prepared to discuss your fatigue.

Doctors tend to attribute symptoms to psychological causes if they are presented in a vague way, especially if the patient is female. The better you articulate your problem, the more responsive your doctor will be. Have answers for the questions I put to you earlier in this chapter. Be as open as possible during the interview, do not be afraid to discuss any topics (as we have seen throughout the book, almost anything can cause fatigue), and take with you notes, a diary, or work you have done in this book to help delineate your fatigue. Give the doctor the message that you would like assistance in solving the problem, whatever the problem turns out to be, not just treating the symptom.

3. Be assertive.

Ask questions. And in particular, ask the following questions:

- What did you find on physical examination?
- What laboratory tests are you going to order and what will they tell you?
- What do you suspect is the cause of my problem at this point?
- If a drug is prescribed, be sure to ask all the

questions discussed in Chapter 8—including what it is, how it is to be taken, what the side effects are (is fatigue one?), and if it interacts with any other drugs or alcohol.

If you really find it difficult to ask these questions and you just cannot seem to get them out of your mouth, try writing them down before you go. Then when the doctor asks if you have any questions, or when he or she is talking with you near the end of the appointment, give the paper to the doctor. That way the list of questions will get answered one by one. If you tend to forget things that are said in the doctor's office, write the answers down.

Or try taking someone with you. Introduce the person to the doctor, and tell the doctor you would like that person to be present. Some doctors will ask the person to leave the room during the physical examination, but most doctors (all, I hope) will allow the person to join you when you discuss your problem at the end of the consultation. Let that person help raise questions that you want answered and think you might have difficulty bringing up. I have accompanied several friends to the doctor and this works very nicely.

4. Get good follow-up.

The symptom of fatigue does not elicit the best follow-up from physicians. If you do not get your answer in the first visit to your doctor and both of you have to wait for the results of laboratory tests, decide with the doctor how and when you will receive follow-up. Tell the doctor you want to know the results of the tests, even if they are normal, and work out a plan of action. Ask the question "Where do we go if the tests are normal?" "What should I do to get rid of fatigue?" Make an appointment for either the next visit or a telephone call.

If you have a positive (abnormal) laboratory test, ask your doctor what it means and what will be done. If you have a battery of negative tests and the doctor says, "From the looks of all the tests, everything seems to be okay," or "Nothing is wrong," do not let this statement pass.

Something is wrong or you would not be so tired. Confront your doctor if you receive this kind of comment. I made a list of several questions you could come back with, depending on how aggressive you can be. Consider these:

- What next?
- Then why do I feel so bad?
- Then what do you think is causing my fatigue?
- What should I do to get rid of my fatigue?
- What do you mean by that comment?
- What you're saying is that you have found nothing physically wrong. Are you implying that something is psychologically wrong?
- Then you are saying the cause is psychological, but not of great concern to you.
- Are you implying that my fatigue is (pick one) "all in my head," "imaginary," "unreal," "made-up"?

Practice going through the scenario in your mind and think of some other ways to handle the comment. If you ever find yourself in a situation where you need to respond, your having practiced the scene will come to your rescue. It will not take you by surprise and you will be ready with a response. Just do not let a comment like that from your doctor end the conversation, and if you do not fire back immediately, it certainly will.

If you lost your chance to ask a question, or you remember one long after you have left the office, it is never too late. Write your questions down and call or write or make another appointment to get them answered. And do not give up until you do.

5. *Be open to the idea of a referral.*

Your doctor may discover you have a special kind of physical ailment that is better dealt with by a specialist, or after talking, your doctor may decide that you are struggling with a difficult life situation and you would do well with a psychological referral. Be open to the suggestion of referral to a private psychiatrist, psychologist, mental-health clinic, or a community program for counseling. If the doctor does not make a referral, ask for one. We all have psychological conflicts in our lives, and sometimes other understanding people can be very helpful in getting us to sort them out. There is no reason not to take advantage of such guidance and help.

In preparation for this possibility and to help your physician decide what would be the best type of service for you, check your insurance plan, if you have insurance, to see what kind of mental-health benefits are covered. There is a wide variety of policies and it would be extremely helpful if you knew that information before going to your doctor's appointment. If you do not have insurance, ask what other mental-health resources are available in your community.

__15__
RECOGNIZE YOUR AILMENT

Veronica was a thirty-three-year-old woman who was admitted to the hospital because of her fatigue. She had been feeling quite well up until about one month prior to admission, when she started getting tired easily and became short of breath whenever she exerted herself. Her appetite had vanished and she lost about ten pounds without trying.[1]

When the doctor examined her, Veronica appeared well nourished despite her weight loss. She looked a bit sallow, though, with the whites of her eyes actually showing a yellow tint. The rest of her physical exam was completely normal, except for a fairly loud heart murmur. In Veronica's case, her physical was not very helpful in providing any clues to the cause of her fatigue.

Her laboratory tests provided the answer. Veronica's complete blood count showed that she had half the normal amount of red blood cells. Her red blood cells and white blood cells were also abnormally shaped. Veronica's fatigue and shortness-of-breath was due to anemia (decreased oxygen-carrying capacity of the red blood cells). What was causing the anemia? Subsequent laboratory tests showed that Veronica's body was severely lacking in Vitamin B_{12}, which is necessary for the development of healthy blood cells.

It is rare for someone to become Vitamin B_{12} deficient through dietary problems, so doctors suspected that something else was wrong. They discovered that Veronica could not absorb Vitamin B_{12} from her intestine because she lacked a substance called intrinsic factor. Veronica's disease is known as pernicious anemia.

The treatment for pernicious anemia is relatively straightforward: Vitamin B_{12} is injected directly into the body, bypassing the need for intrinsic factor. Shots are given monthly for the rest of the patient's life. However, if left untreated, pernicious anemia is fatal within one to three years. So it is important to make the diagnosis and start treatment.

I start this chapter with Veronica's story to illustrate a point. So often, women and doctors automatically assume that fatigue is caused by a psychological problem. It might have been tempting for Veronica's doctor to ignore her fatigue as indicative of some psychological difficulty, such as depression. But it was clearly caused by a physical condition and it was fortunate that a diagnosis was made in time.

The number of physical causes of fatigue is actually much greater than commonly believed, if one considers all physical causes of fatigue, including poor nutrition or dieting, lack of exercise, smoking, use of alcohol and other drugs, pregnancy, menopause, poor sleep, advancing age, diseases, surgery, medical treatments such as radiation, chronic pain, and occupational hazards. Unfortunately, many doctors do not consider all of these diagnostic possibilities when evaluating a patient.

Fatigue is indeed an elusive symptom; it can indicate a variety of physical disease processes. You and you doctor should be persistent in your pursuit of the cause of your chronic fatigue, because fatigue is one of the most common (and often the first) symptoms of an underlying medical problem. In this chapter, I will concentrate on diseases and medical conditions that can cause fatigue.

DISEASES

Infections

An infection is any illness caused by biologic organisms (viruses, bacteria, fungi, parasites) that invade the body and begin to multiply, leading to tissue damage and causing the body to mount an immune response. Infections are common; about one quarter of all people who go to a doctor do so because of an infection.[2] Infections—especially *viral* infections, such as the common cold—are a major physical cause of fatigue. Energy that is usually available for other activities is used to mobilize the body's defense mechanisms to ward off the infectious invader.

The more generalized the infectious process is throughout the body, the more fatigue and malaise you will feel. But even a localized infection, such as a urinary-tract infection, can quietly sap you of your energy. It may take some time to refill your energy coffers after an infection, so do not be surprised if the fatigue lingers after the infection is gone.

Infections can occur anywhere in the body, creating all kinds of symptoms and disorders. Sometimes they can mimic other diseases and lead doctors on a wild-goose chase. Because of the various courses infections can take, it is difficult for me to give you hard and fast rules to determine if you have one. However, there are certain symptoms that are very suggestive of an infectious process:

- abrupt onset of fatigue (and other symptoms)
- fever
- chills
- muscle aches
- swollen glands

The more widespread an infection, the greater your chance is of experiencing these symptoms. If an infection is walled off in a region of the body where it does not affect the rest of the body, you may not experience fever and chills. Two

325

groups of infections extremely common in women often illustrate this: urinary-tract infections and sexually transmitted diseases.

Urinary-Tract Infections (UTI). Infections of the urinary tract (kidney, bladder, and urethra) are very common in women. It is estimated that at least 20 percent of all women have at least one episode of painful urination a year, and that 15 percent of all women will have an acute UTI sometime during their lifetimes.[3] Not everyone with an infection will have overt symptoms (this is why it is important for the doctor to check your urine on a workup of fatigue). However, if you have these symptoms, suspect a urinary-tract infection:

- pain on urination
- urgency of urination
- frequency of urination

Fever and chills are not usually seen in lower urinary-tract infections (bladder and urethra), though these symptoms are common in upper urinary-tract infections (kidney). Kidney infections are usually much worse and the person with this infection knows she is sick. Any of the following symptoms can be present:

- fever
- chills
- nausea
- vomiting
- diarrhea
- pain on or urgency or frequency of urination

Sexually Transmitted Diseases (STD). Unfortunately, these diseases are on the rise in women. And when I speak of sexually transmitted diseases, I mean more than the old standard venereal diseases, such as syphilis and gonorrhea. There are at least twenty-five different infections of the reproductive tract that are spread through sexual contact, caused by such diverse organisms as bacteria, viruses, protozoa, and fungi.

These infections can range anywhere from a low-grade vaginal infection undetected by the woman, to serious pelvic inflammatory disease (PID). PID is an ascending infection that passes from the cervix, up through the uterus and fallopian tubes, and into the abdomen. It can be very serious, resulting in infertility, hysterectomy, and sometimes death. Any of these infections should be treated.

If you have any of the following symptoms, you may have an infection by a sexually transmitted disease (STD) organism.

- increased vaginal discharge
- change in color of discharge
- foul-smelling discharge
- painful intercourse
- vulvar irritation; itching, burning, swelling

Pelvic inflammatory disease is likely when any of the above symptoms are also accompanied with any of these:

- abdominal pain
- pelvic pain
- abnormal menstrual bleeding

Mononucleosis. Mononucleosis is an infectious disease famous for its ability to cause fatigue. It is an infection caused by a herpes virus that reproduces in lymph tissues. During childhood, the infection causes minimal symptoms. However, during the adolescent years and beyond, they can be overwhelming. Mononucleosis usually begins with three to five days of:

- headache
- fatigue
- malaise
- muscle aches

These symptoms are followed by a week to three weeks of:

- sore throat
- swollen lymph glands
- fever

Early in the course of the illness, mononucleosis may be difficult to distinguish from other infections that routinely cause sore throat. A complete blood count will help make the diagnosis by showing elevated levels of monocytes and lymphocytes (white blood cells, which fight infection) in the blood, an SMA-12 will show elevated liver enzymes, and antibodies against the virus will be present in the blood.

There is no treatment for the viral infection. Therapy consists of treating the symptoms of headache, sore throat, achy muscles, and so on, to make the patient comfortable. Rest is important to convalescence, which takes about a month.

Allergies

An allergy is a hypersensitivity reaction mounted by the body to a tiny amount of material. The list of materials capable of causing allergies is a long one indeed, including dust, pollens, molds, animal danders, chemicals, drugs, and food. Many people are only aware of the chronic fatigue that comes from a smoldering allergic reaction, and not the fact that they have an allergy. Since the best treatment for an allergy is avoiding the offending agent or getting desensitization shots—the allergen must be identified.

Allergic Rhinitis. This condition is more commonly known as hay fever, but the name is a poor one because the condition has nothing to do with hay, and fever is not one of the symptoms. The classic symptoms of allergic rhinitis are:

- sneezing
- runny nose and postnasal drip
- stuffed nose
- itching, watering eyes
- dry cough
- dull headache
- fatigue

Allergic rhinitis is often seasonal, triggered by the airborne pollens of weeds, grasses and trees. However, many women develop *perennial* symptoms due to other allergens in the environment that they are constantly exposed to (such as house dust, animal dander, or materials and chemicals used on the job), often without realizing they have allergies. Chronic fatigue and dull headaches, associated with an occasional "cold," might well be allergic rhinitis.

Food Allergies. Allergies to certain foods are very real and can cause a multitude of symptoms, both subtle and not so subtle. The usual offenders are milk, eggs, fish, shellfish, nuts, seeds, chocolate, oranges, and tomatoes. Symptoms of allergies to these foods include:

- fatigue
- headaches
- depression
- itchy skin rashes
- gastrointestinal problems (cramps, bloating, gas, diarrhea)

Food allergies can sometimes be difficult to diagnose. "Elimination diets" are used to search for the offending food or foods. Specific foods are totally removed from the diet for a few weeks. Then, if the symptoms improve, individual foods are slowly added back to the diet while a careful watch is made to see if symptoms return or not. Also, blood tests are available to test for some of the food allergies.

Cardiovascular Diseases

The cardiovascular system is one of the three sytems of the body that is directly involved with oxygen delivery to the tissues. The other two are the respiratory system (lungs) and the hemopoietic system (blood). The lungs draw oxygen into the body and transfer it to the blood which carries it, and the heart pumps the blood so that oxygen is delivered to all the distant parts of the body. A disorder in any one of these three systems can result in poor oxygen transport and ultimately cause fatigue.

Heart disease is very common in this country; it is the leading cause of death. As the strength and health of the heart begin to decline over the decades, a person is capable of less and less activity before fatigue sets in. The shortness of breath and fatigue that a physically fit person experiences after vigorous exercise are similar to the same shortness of breath and fatigue a heart patient will feel after walking up a few steps; the difference is only the amount of activity it took to bring on the exhaustion.

It is only a matter of degree. A lot of Americans, especially women, have allowed their heart to get flabby and out of shape. The heart is a muscle and it must be kept in shape; if it is not, our capacity to perform our daily tasks is diminished. This lack of cardiovascular fitness is probably one of the most common causes of fatigue and heart disease.

Symptoms of heart disease are caused by three basic mechanisms: (1) a lack of oxygen to the heart itself, (2) a disturbance in the muscular contraction of the heart, or (3) an abnormal rate or rhythm of contraction.

A lack of oxygen usually produces the symptom of chest pain, or angina, that is common in heart attacks. The following can also occur:

- numbness or tingling in arm
- tightness or choking in neck
- pressure sensation
- pain in neck, jaw, throat, shoulder

Disturbances of muscular contractions lead to failure of the heart to pump the blood required by the body. This is known as heart failure and can be recognized by the following symptoms:

- fatigue and weakness
- shortness of breath
- difficulty breathing while lying down
- swelling of the extremities
- faintness, headache, anxiety

Sudden disturbances of rhythm cause the following symptoms:

- palpitations
- shortness of breath
- chest pain
- fainting

Two underlying disorders are responsible for causing most heart disease: hypertension and arteriosclerosis.

Arteriosclerosis. Arteriosclerosis, commonly known as hardening of the arteries, is the primary cause of coronary heart disease (CHD). Approximately 5 million Americans have CHD, and it is the leading cause of death in those over the age of forty-five. Males are typically more at risk of developing CHD than females, although women with high blood pressure, diabetes, high fat levels, or premature menopause are also at high risk. Several risk factors make it more likely a person will develop arteriosclerosis and subsequent heart disease:

- cigarette smoking
- hypertension
- obesity
- no physical activity
- emotional stress
- high fat and cholesterol levels
- high blood sugar, as in diabetes

There is no known treatment for arteriosclerosis once present, there is only treatment of the complications that arise from it. All efforts should be made to reduce the risk factors for the disease so as to prevent its development or slow its progression.

Hypertension. Hypertension is an elevation in arterial blood pressure. Initially, it is a disease without symptoms. However, left untreated it will slowly progress until it causes death. People with untreated hypertension often die ten to twenty years prematurely. Death typically results from heart disease, stroke, or kidney failure.

Hypertension is a particularly disturbing disease to doctors because it can be detected and treated so easily. It is extremely important that everyone have their blood pressure taken at least once a year to check for elevations. It can be normal one month and go up the next. No one is exempt from the risk, regardless of sex, race, or age.

Although most people with hypertension do not have any obvious symptoms, symptoms can be present. They are due either to the direct effects of elevated blood pressure or to the organ damage created by the high pressures. The organs most often affected are the heart and kidneys. Elevated pressure can directly cause the following:

- dizziness
- palpitations
- fatigue

Symptoms of organ damage include:

- nosebleeds
- blood in the urine
- blurring of vision
- weakness and dizziness
- chest pain
- shortness of breath

Treatment of hypertension with medication is easy and successful. A word of caution, however: Many of the antihypertensive medications cause fatigue or depression as a side effect (see the drug lists in chapters 8 and 14). Talk to your physician about this possibility before the prescription is written.

Blood Disorders

There are countless disorders of the blood, and with many of them, fatigue is a cardinal symptom. The blood system, along with the cardiovascular and pulmonary systems, is central to delivering oxygen to the tissues. Any condition that compromises the blood's ability to carry or deliver oxygen will cause fatigue. Anemia, in particular, is such a group of diseases.

The classical symptoms of anemia, which are either directly the result of a decrease of oxygen in the blood or indirectly the result of the body's attempt to compensate, include:

- fatigue
- shortness of breath
- weakness
- palpitations

More severe anemia can cause:

- dizziness
- headaches
- faintness
- irritability
- difficulty in sleeping
- hypersensitivity to cold
- loss of appetite
- nausea
- menstrual irregularities

Anemia is not a disease per se; it describes a condition. Anemia is any disorder in which the red blood cells are deficient in number, volume, or hemoglobin content. The word *anemia* does not indicate the cause of the condition. There are over one hundred kinds of anemia, from such causes as: iron deficiency, folic-acid deficiency, B_{12} deficiency, sickle-cell, thalassemia, a bleeding ulcer, heavy menstrual periods, rheumatoid arthritis, chronic inflammation, and cancer. Thus it is not enough to make the diagnosis of anemia by doing only a complete blood count. The doctor must figure out what is causing the anemic condition.

Iron-deficiency anemia is by far the leading cause of anemia in women. It is estimated that in the United States at least 20 percent of women of childbearing age and over 60 percent of pregnant women who do not receive prenatal care are iron-deficient.

Iron is used in the manufacturing of hemoglobin, the protein that carries oxygen inside red blood cells (RBC). If the delivery of iron to the bone marrow falls short, hemoglobin production will fall. Because hemoglobin makes up 90 percent of the protein in RBCs, a lack of it will make the RBCs small and pale. This is exactly what one sees under the microscope in iron-deficiency anemia—small, pale red blood cells.

There are four conditions that can cause the body to become iron-deficient: (1) increased requirement (pregnancy), (2) decreased dietary intake (poor diet or dieting), (3) decreased intestinal absorption (intestinal diseases), and (4) blood loss (menstrual loss). In women, blood loss and decreased dietary intake are the most common causes of iron-deficiency anemia. In many cases, menstrual blood loss cannot be altered (although use of the oral contraceptive pill does tend to decrease menstrual flow), so iron-replacement therapy is usually the best treatment. Before starting iron-replacement therapy, however, the doctor must rule out all other causes of iron deficiency to make sure a correctable problem is not missed.

Sometimes women can be iron-deficient without showing any significant anemia but still experience weakness and fatigue.[4] I think this is an important problem that is not often being diagnosed. Most of the body's iron is found in the red blood cells, but smaller amounts are found in important chemicals in the muscles and the rest of the body.

Perhaps in early iron deficiency, the red blood cells have a priority over muscles and other tissues in competing for the small amount of iron. So, while the red blood cells may still be normal, other tissues could be suffering from an iron deficiency, resulting in fatigue and weakness. Often doctors do not order iron studies unless they see an anemia; I think doctors should check for anemia and iron deficiency at the same time. One can still be iron-deficient without showing a flagrant anemia.

It is imperative that every woman makes sure she is getting enough iron in her diet. This can be done by either increasing the amount of iron-rich food you eat, or by taking a supplement. However, with many women cutting down on the fat and cholesterol in their diet, meat is not being consumed as often. It may be necessary to add an iron supplement.

Premenopausal women should get at least 18 milligrams

of iron a day, while postmenopausal women need about 10 milligrams a day. A woman's iron requirement increases severalfold during pregnancy. The normal diet, however, is often unable to meet the higher demand. Sometimes the use of 30 to 60 milligrams of supplemental iron per day is recommended by doctors during pregnancy and the first three months after birth. Ferrous sulfate is the preferred preparation, as it is more readily absorbed by the body. Check with your doctor if you are pregnant and considering taking iron.

Respiratory Diseases

The pulmonary system's main task is to get oxygen into the body. Oxygen is our most immediate vital substance; we can go without water and food for hours and days, but we can only last a few minutes without oxygen. As we saw in the case of heart disease and anemia, any disease process that directly affects the transport of oxygen to the brain and other body tissues will cause fatigue. When the respiratory system is diseased in any way, oxygen transport is usually affected. It is not surprising then that lung disease is often the underlying cause of fatigue.

Respiratory disease can be the result of a local disease process in the lung, or it can be the result of an illness elsewhere in the body. Unfortunately, many people are developing lung problems because of smoking, environmental pollutants, and occupational exposures, all of which can be controlled. Regardless of the disorder, respiratory conditions tend to exhibit themselves through a few symptoms:

- shortness of breath
- chest pain that is usually localized and related to movement
- cough and sputum production
- coughing up blood
- fatigue

Respiratory disease leads to a decrease of oxygen in the body, which in turn causes the lungs and heart to work harder to get more oxygen in. Ironically, the harder the lungs work at breathing, the more oxygen they consume, leaving little left over for anything else. The work one must do to breathe with some lung diseases can actually require five to ten times more energy than a healthy person uses just breathing normally. It is no wonder one becomes so exhausted when afflicted with a respiratory disease.

Chronic Bronchitis and Emphysema. Chronic bronchitis is one of the most common respiratory diseases. The single most prevalent cause of the disease is cigarette smoking, although environment and occupational exposures are factors. Chronic bronchitis is characterized by:

- mild shortness of breath
- excessive mucous production
- chronic coughing

Emphysema usually occurs with chronic bronchitis, especially in cigarette smokers, although it can occur in isolation. It results in enlargement of the air spaces in the lungs with destruction of the surrounding tissue.

Estimates indicate that one quarter of women (and two thirds of men) will have well-defined emphysema, although not all will complain of symptoms. Emphysema is characterized by:

- severe shortness of breath
- minimal coughing
- small amounts of sputum

Chronic bronchitis and emphysema eventually lead to narrowing of airways, which obstructs the flow of air in and out of the lung. Thus both bronchitis and emphysema act in unison to cause COLD, or chronic obstructive lung disease. Most people with COLD have evidence of both processes going on in the lung.

As mentioned previously, smoking is the most frequent cause of obstructive processes, although other factors, such as air pollution, occupational exposures, infection, and genetics, do play a role. These factors point to ways to decrease the chances of developing COLD; quit smoking and avoid as many toxins as possible—even change jobs if necessary.

Treatment consists of getting patients to exercise and stop smoking. Exercise has been shown to increase work capacity before fatigue sets in and to improve the sense of well-being. Drugs can occasionally alleviate the symptoms, although nothing can reverse the damage that has already been done.

Asthma. About 3 percent of the population suffers from asthma. It is a disease of the airways through which air is carried in and out of the lung. These passageways are extremely reactive to all kinds of stimuli that can trigger the attack: allergens, drugs, environmental and occupational substances, emotional upset, and exercise. An attack results in narrowing of the airways, which leads to the symptoms of:

- shortness of breath
- coughing
- wheezing

The attacks may go away spontaneously or be halted with drug therapy. Occasionally, a mild state of asthmatic attack can persist for weeks, leading to oxygen deficiency and chronic fatigue.

Some people can develop what is called occupational asthma. Exposure to a substance on the job may trigger an attack. These substances are of six types: metal salts, wood and vegetable dust, industrial chemicals and plastics, pharmaceutical agents, biological enzymes, and animal and insect dusts and secretions.[5]

Typically, these people are quite well when away from work and well when they arrive at work. However, toward the end of a shift the symptoms may develop, only to get worse as the person leaves work, but disappear after being away from work a few hours. The clue to the real cause of these attacks may lie in the fact that coworkers have the same symptoms. Asthma and fatigue may well be occupational hazards.

Endocrine Disorders

The endocrine system, in conjunction with the nervous system, controls the metabolic processes of the body. Endocrine glands, for the most part, exert their influence by releasing hormones into the blood. The hormones circulate widely, regulating the activities of other tissues in the body. Thus a malfunction in any of the organs that comprise the endocrine system can result in widespread disruptions throughout the body. Malfunctions generally consist of too much or not enough of a hormone. Fatigue and weakness are common symptoms of almost any metabolic disease.

Diabetes Mellitus. Diabetes, one of the most common of the serious metabolic diseases, is estimated to affect about 1 percent of the population. It is characterized by high levels of glucose in the blood, caused by a deficiency of insulin. Insulin, the hormone produced by the pancreas, helps glucose move from the blood into the cells to be burned for energy. Without insulin, the cells cannot use the glucose, so the glucose stays in the bloodstream; the cells starve in the midst of plenty. Classical symptoms of diabetes include:

- thirst
- excessive urination
- increased appetite
- weight loss
- weakness and fatigue

Long-term complications of diabetes include eye problems (leading to blindness), kidney disease, nerve damage, and blood-vessel damage. Some research suggests that if the diabetes is treated aggressively and glucose levels are kept in good control, the complications of diabetes can be lessened. Although there is debate over this concept, all doctors agree that treatment should be aimed at keeping glucose levels in the normal range, if at all possible.

This can be done in one of three ways. In diabetes that usually begins in middle life or beyond, the so-called non-insulin-dependent, or Type II diabetes, weight reduction and diet alone are often sufficient to manage the disease. Sometimes it is necessary to add an oral agent (pill) to the regimen to help lower blood sugar. In insulin-dependent, or Type I disease, insulin therapy must be given to replace the lack of normal insulin. Individuals with Type I diabetes usually develop it before age forty, often in childhood or adolescence.

About 5 million people in this country are thought to have diabetes (Type II), yet not know of their condition. You could have mild diabetes and not be experiencing anything more than fatigue and a general sense of not feeling well. It is particularly important that your fasting blood glucose (usually the blood is drawn after fasting overnight) be determined. One simple blood test may improve your energy, health, and longevity.

Hypoglycemia. Hypoglycemia refers to a group of symptoms that are usually associated with an abnormally low blood-glucose level. This metabolic disorder is dangerous to the brain because glucose is the primary fuel used by the brain for energy. Without glucose, as with oxygen, the brain begins to function abnormally, and irreversible tissue damage can occur. If the hypoglycemia persists long enough, death can follow.

Years ago, doctors believed that hypoglycemia was a rare disorder. Now, with better tests, it is being discovered that hypoglycemia is much more common. The condition is divided into types: postprandial (after meals) hypoglycemia and fasting hypoglycemia. The first type occurs about two to five hours after eating, while the second type of hypoglycemia occurs only upon fasting. The causes of both types of hypoglycemia are many.

In either type of hypoglycemia, the symptoms are the same. In response to the low level of glucose in the blood, the body releases four hormones to try to drive the level back up to normal. One of them, epinephrine, causes the symptoms many people think of when they speak of hypoglycemia:

- sweating
- tremulousness
- rapid heart beat
- anxiety
- hunger

The deprivation of glucose in the brain leads to nervous-system symptoms:

- fatigue
- dizziness

339

- headache
- clouding of vision
- confusion

When the onset of hypoglycemia is gradual, the nervous-system symptoms far outweigh the epinephrine-caused symptoms.

Many people who have symptoms consisting of nervousness, fatigue, sweating, tremor, and palpitations somewhere between two to five hours after a meal assume that they have hypoglycemia when that is actually not the case. These symptoms may be caused by the release of epinephrine and other hormones after a meal, not by low levels of blood glucose. This syndrome has been called "nonhypoglycemia" or "idiopathic postprandial syndrome" (which translates as "syndrome of unclear origin after a meal"). Most people who have read about hypoglycemia in the lay literature and recognize the symptoms in themselves actually have this syndrome.

Nonhypoglycemia is best treated by diet. You should avoid simple sugars, which create an insulin surge. Most of your diet should consist of protein and complex carbohydrates so the blood-glucose level will remain as level as possible from meal to meal, helping to prevent the discharge of epinephrine.

True hypoglycemia needs to be carefully evaluated, because many conditions can cause it, including some very serious conditions due to gastrointestinal surgery, hereditary disorders, hormone deficiencies, liver disease, drugs, and tumors. Treatment consists of diagnosing the underlying problem and rectifying it.

Hyperthyroidism. Hyperthyroidism is a condition in which hyperfunction of the thyroid gland leads to a state of metabolic overdrive. Hyperthyroidism can be caused by a variety of disorders, however one type, called Graves' disease, is more common than the rest. The onset usually occurs in the patient's twenties or thirties.

The precise cause of Graves' disease is not known, although researchers think it might be due to an abnormal substance in the blood that constantly stimulates the thyroid gland to put out thyroid hormone. Thyroid hormone causes an increase in the metabolic processes throughout the body and leads to more oxygen use. The heart and lungs have to work hard to keep up with the demands. Most of the symptoms of hyperthyroidism can be attributed to this revved-up condition:

- anxiety
- tremulousness
- irritability
- fatigue
- weakness
- insomnia
- excessive sweating
- heat intolerance
- weight loss despite good appetite
- shortness of breath
- palpitations
- loss of menstrual periods

Some people who have hyperthyroidism do not present a picture of hyperactivity, rather they appear apathetic with the predominating symptoms of muscle weakness and general fatigue. Also, in those people who already have heart disease, hyperthyroidism can put them into heart failure.

The diagnosis of Graves' disease is fairly straightforward. It consists of demonstrating an elevated thyroid hormone level in the blood, the presence of an enlarged thyroid gland in the neck, and perhaps changes in the eyes and in the skin on the legs.

Graves' disease can be treated successfully by decreasing the amount of thyroid hormone stimulating the body's tissues. This can be done by chemical blockage with antithyroid agents, removing part of the enlarged gland by surgery, or destroying part of the gland by giving the patient radioactive iodine.

Hypothyroidism. Hypothyroidism is the opposite of hyperthyroidism. It is a decrease in the metabolic rate that is caused by insufficient hormone production by the thyroid gland. Without the hormone circulating in the blood to stimulate the tissues, the body's energy-producing mechanisms slow down. This is why fatigue, weakness, and lethargy are cardinal symptoms of hypothyroidism. These symptoms are among the earliest:

- fatigue and weakness
- constipation
- cold intolerance
- heavy menstrual flow

Other symptoms usually develop as the disease progresses:

- decreased intellectual and motor activity
- decreased appetite
- modest weight gain
- dry hair that falls out
- dry skin
- muscle aches
- voice change

Several conditions can cause hypothyroidism, including iodine deficiency, some drugs, surgery, and pituitary gland problems. It is not enough to simply treat the condition of hypothyroidism; a complete evaluation must be done to determine what is causing the hypothyroidism. Only then is it appropriate to begin therapy with replacement hormone.

Addison's Disease. Addison's disease is an example of a disorder of which fatigue is the main symptom. It is relatively rare, but because fatigue is so central to the disease, it deserves to be included here. In Addison's disease, the adrenal cortex slowly undergoes a degenerative process, and thus loses the ability to make adrenal hormones. The treatment for the condition is to replace the hormones through medication. The symptoms of Addison's disease include:

- fatigue
- weakness
- irritability
- loss of appetite
- weight loss

- abdominal pain
- nausea and vomiting
- pigmentation of skin
- loss of pubic and auxiliary hair

Hormone-replacement therapy seems to be much more effective, especially in alleviating the fatigue, when it is given in split dosages in approximation of the normal circadian rhythms these hormones typically show.

Reproductive System Disorders

Reproductive system problems are commonly sources of fatigue in women not only because of physical disease, but also because the system is intrinsically involved with female sexuality. Many psychological conflicts involving sexuality and relationships can be manifested as disorders of the reproductive system. Any difficulty a woman has in this area should be sensitively and completely investigated. If you have symptoms or difficulties, persist until you find a doctor with whom you can work.

Problems of the reproductive tract can be divided into four categories: menstruation, pelvic pain, sexual dysfunction, and infertility. Abnormal bleeding and pain are the most common physical symptoms, both of which directly cause fatigue. Stress and worry are often symptoms of the last two categories, sexual dysfunction and infertility. These also directly cause fatigue.

In the case of sexual dysfunction, either fatigue can be a cause for failure of arousal, or sexual conflict can cause fatigue. Sometimes it is difficult to figure out which came first. However, in order to treat either disorder, the problems have to be untangled.

Gastrointestinal Disorders

A whole host of diseases has been described which affect the gastrointestinal (GI) system. Many of them start in the GI system itself, while others are the result of disease elsewhere that affects the GI tract. Most of the diseases, however, present one or more of a handful of symptoms that point to the GI tract. One symptom may predominate in a certain

343

disease and be absent in another, which helps the doctor make a diagnosis. Any of the following symptoms suggest a disorder of the GI tract:

- indigestion
- nausea
- vomiting
- constipation
- diarrhea
- appetite loss
- weight loss
- abdominal pain or cramps

Fatigue is usually not a primary symptom of any particular disorder of the GI tract, however, it can result from the effect a disease might have on the entire body, such as malnutrition, fluid and electrolyte imbalance, altered metabolic state, anemia, or chronic pain.

Liver and Gallbladder Diseases

The liver is an extremely complex organ that has an untold number of responsibilities. It is a chemical factory that is involved with digestion, metabolism, blood clotting, detoxifying drugs and alcohol, and manufacturing hormones, among many other things. Any derangement in these functions can lead to widespread changes throughout the body. Fatigue and malaise often accompany liver disease.

Acute Hepatitis. Hepatitis is a viral infection that involves the entire body, although it primarily affects the liver. Vague flulike symptoms precede liver dysfunction by about one to two weeks:

- loss of appetite
- nausea and vomiting
- fatigue and malaise
- muscle and joint aches
- headache
- sore throat
- cough and runny nose

Liver dysfunction is marked by:

- dark urine
- clay-colored stools
- jaundice
- fever
- right-side abdominal pain

There is no specific treatment for acute viral hepatitis. Therapy consists of supportive measures, primarily bed rest and a high-calorie diet. Occasionally, it will take three to four months for complete recovery.

Gallstones. Gallstones are extremely common in women. It is estimated that as many as 20 percent of women may have them. In medical school, I was taught that the typical gallstone patient was the "5 *F*s": female, fat, forty, fertile, with flatulence (gas).

Often gallstones can remain entirely asymptomatic and it is now thought that these are best left alone. Problematic gallstones most often cause:

- severe, steady aching pain on the right side
- episodes of colic on the right side
- nausea and vomiting
- fever or chills

When gallstones are causing symptoms or are picked up on x-ray and expected to cause problems, they can be taken out surgically and sometimes, dissolved away with drugs.

Urinary-Tract Diseases

The kidneys are extremely complex and important organs. They regulate water and electrolyte balance; any disturbance in these finely tuned chemistries can create havoc throughout the body. Slowly developing kidney failure can bring about insidious but profound changes in water load, sodium levels, potassium levels, and toxic waste levels. Fatigue and weakness are common symptoms of altered body chemistries.

Symptoms that suggest a disorder in the urinary tract are:

- decreased volume of urine
- excessive urination
- night urination
- blood in urine
- pus in urine
- pain on urination
- urgency and frequency in urination
- flank tenderness
- difficulty urinating

These disorders range anywhere from urinary-tract infections to hypertension and kidney failure.

Joints and Connective-Tissues Disorders

A vast array of disorders can affect the joints and connective tissues, such as infections, metabolic disorders, immunologic diseases, trauma, degenerative processes, and cancer. However, there are some diseases that primarily affect the joints as well as the rest of the body. Fatigue, weakness, and malaise are very commonly associated with these diseases.

Rheumatoid Arthritis. Rheumatoid arthritis is a chronic disease that affects the entire body, although it primarily attacks the peripheral joints. Other organs that can be affected include the lungs, nerves, heart, and blood.

Rheumatoid arthritis may occur anytime in life in either sex, although it tends to be seen more in women, from the twenties to the sixties. The disease usually starts very subtly; fatigue and achy joints may well be all a person feels. During the first few months, these vague symptoms persist:

- fatigue
- weakness
- joint stiffness
- joint aches
- muscle aches

As the disease progresses, joints become the focal point of the destructive process. At first, the hands, wrists, and feet are usually symmetrically affected; that is, if one wrist is swollen and painful, the other one is at the same time. Joints are:

- swollen
- red
- painful
- warm to the touch

The course of rheumatoid arthritis is hard to predict. It is characterized by flare-ups followed by quiet periods. In 10 percent to 20 percent of patients, the disease may suddenly go away or smolder for years without causing much damage. The crippling form of the disease only occurs in 10 percent of all rheumatoid arthritis sufferers.

There is no cure for rheumatoid arthritis; it can only be treated symptomatically. This usually consists of rest and anti-inflammatory drugs, such as aspirin. Adequate rest is extremely important, and that includes napping when the fatigue becomes great.

All attempts should be made to practice the best of health habits, including good nutrition, plenty of sleep, and adequate activity to keep the joints mobile and the muscles strong. Doctors are learning that strong muscles help protect the damaged joints, and new treatments include weight lifting in graduated amounts to strengthen atrophied muscles.

Exercise is very important to the arthritic patient; it helps beat fatigue and protect the joints. All attempts should be made to make exercise a daily event.

Sjogren's Syndrome. Sjogren's syndrome consists of a triad: dry eyes, dry mouth, and a connective-tissue disease, usually rheumatoid arthritis. The dry eyes and dry mouth are the result of a process that decreases secretions. The lack of secretions may also affect other organs, such as the respiratory tract, vagina, and skin. Sjogren's predominates in women, less than 10 percent with the disease are men.

Anemia is a common finding in this disorder, in which case fatigue is certainly expected. Other symptoms suggesting Sjogren's in someone with joint pain are:

- burning or itching eyes
- blurring of vision
- difficulty swallowing
- decrease in taste
- cracks at corners of the mouth
- nosebleeds
- hoarseness
- pain on sexual intercourse

There is no cure for Sjogren's. Treatment consists of alleviating the symptoms caused by lack of body secretions. This might mean drops for the eyes and lubricants for the vagina. The connective-tissue disease should be treated with appropriate drugs.

Systemic Lupus Erythematosis. SLE—or lupus, as the disease is often called—is an immunological disorder of unknown cause. Patients with the disease have evidence of making antibodies against several of their own tissues, causing damage throughout the body. Multiple organ systems can be involved, including the kidneys, heart, blood, and brain.

SLE occurs in women nine times more frequently than in men. It usually begins sometime between the teens and the forties. Lupus is a chronic disease that can be mild to severe. In some patients, the disease will suddenly disappear; in others, it will respond to therapy; while in some, the disease takes an unremitting course despite therapy and ends with death.

Lupus may begin with a variety of symptoms:

- arthritis of the hands, feet, and large joints
- skin eruptions, especially a facial rash
- fatigue, fever, malaise
- appetite loss, nausea, vomiting, and weight loss

Lupus can go on to exhibit a wide array of symptoms, depending on what organ system is involved in the immune attack. Frequently, involvement of the nervous system causes symptoms suggestive of psychological problems, such as emotional instability or psychosis.

Treatment of lupus usually consists of giving immune-suppressing drugs, such as steroids, to control the flare-ups and prolong life.

Scleroderma. Scleroderma is another immunological disease, usually occurring in women between their twenties and forties. It is characterized by a process of fibrosis that involves mainly the skin, but also extends to a variety of internal organs, such as the gastrointestinal tract, lungs, heart, and kidney. The cardinal feature of the disease is tight, firm skin.

The disease begins insidiously. The first symptom may be what is called Raynaud's syndrome, a vascular spasm of the hands. On exposure to cold or anxiety, the hands (or feet) will first turn white and feel numb, then turn dusky blue, and finally turn red and feel painful. This symptom can actually precede the onset of scleroderma by years (every woman with Raynaud's does not go on to develop a connective-tissue disease; however, Raynaud's is often part of a connective-tissue disease).

Other symptoms that follow include:

- edema of face, hands, and feet
- swelling of fingers and hands
- skin of hands becomes firm and   kened
- skin changes move to arms, face, upper chest, abdomen, and back
- fatigue and muscle weakness
- pain, swelling, stiffness of fingers and knees
- difficulty swallowing
- shortness of breath and dry cough

Unfortunately, there is no cure for this scleroderma, which is a chronic, progressive, unrelenting disease. Management is aimed at treating the symptoms or complications of the various organ systems involved. Exercise, once again, is very important. Regular exercise helps keep the joints flexible and the skin pliable.

Musculoskeletal Diseases

Muscles translate energy into action. They are also the site of metabolic processes. As we saw above in the endocrine system, many metabolic diseases weaken the muscles. Connective-tissue disorders also frequently attack and weaken the muscles.

Weakness is the hallmark of muscle disorders. However, fatigue is a close second. Often people confuse the two symptoms; they may call muscle weakness fatigue. Sometimes it is very difficult to make the distinction, especially when all the body's muscles are involved; however, you should try to discriminate between the two.

Diseases of the muscles often show the following symptoms in various muscle groups (not necessarily the whole body at once):

- decreased strength
- decreased endurance
- paralysis, intermittent
- change in size of muscle
- twitches, spasms, and cramps
- muscle pain

The diagnoses of these diseases are often delayed, because doctors find the complaints of tiredness and weakness—classic symptoms of myasthenia gravis—too vague. Many women who have this type of disease are initially diagnosed as having a psychological problem. If you have any weakness, pay close attention to the timing of it relative to activities and exercises. Such details could be the clue to making the correct diagnosis.

Nervous System Disorders
Any disorder of the nervous system has the potential to bring on fatigue, weakness, and lethargy. Some of the conditions are obvious, such as the drowsiness after a convulsion, or the lethargy after a stroke. Some fatigue and drowsiness, however, can be subtle signs of an impending crisis. For instance, the rapid onset of lethargy, headache, and fever should receive immediate attention because of the possibility of serious brain infection. Mild head injury can cause drowsiness, headache, and nausea a few hours later, indicating a concussion.

Organic brain syndromes—arteriosclerotic and senile dementias—are typically accompanied by fatigue. Sometimes fatigue will appear as an isolated symptom well before the person starts to show the other characteristic signs of dementia. The fatigue is, in part, due to the increased effort required to carry out mental functions in an impaired brain. The person who is becoming demented has a tendency to nap and sleep more.

Degenerative diseases of the nervous system, such as multiple sclerosis, can occur over the course of a lifetime and be a major factor in chronic fatigue. As in other types of chronic conditions, the fatigue should be recognized and planned for in the life of the patient and her family.

Cancer

As our ability to treat diseases increases, so do our individual life spans. Such long life as we are now enjoying, however, makes us vulnerable to developing cancer. Statisticians predict that one out of every four Americans will develop cancer during her or his lifetime.[6]

Cancer is not always a fatal illness, as we once thought. Survival rates are increasing with every passing year. This means that many people and their families must learn to cope with cancer as part of life, to live with it on a day-to-day basis. The fatigue of cancer, just one of the multitude of problems patients must deal with, can have a much more profound effect on the quality of life when cancer becomes a chronic disease.

Cancer is not one disease; there are over one hundred distinct forms. The general term *cancer* refers to an abnormal growth of cells that either results in direct damage to tissues or spreads to distant organs to create damage. There are many mechanisms by which cancerous growths do their damage; they can create pressure on surrounding tissues, obstruct others, perforate tissues, or completely replace some tissue by overgrowing it.

By manufacturing products, tumors can also create very strong effects in the body. For example, an insulinoma, a tumor of the pancreas, manufactures insulin in an uncontrolled fashion, which leads to serious hypoglycemia. Fatigue

351

could be one of the earliest symptoms of this cancer. Anemia is a common condition that is found with several types of cancer, and of course, weakness and fatigue are hallmarks of anemia.

More often, weakness, fatigue, and debility are symptoms that appear as the cancer progresses. The general feeling of feebleness is often instrumental in preventing an individual from living as full a life as possible.

Obviously there are many, many important issues and problems to cope with in the care of the cancer patient, but it is important to attend to such general symptoms as fatigue, pain, and despair. Often doctors take the attitude that these symptoms are "vague" accompaniments to cancer, and nothing can be done about them. All of the guidelines in this book apply especially to the cancer patient. It is mandatory to have as much energy as possible to use in the battle against the tumor; proper nutrition, exercise, plenty of rest, no alcohol, and psychological support will all increase the chances of a person winning the fight against cancer.

TREATMENTS

We tend to think of fatigue as the result of something "wrong," either physically or mentally. However, it is important for you to know that fatigue is often the most frequent side effect of many treatments that doctors use to make patients better. All therapies have the potential of creating some unwanted side effects, although we accept them in belief that the side effects are outweighed by the benefits derived from the treatment. So in the case of fatigue caused by treatment, it may have to be tolerated. However, simply becoming aware that the fatigue is a side effect assists in coping effectively and developing a more supportive plan to combat it.

Surgery
Doctors have long recognized that surgery, although perhaps necessary, is stressful to the body in the short run. Many patients experience profound fatigue, among other symp-

toms, following an operation. This postoperative fatigue, as it has been called, although very common, has not been studied very much. Perhaps that is because doctors take the symptom so much for granted, and think that other symptoms are more distressing to patients, such as postoperative pain. I am not sure this assumption is warranted; fatigue can be the most disturbing aftermath of an operation.

A British study looked at sixteen patients who underwent elective surgery. Surprisingly, two thirds of them still suffered from fatigue one month after uncomplicated surgery, the time doctors usually tell patients they should be fit to go resume all of their normal activities or go back to work. The doctors reported,

> On day 20 [after surgery], when visiting the outpatient clinic, many of the patients had realized how tired they really were. They felt an indefinable weakness throughout the body after doing only minor tasks, such as house cleaning, cooking, shopping, etc. They often felt the necessity of sitting or lying down . . .[7]

I have a feeling that this surgeon did not appreciate just how exhausting household work can be; he refers to household tasks as "only minor tasks." Nevertheless, many of the patients were surprised that they had not returned to their previous level of fitness more quickly.

The study measured several different body functions at different times in the recuperation process. The researchers found small changes in oxygen use, pulse, and muscle performance, but none of these correlated with the patients' fatigue. These researchers then went on to do a more detailed study to see if they could find a factor that did correlate to the fatigue.

This second study turned up some interesting information.[8] The results showed that postoperative fatigue correlated with the amount of fat that was degraded, and the amount of weight loss a patient had; the more weight loss, the greater the fatigue.

Weight loss usually occurs after surgery because the

body increases its energy expenditure in carrying out the reparative process and usually there is a decrease in food intake during recuperation. If this is the mechanism that causes postoperative fatigue, it fits nicely with what is already known about dieting and fasting, and fatigue.

Remember in Chapter 5, when I discussed the body's need for carbohydrates? When the body is forced to use fat and is deprived of its favorite energy food—carbohydrate—fatigue sets in. This suggests that eating the proper diet is not only important in maintaining your normal energy level but that it is especially important during convalescence from surgery. You must accept fatigue after surgery as normal; it can persist for longer than a month. When I had my appendicitis (and I wasn't sixteen, it was just last year), I was considerably fatigued for a good three months. I had to take naps to get through the day. So expect fatigue, but treat it by eating properly, starting moderate exercise, and getting plenty of good sleep.

Chemotherapy

If few studies have investigated the effects of surgery on energy levels, even fewer have looked at the effects of chemotherapy. When I use the word *chemotherapy,* I am referring specifically to the treatment of cancers with potent drugs. As we saw in Chapter 8, fatigue is often a major side effect of medications. It should be of no surprise then to discover that the extremely potent and toxic drugs that are used in the fight against cancer can cause fatigue.

Cancer is not necessarily a fatal disease, although all too often we react to it as if it were. More and more people are being cured of their diseases and others are living much longer with their cancers. Thus, instead of cancer consuming one's entire life, the chronic illness is becoming only a part of life. Consequently more people are receiving chemotherapy treatments in the midst of carrying on their daily activities. In this situation, fatigue can be particularly disturbing.

In one study of fifty women receiving chemotherapy for breast cancer, 96 percent of them reported fatigue as having a major disruptive influence in their life. It was their number-one complaint. The authors of the study write,

"Fatigue, the most commonly reported [symptom], was variously described as being 'generally slowed down,' 'having no ambition anymore,' 'feeling tired all the time,' and so on. This fatigue was often related directly to chemotherapy—many women reported increased energy between . . . treatment cycles."[9]

The fatigue the women experienced stood in the way of their being able to carry on with their normal lives.

We often tend to concentrate on the more dramatic side effects of chemotherapy, such as nausea, vomiting, and hair loss. However, as uncomfortable as these symptoms may be, they do not interfere with normal life as much as fatigue does. Probably no other symptom has such a pervasive nature as does fatigue; it has the potential of affecting every nook and cranny of one's life. The researchers explain,

"The most frequent and marked effect of adjuvant chemotherapy was a reported decrease in both general and work-related levels of activity. A number of women reported that they were now unable to perform activities in which they had regularly participated in the past."[10]

Because the mechanism whereby chemotherapeutic agents cause fatigue is not yet known, the fatigue cannot be abolished. It is a side effect that must be tolerated in the struggle to fight cancer. However, it is important to recognize the symptom and try to institute a supportive plan that will maximize energy and decrease the drain. More attention needs to be paid to fatigue as a side effect of chemotherapy, so that cancer patients can live life as usual.

Radiation

As long ago as 1897, doctors recognized that fatigue was associated with radiation exposure.[11] The use of radiation is becoming increasingly popular in the treatment of some cancers. For instance, some women with breast cancer have the choice of saving the breast and undergoing a series of radiation treatments. This therapy is usually worked into the woman's daily schedule for several weeks, and although it is tolerated quite well, most women complain of fatigue.

Some doctors have hypothesized that the fatigue induced by radiation is "a mechanism which precipitates a slow-down of activity so that available energy is reserved for important reparative needs posttherapy."[12] A second theory postulates that fatigue is the result of the accumulation of toxic substances and cell destruction end products. A third theory suggests that postradiation fatigue is caused by an anemia resulting from radiation destruction of the red blood cell. It is likely that all three mechanisms are playing a role along with several others that have not been identified yet.

In a study of thirty cancer patients being treated with localized radiation, fatigue was related to the length of radiation treatments and the time of day they were received.[13] Fatigue was highest immediately following treatment and tended to decrease over the weekend when the patients did not receive exposure. Those patients who received the most lengthy regimens were the people who had the greatest change in their fatigue levels.

As with the fatigue of chemotherapy, this posttreatment fatigue cannot be eradicated; however, it can be ameliorated. First, being aware of the symptom and expecting it will help reduce any anxieties surrounding a lack of energy or motivation during the posttreatment time. Second, patients and families should be aware that the fatigue will occur consistently after therapy and plan their schedules to accommodate it. The family should understand that the patient will be tired, and activities or outings should be planned carefully. Third, other supportive actions should be taken, such as changing to a high-energy diet; instituting a regular exercise program; getting adequate sleep, including naps; and providing good psychological support during this period.

PAIN

A book about fatigue would not be complete without mentioning pain, especially chronic pain. By some estimates, nearly one third of all Americans have persistent or recurrent chronic pain. Unfortunately, given the magnitude of the problem, modern medicine has not been very successful in treating this symptom. Some of the reasons for this failure are the same reasons fatigue is a relatively ignored problem.

First, as with fatigue, little is known about the mechanism causing pain. And it is one of those complaints that does not fall into any specific medical subspecialty, so it falls between the cracks. Consequently pain research has been ignored and poorly funded. Also, because chronic pain can and often does have a large psychological component, doctors tend to dismiss the complaint altogether as being "in the patient's head." If nothing physical can be found to explain the origin of the pain, the patient is often left to get rid of the pain by her own efforts. Sounds very much like fatigue, doesn't it?

Chronic pain leads to chronic fatigue, as well as anxiety, depression, and sleeplessness, all of which augment the pain, contributing to a vicious cycle. Living with pain of any intensity consumes a tremendous amount of energy. The coping process draws on all of the resources a person has, often leaving the person drained of all energy. Furthermore, the usual treatment of chronic pain, medication, often has fatigue as a side effect. The result is that the person in chronic pain often has a world filled only with suffering, for there is little energy left over for anything else.

Advances in pain treatment are being made. Centers have been established around the country for the sole purpose of dealing with pain. In such centers, doctors of different subspecialties and skills are joined together under one roof to help patients learn about their pain and how to cope.

Treatment consists of an extensive workup that considers both physical and psychological components of a person. Depending on the nature of a person's problem, she is taught new methods of dealing with pain. Physical therapies such as exercise, whirlpools, and massage are used with great success. Also hypnosis, biofeedback, and TENS (transcutaneous electrical nerve stimulation) are proving to be more than faddish attempts at pain control. Thousands to millions are finding relief with these techniques. New methods of drug-delivery systems are also being investigated.

If you are in chronic pain and hooked on potent painkillers that are not doing the trick, consider going to the nearest pain clinic for an (another) assessment. In our culture, we are so accustomed to thinking the answer to our problems, especially pain, comes in the form of a pill or a capsule. You might be surprised to discover that relief can come in another form; you should give it the chance. You have nothing to lose but your pain.

WHAT TO DO

1. View chronic fatigue as a symptom of some ailment.

Chronic fatigue is one of the most common symptoms, if not *the* most common symptom, of physical disease. Most people, including doctors, assume that fatigue is psychologically caused. However, based on doctors' reports, you have at least a 25 percent to 30 percent chance that your chronic fatigue is a symptom of a physical problem—do not ignore it. Those statistics do not include fatigue from a variety of "nondisease physical causes." Chances may even be greater if all possible physical causes are included: poor nutrition or dieting, lack of exercise, smoking, alcohol and other drugs, pregnancy, menopause, poor sleep, advancing age, diseases, surgery, medical treatments such as radiation, chronic pain, and occupational hazards. Many of these physical causes are under your own control; however, with others, you will need the assistance of a good physician.

2. Learn about your ailment.

If you are already aware that you have an illness, or if you should be told so in the future by your doctor, learn as much as you can about your condition. Do not be a passive patient; take control. Find out what to expect from the disease process (symptoms, consequences, length of time, actions you can take) and learn what to expect from the treatment process (side effects, timing, duration). When you know what to expect, you can plan your life accordingly, react when certain situations arise, and help with the therapy.

Knowledge on your part will also help relieve you of a lot of unnecessary worry.

3. Treat your ailment well.

You should take a disease seriously, even if it is not a "serious" disease. So often there are actions that people can take to help themselves get better and yet they do not take those actions because of sheer disregard for their bodies.

Diseases such as diabetes and hypertension do not "hurt" or cause great discomfort in the short run, but in the long run, they can do major damage to several body organs and can even cause premature death. Take your medicines as prescribed, stick to special diets, get exercise, and follow other specific advice from the doctor. You will relieve much fatigue, pain, and long-term suffering if you do. Take care of yourself and do as much as possible to treat your ailment well.

16

FIX YOUR JOB

Most people think that fatigue is a necessary part of work at home or on the job. If I told you that your work can make you tired, you probably would answer, "So what else is new? Isn't work supposed to be exhausting?" No! Work does not have to be as fatiguing as it so often is. As I talk to women around the country, I find that most derive a great deal of satisfaction from their work. Yet they quickly bring up the frustrations they feel or the conditions they endure. Chronic fatigue is so rampant among women in America that almost everyone talks about it as if it were an inherent part of life.

Fatigue is frequently caused by conditions that are not necessary components of working. As in other parts of your life, you do not have to put up with fatigue. You should learn to recognize it as an indicator that something is wrong in your work. If you are excessively fatigued, then something should be changed.

If you become more conscious of the conditions that cause fatigue in your work, then you can begin to make changes that can alleviate the drains on your energy pool. That is my purpose in this chapter—to increase your awareness of the factors within your work that make you tired and to convince you that there are things that you can do to reduce your fatigue.

In the confines of one chapter, I cannot possibly cover all the occupational hazards that can cause fatigue. However, there are five areas that are of particular concern with which you should become familiar: stress, physical exertion, posture, working conditions, and the physical environment (chemicals and toxins). As I discuss each of these five factors, I will provide some examples to illustrate the typical situations that lead to fatigue.

Although many of my examples apply to jobs outside the home, all of the principles apply to work in general—whether inside or outside the home. I consider homemaking a job. When I use the term job, I mean it to include all work, not just paid labor, and I want you to think of all of the work you do, whatever it may be. So when I admonish you to "fix your job," I mean your job at home too!

WORK STRESS

Stress is a great energy drainer. Psychological stress is often the biggest contributor to fatigue on the job, and women seem particularly prone to it. Almost 70 percent of women managers in one survey reported "tiredness" as the main symptom of work-related illness—outranking such other symptoms as irritability, anxiety, physical tension, and frustration.[1] Furthermore, these managers regarded their malady as a symptom of psychological stress. Stress is also a major factor for women who work in the home. A number of studies have shown that homemakers are particularly prone to stress-related diseases. Homemakers are "managers," carrying the major executive responsibilities in the home.

Stress can be the key to whether work exhausts us. A high-stress job that entails little physical exertion can be extremely fatiguing, while a heavy-labor job without stress may make us just pleasantly tired. Tiredness turns into chronic fatigue when the body's stress reaction drains the energy pool. Sometimes it is difficult to get in touch with how much stress you are under and what is causing it. You might consider using your level of work fatigue as a gauge to the amount of stress you are experiencing.

In this space, it is impossible to cover all aspects of work stress—indeed, libraries and bookstores are full of books on the subject—but let us look at a few examples that apply to women today. One of the primary causes of stress and fatigue in women is boredom.

Bored to Fatigue

Relegation to boring work is one of the prices that women pay for cultural stereotyping. For years, people have thought that women were better suited than men for tedious, routine tasks. In factories, women are most often doing the intricate hand assembly that is required to produce high-technology products. And, in the past, women were the primary holders of occupations in industries (such as clothing) where hand-work or repetitive machine operations were typical. In the office, such "thinking work" as data analysis was often given to men, while women were assigned to the menial tasks, such as typing. Women who work in the home are particularly prone to boredom. Many household gadgets have been introduced as labor-saving devices, but they are also boredom-producing devices. Handicrafts and the pride involved in making them have all but disappeared from the homemaker's routine. Now much of housework is tedious and must be done over and over each day or each week. The bed is made only to be unmade again, clothes are cleaned only to be soiled again, the dishes are washed only to get dirty again—there is no end to the vicious cycle of work.

Women are no different from men in terms of their need for fulfillment, self-esteem, or accomplishment—and women's skill with intricate hand-eye movements is more due to training and cultural norms than with inherent physical characteristics. Women put up with repetitive tasks not because they do not have the mind or the interest for doing more, but because they have not had the education, training, or opportunity to do more. And discrimination has kept them in secondary positions.

What can you do if you are faced with a frustrating, boring job, or if you are bored with your work in the home? It is not easy, but you can make some changes, you can take control of your life. Do not assume that you have to accept poor working conditions or that you are stuck for life. You can make changes—and you will feel better if you do.

Change your routine as often as you can. Do not follow the same sequence in doing your tasks. See if your supervisor can help the situation in any way. If at all possible, try to introduce a project into your job that will put some excitement in the routine. For example, if you are bored to fatigue at home, consider taking up a craft (knitting, weaving, sewing) and doing a little each day as the beginning of a cottage industry. I know women who knit at home and sell handknits for fabulous sums of money. Such a project entails a sense of pride and can bring financial reward.

Another solution rests in obtaining new training or education. Many companies offer classes or financial aid for continuing education. High schools, colleges, universities, and other institutions offer after-hours training in a variety of subjects. I know: This adds to your already heavy work load. Once again, think of your priorities. How much is it worth to move around the obstacle to your progress? And remember that much of your fatigue may be due to the feeling that you are stuck and can do nothing about it. When you take action, you will be amazed at how much more energy you can muster to take control of your life. Armed with good qualifications, you can begin to seek new opportunities.

All Dressed Up and Nowhere to Go

"The people that sit next to me have been there five, six years. There is no way they're going to go anywhere. I do not want to sit there and type. I think I am smarter than that. The biggest promotion is, if you're lucky, they might make you a secretary. That's on top of the totem pole . . . and the petty regulations. You have to ask permission to leave the floor to get a box of cigarettes. You have to ask permission to do just about everything that involves leaving your desk. . . . Very few men in this company have any conception of what it's like to sit and type all day, or ask permission to go to the bathroom."[2]

Certainly repetitive, dead-end jobs can frustrate a worker of either gender; but women have more than their share of such jobs. In spite of their massive entry into the work force in recent years, women are still concentrated in particular job categories. Well over half of American women are in service and office work—jobs with a high nurturing content. Certain job categories, such as secretaries, nurses, kindergarten teachers, and dental assistants, are held almost exclusively by women.

The occupations with the highest proportion of females have several characteristics in common. First, they are vocations that seem to have a limited career path. (A "limited career path" is a fancy way to say that these are "dead-end" jobs.) One can argue that teachers can become principals and that sales demonstrators can become managers, but, let's face it: The chances are slim. The pay tends to be low, relative to the amount of education required (consider schoolteachers) and there is little opportunity for career advancement with the attendant increase in salary. Furthermore, these jobs are often made very rigid by overly strict managers.

People who organize work with such rigid rules, as cited in the quotation above, have no sense of the importance of human motivation to the efficient production of goods and services. It is no wonder that workers become angry and contentious when faced with having to "ask permission to go to the bathroom." Women, in fear of the reaction they may get, often let these rules go unchallenged. You must speak up. Maybe if enough women fight to change absurd rules, we can begin to see some rapid movement toward more human considerations in the design of jobs. I contend that if people are given meaningful work, the objectives of their work, the tools and the freedom to carry out their responsibilities, and are rewarded according to their performance, then they do not need rigid, picayunish supervision in order to do their work well.

The answer to the dead-end job dilemma is for women to get more scientific and professional education and training. Consider getting additional training that prepares you for new careers using the latest equipment and techniques. The three most promising areas for jobs in the future are communications, health care, and computers. Do not be afraid of computers! If you can type, you are way ahead of a lot of men. Take advantage of that skill. And encourage your daughters and other younger women to enter scientific and professional fields.

Underworked and Overtired

Madge was a secretary in a large company, working for a manager of a technical organization. It was an active office, with lots of telephone calls, visitors, and correspondence. The office was often visited by high-level managers to review the operations of the technical group. Madge enjoyed the human contact and the prestige of working in such a visible and stimulating environment. Her manager was understanding and pleasant, and he frequently complimented her on the quality of her work.

Although she was "successful in her work," Madge felt anxious and chronically fatigued. She often went home feeling unrewarded and totally drained—she had no incentive to do anything. As time went on, she found herself becoming more and more irritable with her fellow workers.

When Madge examined her feelings closely, she came face-to-face with her smoldering anger about the fact that many of her skills were not utilized. She had worked after hours for several years to get her master's degree in computer science, but the skills that she worked so hard and so long to develop were not being used in her secretarial work. She felt underutilized.

Underutilization can be especially hard for a woman to face after she has worked hard to develop new skills only to have them sit in reserve for some hoped-for moment when a new job will appear. For most people, new jobs do not "just appear." You have to seek assignments in which you can apply the knowledge and capability that you have developed. It may take time and several tries to find the right place, but, in many cases, persistence is rewarded with work satisfaction.

Madge's story had a happy ending. She expressed her frustrations to her manager, who then worked with her to find a job that would make fuller use of her skills. Madge is now working on a special project that uses her special training in computer science and gives her the added opportunity for domestic and foreign travel. She has the chance to meet new people and to receive recognition for her accomplishments.

Madge smiles a lot more now. And we can learn a lot from her style; she did not sit idly by, bite her tongue, and accept her plight—she built up the courage to let her manager know how she felt and what she wanted. It would have been very easy for Madge to say nothing because she did have a good secretarial job. She worked in a good environment, was paid a good salary, had good benefits, and was treated with respect. Many people would have looked at her job and said, "I can't understand why you are unhappy." Madge was in conflict because the "good" job was not using the skills that she worked so hard to develop in computer science. Because Madge expressed her views to her manager, she was rewarded with a solution to her dilemma. If you are underutilized on the job, speak up.

Taking Care of Everyone Else

A characteristic common to many of the professions occupied by women is their high nurturing content. In other words, feelings get managed as a part of one's job; emotions are part of the product for sale or the service to be provided. Think of the number of women you know—perhaps including yourself—who are in jobs that demand a lot of emotional control and nurturing: Pleasantness, congeniality, smiles, and waiting on others are demanded eight or more hours a day.

Many secretaries can attest to the fact that a large part of their job is "taking care" of the boss's needs. Nurses are forever nurturing. Waitresses, counter clerks, bank tellers are all constantly having to provide a "friendly" service to customers. And teachers certainly exercise their share of nurturing; today much of the responsibility of raising children falls on teachers in classrooms.

Airline-flight attendants can tell you many stories of having to be pleasant to obnoxious passengers. My husband

and I saw such a case when we were returning home from Washington several weeks ago. The man behind us seemed to be constantly ringing his hostess call button. When the flight attendant arrived at his seat, he simply wanted attention. "Do you have *Business Week?*" "What kind of airplane is this?" "Where do you fly from?" "Why don't you have French bread and cheese on this flight?"

The flight attendant smiled and answered the man's trivial (yes, even flirtatious) questions in spite of her harried schedule. Was she stressed? You bet! Did she arrive home exhausted? Certainly. The control that the situation demanded (and, I am sure many others do, as well) took a lot of emotional energy. The management of emotions has tremendous costs.

Try to understand how you are using your emotions on the job. Learn to separate your real feelings from the ones you project for show. There are times when it is appropriate to express your real ones—sometimes customers, passengers, patients, and others deserve to be gently reprimanded for their behavior. Be careful about getting in the habit of swallowing your emotions all the time. Those feelings that cannot be expressed on the job should have an outlet elsewhere. Ask your spouse, friends, or associates to lend you an ear. Discuss the fact that your emotions get manipulated and managed.

Furthermore, if you are in a nurturing job—constantly giving to others—make sure you do not let your own needs to be nurtured go unmet. If our needs are not met, we tend to become resentful of having to give to others. So learn to recognize your own needs and to ask for help when necessary.

Sexual Harassment

Many jobs require that we give of our talents and our care. Unfortunately, we also have to take a lot in our working environments. I have yet to meet a woman who has not been sexually harassed. Whether the situation is the aggressive, overtly suggestive sexual approach of the office lecher or the insidious, condescending attitude of a male boss, sexual harassment takes its toll in internal stress, frustration, intimidation, and fatigue. Too often people tend to get tangled up in the definition of the term without considering that it is the effect on women about which we should be concerned. The male passenger on the airline who kept asking silly questions of the flight attendant was, in my view, engaging in a form of sexual harassment. He certainly would not have behaved in the same manner toward a male flight attendant. His flirtatious manner was no compliment to the young woman, and I could see her tension as she attempted to exercise courtesy and discretion in dealing with him. Many of us encounter similar experiences every day.

Maybe the national laws are finally beginning to have an effect on overt sexual suggestions and demands for sexual favors in return for promotions; but, if anything, derogatory or suggestive comments toward women have increased. Women entering a room filled with men still have to put up with some comment regarding the role of women, or such remarks as "Well, we can start the meeting now; the beauty has arrived." Such comments have no place in business (or society, for that matter); they add to women's stress levels and create uncomfortable working environments.

One of the reasons that sexual harassment takes such a toll on women is because they absorb it and bury their fury. The best way to deal with it is to make your feelings about the incident known—to the perpetrator—as soon as possible so that you do not harbor them. If you are the victim of sexual intimidation, do something about it; do not let nonaction eat away at your self-esteem. It takes a lot of courage to fight what seems to be society's accepted system of male behavior. Yet you will find that you can get support for your position and you can make changes—and you will feel better in the end.

Work-related stress has many faces. As you learn to detect the sources of your pressures, you can begin to understand the relationship between your individual stresses and the resulting fatigue. Remember: Fatigue is the third and final stage of the stress reaction. Listen to it. There are always options in life. Identify them and know that you can make some changes, you can take control of your work and lead a more peaceful, energetic life.

PHYSICAL EXERTION

Although we often think that the work of women requires only light physical exertion, many occupations involve extensive use of muscles. Homemaking and a number of vocations held by women require a great deal of muscular movement and strength. Physical exertion can run the gamut from muscle strain caused by lifting to tired muscles due to repetitive motions. Let us take a look at some physical exertion that can cause fatigue and other more serious conditions.

Lifting and Fatigue

Strain due to physical exertion is often manifested in injuries to the back. As with other conditions, fatigue is often a precursor to or a result of an injury. Back injuries are a leading cause of lost time and disability, resulting in an estimated 100 million lost workdays per year.[3] As you might expect, women are particularly susceptible to strained back muscles. Men, because they tend to be taller and stronger than women, have the advantage of better mechanical leverage. Women's bodies are structurally different; the hip joint is angled differently and the legs are shorter relative to the torso, both of which create more strain on the back when lifting a given object. Therefore, women need to be particularly careful when a job requires lifting.

Homemakers do a great deal of lifting—furniture, corners of mattresses, the laundry, the vacuum cleaner, groceries, children, hundreds of items get lifted every day. Yet most women seem to pay little attention to the weight of the object or whether or not they are twisting or straining when they lift. Too many women lift heavy items using their back rather than their leg muscles. Tired and injured back muscles are a plague for women who work in the home, and lead to easy fatigability. How many times have you said, "Oh, my aching back"?

369

Nurses and hospital aides are also good examples of people who often use muscular strength and leverage. Many times I have helped nurses move a limp, helpless patient into a hospital bed. We avoided muscle strain by carefully planning such a lift and executing it slowly with an adequate number of people.

The best possible way to avoid injury is to make sure that you are physically fit. Women do not have to accept muscle weakness as inherent to our gender, and yet so many do. It has been proved over and over again that people who are fit become less tired and suffer less injuries as a result of muscle exertion. Exercise.

Another way to avoid back injuries is to change the nature of the job. Can the object be divided into smaller pieces? Can another person help you with occasional lifting? (Do not be afraid to ask.) Can a change in the orientation of the work objects reduce the need for lifting? Could pulleys or other devices help in the lifting task? If levers, pulleys, or machines are available, use them. Take a little extra time if necessary. If you must lift heavy objects, keep your back straight and lift with your legs rather than with your back muscles. Avoid lifting and twisting or stretching at the same time. Pay attention to your lifting and save your back.

Hand and Wrist Fatigue

In factories, women are often relegated to repetitive jobs that require intricate hand skills and precise eye-hand coordination. Repetitive motions can be extremely fatiguing and have profound physical effects. You need to be particularly aware of fatigue in the hands, wrists, or lower arms. Several diseases, including tendonitis, bursitis, Raynaud's phenomenon, tenosynovitis, and carpal tunnel syndrome, are directly related to repetitive physical motion.

The human hand is a complex and delicate instrument consisting of numerous bones and joints. The bones in the hand are controlled by muscles in the forearm through connectors called tendons. These tendons are covered by sheaths, which provide protection and lubrication as the tendons move to do their job. Excessive movement of the tendon or a blow to it can cause inflammation of the tendon's important sheath. This is called tenosynovitis.

Workers who perform repetitive hand motions are particularly susceptible to tenosynovitis of the wrist or the back of the hand. Studies have indicated that people involved in tasks requiring repetitive arm or hand motions are up to three times more likely to suffer tenosynovitis than the general population. They include musicians, painters, and haircutters.

Severe tenosynovitis can also cause carpal tunnel syndrome. The carpal tunnel is the passageway in the inside of the wrist through which many of the tendons, blood vessels, and nerves pass from the forearm to the hand. When the tendon sheaths become inflamed, they may swell, constricting the carpal tunnel. This usually results in numbness, tingling sensations, or burning sensations in the fingers. Similar sensations can be caused by any force that compresses the important median nerve, which passes through the carpal tunnel. Poorly fitting tool handles or other devices that apply excessive pressure to the palm of the hand can create this effect.

Studies have found that women have a higher incidence of hand or wrist injuries. Carpal tunnel syndrome is much more likely to be found in women workers than in men workers. One reason is probably that women have smaller carpal tunnels than men. Another is that they are concentrated in work that involves repetitive motions.

Fatigue is the precursor to such syndromes. Jobs that are tiring to certain muscle groups are likely to cause such physical problems. If you are having excessive localized fatigue in your work, do something about it. Look for ways to reduce repetitive hand motions. Perhaps a task can be done by alternating hands. See if another position of the workpiece or the tools would help. Try to keep your wrist straight. (Different kinds of tools may be necessary in order to accomplish this.) Use tools with padded handles and be careful of exposing the palm of your hand to sharp tool handles. Make sure that your tools fit your hand. Suggest new ways of structuring the work to your manager. Is your training adequate for the job? Perhaps a more experienced worker could help explain a better way of doing the job. Work to get a change.

Poor Workplace Design and More Fatigue

Workplaces that are designed for men often subject women to unsafe or tiring movements and positions. When a woman has to reach too high, lift loads that are too heavy, move items in ways that require uncomfortably longer reaches, or work from positions designed for men, she undergoes a lot more physical and psychological stress than would a man in the equivalent position.

My husband recently had the opportunity to visit the factory of a famous appliance manufacturer. Although much of the plant was automated, there were still many manual jobs. He told me of seeing a workplace that was shared between a six-foot-plus man and a woman of average height. Apparently, one of the two workers was being trained to take over the job. As the appliances went by on a conveyor, the workers took turns attaching small mechanical parts to the appliances; the man would work on one appliance, then the woman would work on the next. The appliances on the conveyor were within easy reach of the man; he could attach the parts with little twisting of his body or excessive arm motion. The much shorter woman had to stretch and twist her body, then reach upward with her arms in order to do the work. The engineer who designed the job must have had the male physique in mind; the conveyor was much too high for the average female.

Nevertheless, the woman's job could be made much easier with some simple changes. For instance, a small platform for her to stand on could be designed. I wonder if the woman ever considered that something could be easily changed to make her less tired? More than likely, she accepted the conditions as being part of the job; furthermore, she probably would not want to emphasize that she needed special consideration to make her more effective in the job. The result was that she was putting up with conditions that unnecessarily added to her physical and mental fatigue.

FATIGUE AND POSTURE

We all remember our mother's plea to "stand up straight" and many of us implore our children to do the same thing (even if we ourselves do not set so good an example). In work, posture has a broader meaning than just standing up straight. The position of your body during a sustained period of work has a lot to do with the feeling at the end of the day. If you have to work in a consistent stooped position or if you have to stay in any one position for a long time, you know how tired you get.

The body must expend a tremendous amount of energy to maintain one position. It takes muscle strength not to move or to limit movement. Not moving is a big energy drainer. The body is designed so that movement—especially of the legs—aids blood circulation. When leg or body movement is restrained for long periods of time, circulation is reduced, which causes fatigue and sometimes dizziness.

In most jobs, you have control over your posture. When you work from a standing position, learn to pay attention to it—watch whether you are straight or not. Try to work from a straight, not leaning or twisting position. Change your position often so that you will not be tired from holding a sustained posture for too long. Take a short break every hour. Light stretches can help relax muscles and improve circulation.

If sustained standing is part of your work, get comfortable shoes with sufficient cushioning and support, and get a pad on which to stand. High-heeled shoes are the scourge of womanhood; they are bad for the feet, make walking or standing more exhausting, and expose women to falling or twisting their ankles. I have heard women say that they are more comfortable in high heels; that can only be because their feet and legs are so distorted from years of mistreatment that they have difficulty adapting to ordinary flat shoes. Wear low-heeled, comfortable shoes—and make sure that they give your feet the proper support.

Many women work in offices or factories where they have to spend most of their time in a sitting position. Although the office worker may have a comfortable chair and even sit with good posture, she may become quickly fatigued because she has little chance to change her posture. If she sits in a hunched position while working, or if her chair and desk are not suited to her physique and the work required, she compounds the effect.

Sitting is not necessarily resting. Even if you have the correct posture, sitting can actually put more stress on the spine than standing. If you have a poor chair or sit improperly, the effect is multiplied. Slumping often makes it harder to breathe fully and evenly. A bad chair can even restrict blood flow to certain parts of your body, creating a "pins-and-needles" feeling in your appendages. Beware that a poor sitting position or an inadequate chair can induce fatigue in at least three ways: by putting physical strain on the spine and muscles, by impairing effortless breathing, and by taxing the circulatory system.

One of the fundamentals of reducing the fatigue from sustained sitting is to have the proper chair. The chair should be adjustable to your body and provide the proper support to your back and seat. Feet should be firmly on the floor or on a footrest so that there is no pressure under the legs (that could impair circulation). The chair or the worktable should be adjustable so that the proper relationship of height can be maintained. If you need to turn often, the chair should swivel.

When I go into offices, I am appalled at the kind of chairs and seating positions that I see. Good ergonomically designed chairs are on the market, but seem to be invading the offices too slowly. Insist on a good chair and have it adjusted properly. Get the proper adjustment between the height of the table on which you work and the chair, and sit up straight. Change your position often; move your legs, get up and walk, do simple exercises, move your arms, take several deep breaths.

WORKING CONDITIONS

Women often tolerate poor working conditions because of the nature of their jobs. Many clerical jobs are the epitome of repetitive tasks. Clerks and typists sit in one place, stare at one spot (usually a piece of paper or a video display terminal), and move only their fingers. When women are assigned repetitive tasks that tax few of their many skills as human beings, they suffer overuse of selected muscles and brain cells while the rest are relatively idle.

Women who have used manual typewriters understand that typing for eight hours tires the fingers, arms, back, legs, neck, shoulders, and eyes. Typing or using a keyboard all day is hard, tiring work. (I can particularly sympathize with women clerical workers after spending so much time at my keyboard while writing this book.) Electric typewriters may decrease the amount of pressure required to depress the keys, but do not change the content of the work, the effect on the body and the eyes, or the need to sit in one position all day.

Clerical work is fatiguing for several reasons. First, only limited physical motions are employed in performing the work, and they occur over a sustained period of time. Second, the work is done within a restricted posture and seating position. Third, the work requires sustained use of visual skills.

Fatigue is a frequent outcome of work that requires concentrated visual effort, because much energy is consumed through the use of the eyes and visual system in the brain. In fact, prolonged visual work is one of the primary causes of fatigue for women on the job.

As new computers and other automated equipment have been installed in American businesses, companies have attempted to systematize office procedures by breaking down the processing of clerical and informational tasks into finer and finer pieces. The introduction of automation in the office has often served to further narrow already-boring jobs. Women, concentrated in the office environment, find themselves in production-like jobs, having to process many repetitive items at relatively high rates of speed.

Although the designers of such organizations seem concerned about production and efficiency, studies have consistently shown that production is improved when jobs and organizations are designed with the best interests of the worker in mind. I am amazed at how companies ignore these facts in the design of organizations and jobs. The new office technologies could actually be used to make jobs more, not less, interesting. Machines should be used to eliminate fatigue and human drudgery, not to further dehumanize women office workers' jobs. A growing number of women are working with such a machine, the VDT.

Video Display Terminals

Millions of video display terminals (VDTs) have been installed in offices over recent years. The VDT is a television-like screen that displays writing or graphical data to the user of a computer or other office equipment. VDTs are used as a way of entering information into or retrieving information from a computer. VDTs are also used on word processors, which have replaced typewriters in many organizations. Such machines promote large increases in office productivity because they allow easy correction of mistakes, easy manipulation of written text, and automatic handling of many clerical tasks.

Small computers, which use VDTs, are being found in more and more homes, small businesses, schools, and offices of various types. It is almost hard to imagine an occupation that has not been affected in some way by computers or VDTs. So almost all of us will be at least part-time users of VDTs. Believe me, I have become quite familiar with one since writing this book.

VDTs have recently received a lot of coverage in the media. One of the primary motivations for the study of the effect of VDTs on workers is that the device emits electronic signals. This has raised concern about the possible effects of electronic radiation on people who are exposed to VDTs for long periods of time. Studies have indicated that there is little risk of sickness due to radiation; the machines in the studies were well below radiation levels considered safe by the U.S. Government Occupational Safety and Health Administration (OSHA). However, a variety of other health complaints have been described by operators. These include fatigue; headaches; eye problems; dizziness; nausea; and neck, back, and arm pain.[4]

Lea, a secretary I know, told me about her fatigue and the VDT. She had worked with electronic typewriters for years. Although she realized that clerical work was tiring, she loved her work. She enjoyed the fast pace of working for a high-level manager in a large corporation. Lea was a skilled secretary; her typing speed was exceptionally high and she was a fast and accurate stenographer. When she was offered the chance to use a new word-processing machine in her work, she jumped at it, thinking that the device would improve her efficiency, accuracy, and skills.

Lea learned rapidly; within a few days her productivity had exceeded the highest level that she had ever been able to achieve on the electric typewriter—and she was pleased. But after a few weeks, she began to notice her patience with fellow workers had diminished, and several coworkers commented on her short temper. In addition, Lea noticed that she was unable to read or watch television when she got home; she was exhausted. When she began to focus on the problem, Lea realized that her eyes were the source of her fatigue and that she was having trouble reading the VDT screen that was attached to the word processor.

Lea's first reaction was to go back to the typewriter, but she quickly decided against that. She did not want to give up the advantages of the new machine. She got the help of her manager. He checked to make sure that the adjustment of the machine, the surrounding light, and the relationship of the chair to the machine were correct—no problem was found. Then, they consulted the company physician, who suggested an eye examination.

The eye doctor prescribed special glasses to help Lea focus at the distance from her head to the VDT. Although it took a little time for her to get accustomed to the new glasses, Lea's eyestrain and headache substantially decreased so that she was able to use the new machine comfortably. Her fatigue vanished. Lea's company has now instituted a policy to provide free special eye correction devices to VDT operators who require them.

Several government studies have indicated that a number of workplace and physical conditions, such as screen glare, poor lighting, and lack of rest breaks, are major factors in VDT problems. Based on present studies, it appears that this new technology is not inherently dangerous or necessarily tiring; rather, the job and the physical characteristics of the workplace are responsible for the resulting fatigue and other ailments. With the proper working conditions and an emphasis on breaks and exercise, VDT operators can have much less tiring jobs.

If your work involves the use of VDTs, typewriters, or other similar equipment, there are several things that you can do to reduce your fatigue. Almost every study has supported the need for frequent rest periods. Several studies have recommended short rest periods every fifty minutes. The data indicate that such a regimen is more effective in reducing fatigue and maintaining productivity than longer breaks taken less frequently. While you are taking your break, do some gentle exercises: Move your head, arms, legs, and back. Close your eyes and massage your temples and forehead.

When you are using a VDT, remember to look away from the screen every few minutes; that will help relieve eye-muscle strain. Change the focus of your eyes by glancing around the room, focusing first on far-off objects, then on close ones. Close your eyes for a few minutes and think some nice thoughts.

Make sure that you have the right kind of eye correction. Many people who wear bifocal glasses find that they cannot focus properly on a VDT screen through either lens of their glasses. Also, make sure that you have the right light and that the screen is free of glare. The face of the screen should be at right angles to windows or other direct light, and the room light should be diffused (indirect). The top of the VDT screen should be at or below eye level. If the screen is above eye level, you will experience increased eye fatigue.

The layout of your desk space can help you eliminate tiring positions and sore necks. A copy holder can display the document that you are typing from so that you do not have to crane your neck. Attempt to identify any other aspects about your personal situation that could make your job easier and less tiring.

Sometimes correcting a tiring work situation will take an

action from management or the company for whom you work. Do not be afraid to approach your boss with suggestions for improving your workplace. Point out that you will be able to do your work better and produce better results for the company if you are less tired and the work is more pleasant.

PHYSICAL ENVIRONMENT

In all jobs, women encounter a variety of physical conditions that can dramatically affect their energy. Lighting conditions, colors, layout and design of the work space, temperature, noise, and a variety of other environmental conditions can have a profound effect on your morale, your productivity, and your level of fatigue.

Once again, you have to adopt an attitude that you can take charge and make some changes. Your employer may initially resist your request to improve your working environment. However, that attitude will change when your employer starts to realize that changes which reduce fatigue also improve effectiveness.

Some countries, such as Sweden and Germany, have sponsored a great deal of research on ways to make working environments, including offices, safer and more pleasant places to work. This has resulted in a variety of laws that set requirements for lighting, noise, physical space, and equipment design. For instance, Germany has set limits on the maximum amount of noise that office machines are allowed to generate, the size and shape of keyboards, and other "ergonomic" factors (ergonomics is the science of the relationships of people to their equipment and their working environment). The United States has lagged behind in this area. Yet studies have proven that properly designed equipment and work spaces can substantially reduce fatigue. Although new ergonomically designed chairs, desks, and other equipment are starting to appear on the American market, woefully few American office workers have access to them.

It is interesting that as more managers in business are using VDTs and terminals, we are starting to see increased emphasis on office layout, comfortable chairs, and other ergonomic considerations. It is too bad that managers have not paid attention to these details before—they could have done much to decrease their workers' fatigue.

Take a look at your working environment. Do you have enough light and does it come from the right direction? Is your work area properly ventilated? Is the temperature comfortable? Is there excessive or distracting noise? Are there odors or fumes that are irritating? Insist on a good working environment, and your reward will be less fatigue at the end of the day.

Chemicals and Toxins

Chemicals and toxins can exert a subtle influence on your energy level. Fatigue is usually the first sign of problems caused by chemical agents—a cause that is usually missed. I think that all women, no matter what their occupation, should be acutely aware of the risks of chemicals and toxins in their workplaces.

Although most places where women work seem relatively safe, chemicals can be found in almost all of them, including the home. Homemakers use a myriad of chemicals to clean, to kill insects, to help things grow, to repair, to decorate. You are exposed to toxins (any substance that is harmful to the human body) in many work situations, often without knowing it.

Toxins can take the form of dust, fumes, mists, vapors, or gases. They can enter the body through the lungs, the skin, or the digestive tract—and cause a variety of short- or long-term damage. Some toxins are known to directly cause a variety of acute or chronic diseases. The list of substances that are known to have harmful effects grows every day. Carbon tetrachloride was a common cleaning fluid in my mother's day; almost every household had a bottle of it readily available. Yet we now know that "carbon tet" is carcinogenic, that is, a substance that causes cancer if absorbed through the skin over a long period of time.

Even though our knowledge of occupational hazards is growing, relatively speaking, we know so little about most of the substances to which workers are exposed. I have no doubt that in many cases, workers are suffering from a variety of ailments—fatigue a primary one—due to some unidentified toxin in the workplace. Yet we do not have the time, investigators, or finances to do all the studies that need to be done. For the most part, the fatiguing effects of chemicals are not (and will not be) known. Assume the worst.

Fatigue can be a direct result of exposure to certain chemicals. A Finnish study of 102 car painters reported that fatigue and concentration difficulties were frequent complaints voiced by the workers.[5] Investigators determined that the symptoms were directly related to the painters' exposure to a wide-ranging variety of chemicals and solvents.

Often the subtle sensations of fatigue or similarly vague symptoms were not recognized by workers, family doctors, or management as being related to exposure to toxic substances on the job. However, more serious symptoms such as nausea, vomiting, and dizziness were quickly recognized as being caused by chemical intoxication and prompted quick action. This demonstrates that the "quiet" complaint of chronic fatigue can easily get lost in everyday living, and the connection between it and toxins on the job can be easily missed. In the Finnish study, it took trained investigators with their questionnaires to help both workers and management become aware of the problem.

Fatigue may be the first—and sometimes only—indicator of overexposure to a toxin. Toxic exposure is not limited to the exotic occupations of chemical workers or car painters. You should be cautious about your everyday use of chemicals or work you do around excessive dust or vapors. Foreign substances should be treated with caution, and you should carefully examine your workplace in an attempt to identify the substances to which you are exposed.

Tracking down the cause of fatigue due to occupational exposure to foreign agents often requires the talents of experts in the field, such as epidemiologists or toxicologists. If you suspect that your problems may be related to substances on the job, go to your management, company physicians, or your own doctor (but beware that many doctors are not attuned to occupational health risks). If you need additional help in an emergency or a difficult-to-define situation, the

WOMEN AND FATIGUE

National Institute for Occupational Safety and Health (NIOSH), an institute of the federal government, can be called for help. In certain cases, an investigator from the institute will be made available for study of the problem.

The most important thing to remember about your working life is that it does not have to be excessively fatiguing. There are many ways that you can change your work to make it more rewarding and less tiring. If you make a strong effort to change the way you work, you will probably be pleased with the result; and so will your supervisor, your coworkers, and your family. Your fatigue can be reduced, your productivity can be improved, and you can take more pleasure in your work.

Many people often avoid bringing up problems on the job for fear that they will be called "just another complaining woman" (or worse). So, simple things that could be changed do not get fixed. You have to learn to speak up. You may be surprised by the reception you get from your supervisor when you make suggestions.

The way a problem is presented can have a big effect on your supervisor's reaction. If you identify a problem, think of ways that it can be solved. If you cannot fix it alone, go to the supervisor with some suggestions. Do not just complain about a problem; have some solutions in hand. In that way you will be seen as having a positive, helpful attitude. The same applies to working with your coworkers or family. Be positive! And you will receive positive results.

WHAT TO DO

1. Change your attitude.
Adopt the attitude that you do not have to accept excess fatigue from your work. Learn to recognize what contributes to your fatigue in the home and out of the home. When you start being aware of the fatiguing situations in your work, then you can begin to figure out ways to make your work easier.

2. Analyze your work.

Analyze how you are doing your jobs, both at home and out of the home, with the factors discussed in this chapter in mind.

How much stress is in your work? What are the causes of stress? Are you engaged in boring, repetitive work? Are you underutilized? Are you frustrated by job conditions?

How much physical exertion is needed to perform your duties? Do you need to lift, twist, or use certain muscles over and over?

Do you maintain good posture in your work? Do you change positions often? Do you have to lean or hold a given posture for a long period of time? Do you have a good chair?

Are your working conditions conducive to conserving your energy and comfort? Do you engage in repetitive work with a great deal of eyestrain? Is the work space arranged to make your work easy?

Is your physical environment safe, pleasant, and free of distractions? Is the light adequate for your tasks? Is there excess noise or heat? Do you work with machines that expose you to vibration? Do you work with chemicals or toxins?

3. Develop a fatigue-elimination plan.

The way you do each of your jobs can have a significant effect on your fatigue. Do not just assume that jobs have to be done in the same old way. Let your imagination wander, and look for creative ways to do things better and easier. Would new methods of doing the work help? How about new tools or equipment? Could rearrangement of the desk, table, or work space help? Are all the items that you need readily accessible?

After you have identified the fatiguing situations and the list of things that can be done, figure out the steps (including political steps) that must be taken to bring about the changes. What has to be done to make the changes? Who do you have to convince that a change is needed? Who has responsibility to make the change? Set some goals. What do you want to accomplish and by when?

4. *Enlist help.*

Develop a game of eliminating fatiguing situations with the help of others. Talk to your coworkers and family about the tasks that make all of you tired. Several brains are better than one, especially when the ideas start flowing. Make a list of all the ideas, no matter how wild they are, of how to bring about the needed changes. Then go back to the list and check the ones that will have the greatest impact.

5. *See your supervisor.*

Confronting a supervisor to get help in making changes is difficult for most of us. If necessary, enlist the psychological support of family and coworkers as you prepare for the discussion. Then show the supervisor your plan. Be positive, state why you would like to minimize fatigue on the job. Point out that people are more productive and produce better quality work if fatigue is decreased. Demonstrate your proposed solution to each of the problems and offer to help implement any changes needed. You will probably be pleased with the reaction.

Epilogue

During the writing of *Women and Fatigue,* countless women and men who were aware that I was working on the book approached me and asked the same question: "Well, so why are women tired all the time? What's the bottom line?"

In the early phases of researching the book, I always stopped a moment and pondered the question, not quite knowing how to answer; then I most likely responded by talking about the issue with which I was consumed at the moment—women and food, or women and exercise, or women and drugs. Early on, I didn't have a clear answer to the question. But slowly, as I spoke to women and experts, read studies, thought about concepts and spelled them out, the answer began to crystallize. The big picture was growing clearer and clearer to me—and suddenly, it came into focus.

For the most part, women's fatigue (as well as many other problems) is caused by the very conditions of our lives that result from our being female. Some of the fatigue is from personal problems, while much of it is "structural"—it is built into our social institutions (women's jobs, wage discrimination, the consequences of divorce, et cetera).

We are in a great social transition, and although it is an exciting time, it is also a very stressful time. With the old image of the "ideal" woman shattered and the new images not quite formed, women are struggling to achieve an identity in a society fraught with conflicting values. Everywhere women turn they are confronted by a mess of contradictions.

Many women are caught between the two worlds—they are left with the responsibilities but not the protection of the traditional world, and are burdened with new responsibilities but lack the skills necessary for survival in the "new" work world. Women are overburdened with too much responsibility and too much work, without enough appreciation and support.

Women are struggling—to better themselves, to survive a divorce, to achieve, to gain a sense of self, to make ends meet, to "do it all." Regardless of the details of each of our own personal struggles, most women are grappling with some issue that stems from the conflict between the old and new roles for women. Struggle consumes energy. Chronic fatigue is a symptom of all the work women are doing—psychic work and physical work—in an effort to gain a place in what has been called a "man's world." Women have paid great prices, but I believe, overall, we have made great gains in achieving personal freedom and making the world a more equal and humane place.

Fatigue should be only a transitory part of our day—at the close—not a permanent way of life. And yet, so many women have come to accept it as a given; just one of the many prices they must pay. Indeed, it is a price. Fatigue causes a lack of well-being, and I believe, heralds subsequent illness if ignored for too long.

Perhaps we should use the fatigue in our lives, both individually and collectively, as one of the measures of how we women are doing. It is a reliable symptom; its presence indicates that the individual is failing to cope with some demand in life. It also signals that there is great potential for personal growth. Furthermore, fatigue is a symptom that is extremely hard to mask. We have pills that will cover up or treat many "vague" conditions, such as anxiety, pain, depression. We do not have a pill to alleviate chronic fatigue. Getting rid of it means treating the cause. For these reasons, it can be an excellent indicator of well-being.

Our well-being, to a great extent, lies within our control or in the act of taking control. I am reminded of what one of the women with whom I spoke said to me. After years of struggling with the image of the "ideal" woman, she came to terms with herself, rejected the homemaker role, and sought an education and employment. Now she is at peace. "What a difference my life would have been had I known all along that I had absolute control over how I feel."

In order to gain control of your life, you must simply take it, for nobody can give it to you. Once you know that you are in control, there are numerous changes in your life that can be made that will alleviate fatigue and other problems. I hope this book has provided you with useful suggestions on what changes to make in certain dilemmas. Some of them are little changes, some are big changes; some are easy, some are difficult; some changes will take years and an effort on the part of all of us. For there does come a point where individual effort is not enough and the answer lies in institutional and societal changes.

Many women are carrying burdens and struggling with conditions that defy any one individual's greatest attempt to solve them: poverty, lack of adequate child care, wage discrimination, and so on. We must forge ahead—not go back to traditional ways—to change the institutions (schools, business, child care) that create "structural" fatigue and stress in women's lives and that still erect barriers to achieving a satisfying life.

We cannot go back. Going back to the "traditional role" in this day and age is not good for women's mental health, or subsequently, our children's mental health and, economically, it can't be done anyway. The traditional life-style will not solve the problems of work and family today. Specifically, what will solve these problems? I foresee two phases of change in the "family" structure beyond the two that have already occurred.

In the first phase, men left the home to work; in the second phase, women left the home to work. The third phase of change, which we are entering, is that the children will leave the home for day care on a much wider scale than presently occurs. As day-care centers spring up in schools, churches, temples, businesses, and government facilities, most of our young will be cared for, for a large part of the day, by specialists in a group setting.

The lack of child-care facilities in this country is appalling when compared to other industrialized nations, and is probably the biggest impediment today to women's access to good health care, good education, and competitive jobs. This third phase is one to fight for and one to look forward to, but it is only a step to the fourth phase.

The fourth phase will take place at the passing of the industrial revolution and the coming of the information revolution. The economy will no longer be based on energy; rather, it will be based on information. Of course, it is the computer that will allow for this shift to take place. Few women yet realize that the computer is actually our ally. Computer technology may be the very key to balancing our lives between home and work in the future.

How so? In the fourth phase of change, hopefully, men, women, and children will come back to the home as the center of work and family life. The realms of work and home will be more easily integrated, allowing women greater access to work and men greater involvement with the family. The computer will replace the auto or the bus as a means of "getting to work." As one social scientist has predicted:

> Twenty years from now—probably even sooner—we are likely to consider it a fundamental improvement in [the] standard of living that large numbers of people do not commute to work over long distances but work instead in office clusters near their homes and let information travel rather than travel themselves.[1]

The information economy will allow people to build communities that can provide the solution to some of our deep-seated problems today. Cluster communities can provide communal housing, support, and friendship for the ignored of today's world: the old, the widowed, the single women heads of household, the divorced. With offices and homes near one another, programs such as flextime and job sharing will be easier to institute. Day care can be provided within the community setting, not very far from either mother or father. Likewise, such reforms as maternity leave, paternity leave, and parental sick leave will be easier to institute because absent workers need not totally lose touch with their jobs if they are close to home. Furthermore, much work can actually be done in the home and sent to the appropriate office with the push of a terminal key.

Two years ago, I never would have foreseen that I would regard the computer as woman's ally. The writing of this book—not just the subject matter, but also the literal writing of it—has opened my eyes. This entire book was written using a word-processing program on a personal computer at home. Much of the research was initially done by searching a variety of electronic information bases to which I subscribe. For example, I have at my fingertips the entire database of the National Library of Medicine in Bethesda, Maryland. Before I had this research capacity, I had to go to a medical library and search volumes and volumes of indexes by hand, which took days upon days. I cannot begin to estimate how much time and travel my computer has saved me—time I have spent at home instead.

My husband occasionally works at home on his computer (he'd like to spend more time working at home, but managers frown upon it because they don't know how to "manage" workers at home yet, and this makes them nervous) and when he does, we have a wonderful day. It is truly a balance of home and work. Actually I think we both get more done and work longer hours when we are at home together than at the office. I work around meals, household chores, naps, errands, sickness, and appointments very efficiently—and without guilt. In a society that has not changed to accommodate working mothers or egalitarian couples, the computer has to be the single most important item that has allowed me (and my husband) to integrate home and work.

The impetus for change to bring about such integration will have to come primarily from women—we must provide the leadership and take the responsibility. In order to solve the problems of work and family, we will have to devote our energies to fighting for new child-care programs and restructuring the workplace. Only then will we have suitable conditions under which women can be mothers and equal people, too. To fall short of the goal will be damaging not only to women but to the very future of the human race. It is time that women's cherished values—of love, nurturing, and connectedness to others—are integrated into the basic institutions of our society. This will be a long and difficult struggle, but at the end, we will know where our exhaustion came from and we will be able to take delight in our accomplishments. And it is only then that women will be able truly to rest.

NOTES

1. FATIGUE IS REAL

1. Patricia K. Riddle, "Chronic Fatigue and Women: A Description and Suggested Treatment," *Women and Health* 7(1) (spring 1982): 37.

2. Cary L. Cooper and Marilyn J. Davidson, "The High Cost of Stress on Women Managers," *Organizational Dynamics* 10(4) (spring 1982): 49.

3. George L. Engel, "Nervousness and Fatigue," in Cyril Mitchell MacBryde and Robert Stanley Blacklow, eds., *Signs and Symptoms*, 5th ed. (Philadelphia: J. B. Lippincott Company, 1970), p. 637.

4. Robert G. Petersdorf, Raymond D. Adams, Eugene Braunwald, Kurt J. Isselbacher, Joseph B. Martin, and Jean D. Wilson, eds. *Harrison's Principles of Internal Medicine*, 10th ed. (New York: McGraw-Hill Book Company, 1983), p. 71.

5. George L. Engel, "Nervousness and Fatigue," p. 641.

6. Harold Merskey, "Diagnosis of the Patient with Chronic Pain," *Journal of Human Stress* 4(2) (June 1978): 6.

7. John D. Morrison, "Fatigue as a Presenting Complaint in Family Practice," *The Journal of Family Practice* 10(5) (1980): 795.

8. A. Whiren, "Reducing Stress for Working Parents," *Day Care and Early Education* 9(3) (spring 1982): 35–36.

9. As reported in Patricia K. Riddle, "Chronic Fatigue and Women": 38.

2. CYCLES OF FATIGUE

1. Nancy Fagley, Paul Miller, and John Sullivan, "Stress, Symptom Proneness, and General Adaptational Distress During Pregnancy," *Journal of Human Stress* 8(2) (June 1982): 15–22.

2. Penny Wise Budoff, *No More Hot Flashes* (New York: G. P. Putnam's Sons, 1983), p. 17.

3. Jean Coope, "Problems around the Menopause," *The Practitioner* 227 (May 1983): 793.

4. Penny Wise Budoff, *No More Hot Flashes,* p. 40.

3. WAVES OF FATIGUE

1. This approach is an extension of work by S. Howard Bartley, *Fatigue: Mechanism and Management* (Springfield, Illinois: Charles C. Thomas, 1965).

2. Adapted from Ernst Simonson, *Physiology of Work Capacity and Fatigue* (Springfield, Illinois: Charles C. Thomas, 1971).

3. S. Howard Bartley, *Fatigue: Mechanism and Management,* p. ix.

4. Berton Roueche, "The Hoofbeats of a Zebra," *The New Yorker* LX (16) (June 4, 1984): 72.

5. S. Howard Bartley, *Fatigue: Mechanism and Management,* p. 37.

6. George L. Engel, "Nervousness and Fatigue," in Cyril Mitchell MacBryde and Robert Stanley Blacklow, eds., *Signs and Symptoms,* 5th ed., (Philadelphia: J. B. Lippincott Company, 1970), p. 641.

7. W. F. Ganong, *Review of Medical Physiology,* 11th ed. (Los Altos, California: Lange Medical Publications, 1983), p. 233.

8. Hans Selye, *Stress without Distress* (New York: New American Library, 1974), p. 14.

9. Hans Selye, *Stress without Distress,* p. 16.

10. Hans Selye, *Stress without Distress,* p. 26.

11. Hans Selye, *Stress without Distress,* p. 26.

12. A. Poteliakhoff, "Adrenocortical Activity and Some Clinical Findings in Acute and Chronic Fatigue," *Journal of Psychosomatic Research* 25(2) (1981): 91–95.

13. A. Poteliakhoff, "Adrenocortical Activity": 95.

14. George L. Engel, "Nervousness and Fatigue," p. 646.

4. KNOW YOUR SELF

1. H. Yoshitake, "Relations between the Symptoms and the Feeling of Fatigue," *Ergonomics* 14(1) (1971): 176.

2. This test was developed from concepts from H. Yoshitake, "Relations between the Symptoms and the Feeling of Fatigue": 175–186.

3. Adapted from Blue Cross and Blue Shield Associations, *The Blue Cross & Blue Shield Guide to Staying Well* (Chicago: Contemporary Books, 1982), pp. 57–59.

4. These questions were developed by adapting information from the following:

"Could You Be an Alcoholic," *Harper's Bazaar* (September 1982): 159, 162, 164; Blue Cross / Blue Shield of Greater New York, "Think before You Drink" (June 1984), pamphlet DDP-3; U.S. Department of Health, Education, and Welfare, Public Health Service Alcohol, Drug Abuse and Mental Health Administration, "Deciding about Drugs: A Woman's Choice," 1979 DHEW Publication No. (ADM) 80–820: 10; Clark Vaughn, *Addictive Drinking: The Road to Recovery for Problem Drinkers and Those Who Love Them* (New York: Penguin Books, 1984), pp. 6, 7.

5. U.S. Department of Health, Education, and Welfare, "Deciding about Drugs": 10.

6. Adapted from Grace Baruch, Rosalind Barnett, and Caryl Rivers, *Lifeprints: New Patterns of Love and Work for Today's Woman* (New York: New American Library, 1984), pp. 269, 271.

7. Grace Baruch, et al., *Lifeprints*, p. 268.

8. Grace Baruch, et al., *Lifeprints*, pp. 266, 267.

5. EAT FOR ENERGY

1. Susie Orbach, "Food, Fatness and Femininity," *Practitioner* 227 (May 1983): 861.

2. Dr. Charles F. Ehret and Lynne Waller Scanlon, *Overcoming Jet Lag* (New York: Berkley Books, 1983), p. 60.

3. Chester F. Cullen and Roy L. Swank, "Intravascular Aggregation and Adhesiveness of the Blood Elements Associated with Alimentary Lipemia and Injections of Large Molecular Substances," *Circulation* 9 (March 1954): 335–346.

4. Nathan Pritikin, "Food Poisoning: A Major Health Problem in the United States," *The Humanist* (September/October 1984): 5.

5. Robert G. Petersdorf, Raymond D. Adams, Eugene Braunwald, Kurt J. Isselbacher, Joseph B. Martin, and Jean D. Wilson, eds., *Harrison's Principles of Internal Medicine,* 10th ed. (New York: McGraw-Hill Book Company, 1983), p. 1850.

6. William A. Nolen, "What that Tired Feeling May Actually Mean," *McCall's* (March 1981): 88.

7. William T. Jarvis, "Food Faddism, Cultism and Quackery," *American Review of Nutrition* 3 (1983): 46.

8. Myron Winick, "Making Every Calorie Count—Especially If You Are a Woman," *Columbia Magazine* (November 1983): 31.

9. William T. Jarvis, "Food Faddism": 40.

6. EXERCISE FOR FITNESS

1. Evalyn S. Gendel, "Women: Fitness and Fatigue," *The West Virginia Medical Journal* 69(5) (May 1973): 114.

2. Carlyle H. Folkins and Wesley E. Sime, "Physical Fitness Training and Mental Health," *American Psychologist* 36(4) (April 1981): 373–389.

3. Ralph S. Paffenbarger, Robert T. Hyde, Alvin L. Wing, and Charles H. Steinmetz, "A Natural History of Athleticism and Cardiovascular Health," *The Journal of the American Medical Association* 252(4) (July 27, 1984): 491–495.

4. Ralph S. Paffenbarger, et al., "A Natural History": 494.

7. QUIT FOR GOOD

1. U.S. Department of Health and Human Services, Public Health Service, Office of the Assistant Secretary for Health, Office on Smoking and Health, *The Health Consequences of Smoking for Women, a Report of the Surgeon General* 1980.

2. *Health Consequences of Smoking*, p. 307.

8. ABSTAIN FOR SPIRIT

1. As defined by the National Institute on Alcohol Abuse and Alcoholism (NIAAA), a problem drinker is an individual whose use of alcohol creates health, social, financial, or emotional problems for herself or another, but who is not necessarily alcoholic. A problem drinker is often at risk for becoming an alcoholic.

2. U.S. Department of Health and Human Services, Public Health Services, National Institute on Alcohol Abuse and Alcoholism, *Spectrum: Alcohol Problem Prevention for Women by Women* 1981, DHHS Publication No. (ADM) 81–1036.

3. U.S. Department of Health and Human Services, *Spectrum: Alcohol Problem Prevention*, p. 8.

4. Marian Sandmaier, *Alcohol Programs for Women: Issues, Strategies, and Resources*, National Clearinghouse for Alcohol Information, National Institute on Alcohol Abuse and Alcoholism.

5. L. S. Fidell, "Sex Role Stereotypes and the American Physician," *Psychology of Women Quarterly* 4(3) (1980): 313–330.

6. R. Cooperstock, "Sex Differences in Psychotropic Drug Use," *Social Science and Medicine* 12(3B) (1978): 179–186.

7. L. S. Fidell, "Sex Role Stereotypes": 313–330.

8. R. Cooperstock and H. L. Lennard, "Some Social Meanings of Tranquilizer Use," *Sociology of Health and Illness* 1(3) (1979): 331–347; as reported in Thomas J. Glynn, Helen Wallenstein Pearson, and Mollie Sayers, eds., *Women and Drugs*, Research

Issues 31, 1983, U.S. Department of Health and Human Services, Public Health Service, Alcohol, Drug Abuse and Mental Health Administration, DHHS Publication No. (ADM) 83–1268: 52.

9. D. B. Kandel, M. Davis and V. H. Raveiw, "Women and Drug Use: Social Strains, Coping and Psychological Functioning: A Pilot Study," Final Report of NIDA Grant No. DA 01931, 1981 (New York: Columbia University and New York State Psychiatric Institute).

10. L. S. Fidell, "Sex Role Stereotypes": 98.

11. National Institute on Drug Abuse, U.S. Department of Health, Education, and Welfare, *Deciding about Drugs: A Woman's Choice* 1979, DHEW Publication No. (ADM) 80–820.

9. SLEEP FOR VITALITY

1. Gay Gaer Luce, *Biological Rhythms in Psychiatry and Medicine* 1978 (National Institute of Mental Health, U.S. Department of Health, Education and Welfare), p. 49.

2. Robert G. Petersdorf, Raymond D. Adams, Eugene Braunwald, Kurt J. Isselbacher, Joseph B. Martin, and Jean D. Wilson, eds., *Harrison's Principles of Internal Medicine,* 10th ed. (New York: McGraw-Hill Book Company, 1983), p. 119.

3. William C. Dement, *Some Must Watch While Some Must Sleep* 1972 (Stanford, California: The Portable Stanford, Stanford Alumni Association), p. 74.

4. William C. Dement, *Some Must Watch,* p. 86.

5. William C. Dement, *Some Must Watch,* p. 80.

6. Robert G. Petersdorf, et al., *Harrison's,* p. 120.

7. Lynne Lamberg, "Circadian Rhythms, Punching Your Body's Time Clock," *American Health* 3(8) (November 1984): 84–89.

8. T. Akerstedt, "Work Schedules and Sleep," *Experientia* 40 (1984): 417–421.

9. T. Akerstedt, "Work Schedules and Sleep": 417–421.

10. Jane E. Brody, "Personal Health," *New York Times* (August 15, 1984): p. C10.

10. RESOLVE YOUR CONFLICTS

1. Alan Jay Lerner and Frederick Loewe, "A Hymn to Him," *My Fair Lady,* 1956.

2. Susan Price, *The Female Ego* (New York: Rawson Associates, 1984), p. 70.

3. Susan Price, *The Female Ego,* pp. 5, 6.

4. Elaine (Hilberman) Carmen, Nancy Felipe Russo, and Jean

Baker Miller, "Inequality and Women's Mental Health: An Overview," *American Journal of Psychiatry* 138(10) (October 1981): 1321.

    5. Alice Walker, *In Search of Our Mothers' Gardens* (New York: Harcourt Brace Jovanovich, 1983), p. 58.

    6. Elaine Carmen, et al., "Inequality and Women's Mental Health": 1321.

    7. Elaine Carmen, et al., "Inequality and Women's Mental Health": 1323.

    8. Elaine Carmen, et al., "Inequality and Women's Mental Healthy": 1323.

    9. Susan Price, *The Female Ego*, p. 89.

    10. Grace Baruch, Rosalind Barnett, and Caryl Rivers, *Lifeprints: New Patterns of Love and Work for Today's Woman* (New York: New American Library, 1983), p. 28.

    11. Elaine Carmen, et al., "Inequality and Women's Mental Health": 1325.

    12. Grace Baruch, et al., *Lifeprints*, p. 15.

    13. Grace Baruch, et al., *Lifeprints*, p. 2.

11. LIGHTEN YOUR WORK LOAD

    1. Linda Wolfe, "The New York Mother," *New York* 17(36) (September 10, 1984): 38.

    2. Patricia K. Riddle, "Chronic Fatigue and Women: A Description and Suggested Treatment," *Women and Health* 7(1) (spring 1982): 37.

    3. Suzanne M. Bianchi and Daphne Spain, *American Women, Three Decades of Change* 1983 (U.S. Department of Commerce, Bureau of the Census, CDS-80-8), p. 15.

    4. Claire A. Scott Miller, "Dual Careers: Impact on Individuals, Families, Organizations," *National Association of Bank Women Journal* 60(3) (March/April, 1984).

    5. John M. Rhoads, "Overwork," *The Journal of the American Medical Association* 237(24) (June 13, 1977): 2617.

    6. Ruth Schwartz Cowan, *More Work for Mother* (New York: Basic Books, Inc., 1983), p. 213.

    7. Janice Radway, "Interpretive Communities and Variable Literacies: Functions of the Romance Reading," *Daedalus* (summer 1984): 63.

    8. Philip Slater, *The Pursuit of Loneliness* (New York: Beacon Press, 1970) as quoted by Karen Barrett, "Two-Career Couples, How They Do It," *Ms.* (June 1984): 39.

    9. Edward Wakin, "Career and Family: The Juggling Act of the '80's," *Today's Office* 18(3) (August 1983): 44.

    10. Grace Baruch, Rosalind Barnett, and Caryl Rivers, *Life-*

prints: New Patterns of Love and Work for Today's Woman (New York: New American Library, 1984), p. 144.

11. A. Whiren, "Reducing Stress for Working Parents," *Day Care and Early Education* 9(3) (spring 1982): 35–36.

12. Patricia K. Riddle, "Chronic Fatigue and Women": 38.

13. Arlie Hochschild, "Dual Work Families: New Sex Roles," National Institute of Mental Health, report no. NIMH-83-331 (September 28, 1983): p. 4.

14. Edith M. Netter and Ruth G. Price, "Zoning and the Nouveau Poor," *Journal of the American Planning Association* 49(2) (spring 1983): 171–181.

15. Andrew Hacker, ed., *U/S; A Statistical Portrait of the American People* (New York: The Viking Press, 1983), p. 111.

16. Andrew Hacker, *A Statistical Portrait*, p. 134.

17. Katherine Bouton, "Women and Divorce: How the Law Works against Them," *New York* 17(40) (October 8, 1984): 37.

18. Katherine Bouton, "Women and Divorce": 39.

19. Kathleen Gerson, "Changing Family Structure and the Position of Women, A Review of Trends," *Journal of the American Planning Association* 49(2) (spring 1983): 141.

20. Sylvia Ann Hewlett, "Child Carelessness," *Harper's* (November 1983): 21.

21. ———, "Readings, RE: Smiles," *Harper's* (March 1984): 21.

22. Andrew Hacker, *A Statistical Portrait*, p. 135.

23. Andrew Hacker, *A Statistical Portrait*, p. 134.

24. Sylvia Ann Hewlett, "Child Carelessness," *Harper's* (November 1983): 21.

25. Iria Lee Zimmerman and Maurine Bernstein, University of California at Los Angeles, as quoted by Kathleen Doheny, "Children Not Hurt by Mothers Working," *Litchfield County Times* (January 27, 1984): 21.

26. Sylvia Ann Hewlett, "Child Carelessness": 25.

12. SURVIVE YOUR LOSSES

1. Sigmund Freud, "Mourning and Melancholia," in John Rickman, ed., *A General Selection from the Works of Sigmund Freud* (New York: Liveright Publishing Corporation, 1957), p. 125.

2. George L. Engel, "Nervousness and Fatigue," in Cyril M. MacBryde and Robert S. Blacklow, eds., *Signs and Symptoms*, 5th ed. (Philadelphia: J. B. Lippincott Company, 1970), p. 643.

3. Sigmund Freud, "Mourning and Melancholia," p. 126.

4. James Pennebacker, "Confiding in Others and Illness Rates

among Spouses of Suicide and Accidental Death Victims," *The Journal of Abnormal Psychology* 93(4) (winter 1984): 473–476.

13. BEAT YOUR BLUES

1. Robert G. Petersdorf, Raymond D. Adams, Eugene Braunwald, Kurt J. Isselbacher, Joseph B. Martin, and Jean D. Wilson, eds., *Harrison's Principles of Internal Medicine,* 10th ed. (New York: McGraw-Hill Book Company, 1983), p. 2205.

2. John F. Burnum, "Diagnosis of Depression in a General Medical Practice," *Postgraduate Medicine* 72(3) (September 1982): 71.

3. Robert G. Petersdorf, et al., *Harrison's,* p. 2205.

4. Elaine (Hilberman) Carmen, Nancy Felipe Russo, and Jean Baker Miller, "Inequality and Women's Mental Health: An Overview," *American Journal of Psychiatry* 138(10) (October 1981): 1322.

5. George L. Engel, "Nervousness and Fatigue," in Cyril Mitchell MacBryde and Robert Stanley Blacklow, eds., *Signs and Symptoms,* 5th ed. (Philadelphia: J. B. Lippincott Company, 1970), p. 642.

6. Adapted from Bonnie Kawczak Hagerty, *Psychiatric-Mental Health Assessment* (Saint Louis: C. V. Mosby Company, 1984), p. 98.

7. A. T. Beck, C. H. Ward, M. Mendelson, J. Mock, and J. Erbaugh, "An Inventory for Measuring Depression," *Archives of General Psychiatry* 4 (1961): 561–571.

8. George L. Engel, "Nervousness and Fatigue," p. 642.

9. Leonard M. Giambra, "Independent Dimensions of Depression: A Factor Analysis of Three Self-report Depression Measures," *Journal of Clinical Psychology* 33 (4) (October 1977): 928–935.

10. Katharina Dalton, *Depression after Childbirth: How to Recognize and Treat Postnatal Illness* (Oxford, U.K.: Oxford University Press, 1980).

11. Elaine Carmen, et al., "Inequality and Women's Mental Health": 1322.

12. Myrna M. Weissman and Eugene S. Paykel, *The Depressed Woman: A Study of Social Relationships* (Chicago: The University of Chicago Press, 1974), p. 7.

13. Grace Baruch, Rosalind Barnett, and Caryl Rivers, *Lifeprints: New Patterns of Love and Work for Today's Woman* (New York: New American Library, 1983), p. 21.

14. Elaine Carmen, et al., "Inequality and Women's Mental Health": 1322.

15. P. M. Miller and J. G. Ingham, "Friends, Confidants and Symptoms," *Social Psychiatry* 11 (2) (April 1976): 51–58.

14. DISCUSS YOUR FATIGUE

1. L. S. Fidell, "Sex Role Stereotypes and the American Physician," *Psychology of Women Quarterly* 4(3) (1980): 313–330.

2. L. S. Fidell, "Sex Role Stereotypes": 313–330.

3. R. Cooperstock, "Sex Differences in Psychotropic Drug Use," *Social Science and Medicine* 12(3B) (1978): 179–186.

4. Karen J. Armitage, Lawrence Schneiderman, and Robert Bass, "Responses of Physicians to Medical Complaints in Men and Women," *The Journal of the American Medical Association* 241(20) (May 18, 1979): 2186.

5. L. S. Fidell, "Sex Role Stereotypes": 313–330.

6. John D. Morrison, "Fatigue as a Presenting Complaint in Family Practice," *The Journal of Family Practice* 10(5) (1980): 798.

7. John D. Morrison, "Fatigue as a Presenting Complaint": 800.

15. RECOGNIZE YOUR AILMENT

1. This case was adapted from a clinical case reported by D. W. Foster and J. F. Barlow, "Thirty-Three-Year-Old Caucasian Female with Easy Fatigability," *South Dakota Journal of Medicine* 33(9) (September 1980): 5–12.

2. Robert G. Petersdorf, Raymond Adams, Eugene Braunwald, Kurt J. Isselbacher, Joseph B. Martin, and Jean D. Wilson, eds., *Harrison's Principles of Internal Medicine,* 10th ed. (New York: McGraw-Hill Book Company, 1983), p. 839.

3. Robert G. Petersdorf, et al., *Harrison's,* p. 1649.

4. Robert G. Petersdorf, et al., *Harrison's,* p. 1850.

5. Robert G. Petersdorf, et al., *Harrison's,* p. 1514.

6. Robert G. Petersdorf, et al., *Harrison's,* p. 751.

7. T. Christensen, T. Bendix, and H. Kehlet, "Fatigue and Cardiorespiratory Function following Abdominal Surgery," *The British Journal of Surgery* 69 (1982): 418.

8. T. Christensen and H. Kehlet, "Postoperative Fatigue and Changes in Nutritional Status," *The British Journal of Surgery* 71 (1984): 473–476.

9. Beth E. Meyerowitz, Frank C. Sparks, and Irene K. Spears, "Adjuvant Chemotherapy for Breast Carcinoma," *Cancer* 43(5) (May 1979): 1616.

10. Beth E. Meyerowitz, et al., "Adjuvant Chemotherapy": 1616.

11. H. Yoshitake, "Relations between the Symptoms and the Feelings of Fatigue," *Ergonomics* 14 (1971): 175–196.

12. Pamela Haylock and Laura K. Hart, "Fatigue in Patients Receiving Localized Radiation," *Cancer Nursing* (December 1979): 461.

13. Pamela Haylock and Laura K. Hart, "Fatigue in Patients": 461–467.

16. FIX YOUR JOB

1. Cary L. Cooper and Marilyn J. Davidson, "The High Cost of Stress on Women Managers," *Organizational Dynamics* 10(4) (spring 1982): 49.

2. J. Tepperman, *Not Servants, Not Machines: Office Workers Speak Out* (Boston: Beacon Press, 1976), as quoted in Frederick P. Spouris and Larry M. Miller, "The Context of Work in America," in Barry S. Levy and David H. Wegman, eds., *Occupational Health, Recognizing and Preventing Work-Related Disease* (Boston: Little, Brown and Company, 1983), p. 21.

3. Anonymous, "Sitting Down on the Job: Not as Easy as It Sounds," *Occupational Health and Safety* (October 1981): 24–25.

4. Melanie Brunt and Andrea Hricko, "Problems Faced by Women Workers," *Occupational Health* (Boston: Little, Brown and Co., 1983), p. 407.

5. Kaj Husman, "Symptoms of Car Painters with Long-term Exposure to a Mixture of Organic Solvents," *Scandinavian Journal of Work, Environment and Health* 6 (1980): 19–32.

EPILOGUE

1. Peter F. Drucker, "Out of the Depression Cycle," editorial in *The Wall Street Journal* (Journal 9, 1985): 26.

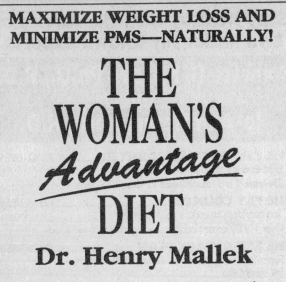